NERVOUS DISEASE IN LATE EIGHTEENTH-CENTURY BRITAIN: THE REALITY OF A FASHIONABLE DISORDER

NERVOUS DISEASE IN LATE EIGHTEENTH-CENTURY BRITAIN: THE REALITY OF A FASHIONABLE DISORDER

BY

Heather R. Beatty

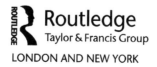

Routledge
Taylor & Francis Group

LONDON AND NEW YORK

First published 2012 by Pickering & Chatto (Publishers) Limited

Published 2016 by Routledge
2 Park Square, Milton Park, Abingdon, Oxfordshire OX14 4RN
711 Third Avenue, New York, NY 10017, USA

First issued in paperback 2015

Routledge is an imprint of the Taylor & Francis Group, an informa business

© Taylor & Francis 2012
© Heather Beatty 2012

BRITISH LIBRARY CATALOGUING IN PUBLICATION DATA

Beatty, Heather, 1979–
Nervous disease in late eighteenth-century Britain: the reality of a fashionable
disorder. – (Studies for the Society for the Social History of Medicine)
1. Neuroses – Great Britain – History – 18th century.
I. Title II. Series
616.8'52'0941'09033-dc23

ISBN-13: 978-1-138-66460-9 (pbk)
ISBN-13: 978-1-8489-3308-8 (hbk)

Typeset by Pickering & Chatto (Publishers) Limited

CONTENTS

ACKNOWLEDGEMENTS

It is with much gratitude that I wish to thank the people that helped to make this book possible. Many thanks to the librarians at the Bodleian Library, and to Iain Milne and Estela Dukan at the Royal College of Physicians in Edinburgh, whose warm welcome made my time in their beautiful archives even more magical. I am grateful to Margaret Pelling, whose helpful advice and consistent encouragement guided me through my DPhil years and the many years since. Likewise, I am indebted to Perry Gauci for his abiding cheerfulness and remarkable ability to help me find clarity amidst my piles of notes and flurries of ideas. Many thanks to Erica Charters for her academic advice and cherished friendship, and to Norman Ansley for building my love of history and a most treasured library. Thanks most of all to my family, and especially to my parents, for their unfailing support and loving words throughout the years.

INTRODUCTION: EXPLAINING A
FASHIONABLE DISORDER

In his *Lectures on the Duties and Qualifications of a Physician* (1770) Doctor John Gregory sympathized with students who were forced to study medical history, claiming, 'It is indeed an unpleasant task, and, at first view, seems a useless one, to enquire into the numerous theories that have influenced the practice of physic in different ages'. Nevertheless, he maintained, the subject did have some redeeming value; certain forgotten historical remedies could have real therapeutic importance, and the study of 'fanciful hypotheses' adopted by physicians of earlier ages could encourage modern practitioners to be more discerning in their own adherence to new medical theories.[1] To historians, the study of medical history has yet a greater significance. As Gregory noted in his earlier publication, *A Comparative View of the State and Faculties of Man with Those of the Animal World* (1765), doctors create medical theories by drawing upon all avenues of knowledge. Consequently, Gregory explained, 'the history of Medicine does not so much exhibit the history of a progressive art, as a history of opinions'.[2] As many historians have argued, when viewed in a cultural context, medical theory can tell us much about the ideas, beliefs and prejudices of the society in which it was born. Nervous disease – including the conditions of hysteria, hypochondria and melancholy – has proven a virtual goldmine for historians who have successfully proven its relationship to larger themes including fashion, literature, gender and class.[3]

Despite this wealth of literature, surprisingly little is known about the actual experience of treating or suffering from this socially significant malady. Was nervous disease a serious pathological entity? Who treated nervous disease, and what modes of treatment were employed? How prevalent were nervous patients in eighteenth-century Britain? What symptoms did patients exhibit, and how did they think about their illness? The answers to these questions reveal surprising discontinuities between popular perceptions about nervous disease and its lived reality. By exposing these differences and investigating the reasons behind them, this study further develops our understanding of the relationship between medicine and culture, and allows nervous patients and their physicians to offer very personal accounts of a supposedly national malady.

Nervous disease first achieved widespread attention as a nationally significant disorder early in the eighteenth century, with the work of the Bath physician, George Cheyne. Composed for a public audience, Cheyne's enormously successful *English Malady* (1733) sketched a stereotypically defining image of nervous disease and its sufferers, which persisted for much of the century. First, Cheyne explained, nervous disease most commonly affected English citizens. The reasons behind this civic susceptibility were many:

> *The* Moisture *of our* Air, *the Variableness of our* Weather, (*from our Situation amidst the* Ocean) *the* Rankness *and* Fertility *of our Soil, the* Richness *and* Heaviness *of our Food, the* Wealth *and* Abundance *of the Inhabitants (from their universal Trade) the* Inactivity *and* Sedentary *Occupations of the better Sort* (*amongst whom this* Evil *mostly* rages) *and the* Humour *of living in great, populous and consequently unhealthy Towns, have brought forth a* Class *and* Set *of Distempers, with atrocious and frightful* Symptoms, *scarce known to our Ancestors, and never rising to such fatal* Heights, *nor afflicting such* Numbers *in any other known Nation. These* nervous *Disorders being computed to make almost one* third *of the Complaints of the People of* Condition *in* England.[4]

Historians have effectively illustrated how Cheyne's discussion of the nation's proclivity to nervous disease was tinged with conspicuous pride. As perhaps the most prolific author on the subject, Roy Porter explained that 'Cheyne's drift' was that all 'disease symptoms should also be read as symptomatic of something else: an economic and social success story of which the English could justly be proud'.[5] Luxury, laziness, gluttony and flashy city living were vices only the wealthy could afford. Hence, the consequences of these vices – delicate health and strained nerves – were equally indicative of a person's wealth, implying their ability to afford the offendingly opulent lifestyle. The effect of these implications was, as Porter suggested, to 'glamorise the condition of being nervously ill'.[6]

Further glamorizing the condition, Cheyne introduced a class-oriented nervous physiology:

> Persons of slender and weak Nerves are generally of the first Class ... *The Truth is, it* [ie., affliction with nervous disorders] *seldom, and I think never happens or can happen, to any but those of the liveliest and quickest natural Parts, whose Faculties are the brightest and most spiritual, and whose Genius is most keen and penetrating, and primarily where there is the most delicate Sensation and Pain.*

Thus, it was only in a prosperous, well-educated, modernized and highly civilized consumer society that nervous disease could plague so many. Cheyne's 'English Malady' was, as Porter has explained, a fashionable 'disease of civilization'.[7]

Because nervous disease was adorned with such flattering implications, critics of the medical profession expressed concern that patronage-dependent physicians would indiscriminately bestow the complimentary diagnosis upon anyone willing to pay. Even Thomas Beddoes, a well-respected physician and nerve doctor, admitted to the influence that lucrative patients could wield over their diagnosing physicians. Noting the way in which some doctors listened with 'obsequious attention to the medical nonsense of fashionable ladies', Beddoes lamented that the art of healing was often secondary to 'the art of pleasing'.[8] Historians have effectively explored nervous disease within this context of patronage and consumer society, revealing how medical theory and diagnoses often bent to accommodate cultural whim.[9]

Indeed, as the following chapters will show, historians have examined nervous disease in an impressively wide range of frameworks. Beyond its roles as a supposed disease of the nation, symptom of consumer society, gauge of civilization, arbiter of fashion and indicator of the power of patronage and professional integrity, nervous disease has also been explored in terms of gender. As weak nervous systems were most often associated with delicate women, historians have demonstrated how medical theory both responded to, and prescribed, 'proper' female behaviour, and contributed to the late eighteenth century's frenzied concern with effeminate men.[10] Nervousness has also been fruitfully discussed in terms of Scottish Enlightenment philosophy, in which the work of David Hume and Adam Smith contributed to medical theories relating a person's moral fibre to the state of their nerves.[11] Sensitive people possessed delicate nerves. Hence, delicate health was a physical manifestation of admirable emotional depth and sensibility. Historians have studied nervous disease in the context of sensibility extensively, revealing how this term became the shared territory of physicians, philosophers, politicians and authors of fiction.[12]

These histories, demonstrating the many ways that nervous disease was contextualized and understood, are crucial to this study's investigation of the disease experience. Nervous patients and their practitioners were an indelible part of the culture that attributed such strong connotations to disordered nerves. Likewise, as this study will show, the way that patients coped with their ailments was heavily dependent upon these cultural narratives. For instance, some patients revelled in their nervous complaints, confident that they were indicative of mental superiority while others suffered in embarrassed silence, believing that their malady signified their degenerate masculinity. Yet just as these narratives are crucial to understanding the disease experience, so too are the ways in which patients physically suffered from, and treated, their disorders on a daily basis.

To date, learned and literary figures have served as history's most reliable informants on the experience of nervous disease; the prolific pens of such high-profile sufferers as James Boswell, Samuel Johnson, David Hume, Adam Smith and Samuel Taylor Coleridge have left historians with useful personal accounts of their nervous maladies.[13] Yet aside from these shining stars, little has been said about the constellation of 'ordinary' citizens who suffered in such supposed quantity as to qualify nervous disease as 'the' English malady.[14] Through an exploration of hospital registers, medical society records, medical school lectures and dissertations, letters composed by sufferers and private writings and case notes from medical practitioners, this study investigates the experiences of these patients and their doctors, complementing our understanding of the disorder's cultural baggage with a greater understanding of those that carried it.

The bulk of patient examples employed in this study come from the surviving postal correspondence of the famed Edinburgh physician and nerve expert, William Cullen. Like many renowned physicians of his time, Cullen conducted a significant amount of his practice by mail. Housed at the Royal College of Physicians in Edinburgh, thousands of these consultation records survive, spanning from the early years of Cullen's private practice in 1755 to his death in 1790.[15] As a guiding light in eighteenth-century nerve theory and the founding father of the 'neuroses', Cullen's correspondence includes a wealth of letters to and from nervous patients. The blunt descriptions of symptoms, treatments and patient concerns exhibited in these letters offer historians a thrillingly unguarded glimpse into the experience of treating and living with nervous disease in late eighteenth-century Britain.

The chronological focus of this study, spanning from the 1760s to the beginning of the nineteenth century, is significant and strategic. As will be discussed at length in the following chapters, nervous disease reached its height in popularity in the 1760s, following the publication of Robert Whytt's treatise *On Nervous, Hypochondriac, or Hysteric Diseases* (1764). As a physician and professor of medicine at the University of Edinburgh, Whytt's emphasis on the primacy of the nervous system influenced an entire generation of medical minds who inherited belief in its role as the physiological bridge between mind and body. This period also marked, as other historians have shown, the peak in the fashionable nature of nervous sensibility.[16] By the turn of the nineteenth century, the flattering implications of disordered nerves were tempered with moral concern over the apparent ethical and political dangers posed by nervous debility. Thomas Trotter's *View of the Nervous Temperament* (1807) is highly representative of this ideological juncture, and therefore marks the end of this study's chronological focus. The shift in medical and cultural perceptions of nervous suffering witnessed from 1764 to 1807 makes it a particularly useful period for examining the relationship between the stereotyped and lived experiences of nervous disease.[17] On a practical level, Cullen's consultation records fit remarkably well with this timeframe, offering a stream of patient examples spanning the second half of the century.

The first chapter of this study necessarily covers a much longer time span than the rest. Through an exploration of the origins and evolution of medical, literary and philosophical discussions of the nerves, this chapter illustrates the degree to which disordered nerves were laden with cultural meaning by the middle of the eighteenth century. It also demonstrates the enormity and arguable futility of the struggle by medical academics to achieve a clinical definition of nervous disease. Together with the widespread confusion over the structure and workings of the nervous system, the symptoms of nervous disease were, as the seventeenth-century physician Thomas Sydenham described, as 'varied as the colours of a chameleon'.[18] As this chapter reveals, the socially charged yet scientifically vague definition of nervous disease made it a constant source of debate. While countless physicians and nervous patients insisted on the horrid reality of the disease, sceptics argued that it was merely a social construction, designed for deceptive 'sufferers' to feign fashionable sensibility. This chapter explains the reasons behind these suspicions while also exploring how the nerves and nervous disease came to dominate academic medical theory by the middle of the eighteenth century.[19]

Chapter 2 explores the medical practitioners who developed nerve theory and diagnosed nervous disease in the second half of the century. Popular portrayals of nerve doctors during the period commonly depicted them as ostentatious money-grubbing quacks. The tendency of historians to contextualize nervous diagnoses in terms of a competitive consumer society has inadvertently perpetuated this stereotype. Although some doctors did diagnose nervous disease in an effort to make money, compete with professional rivals and improve their own status, this chapter argues that they were not representative of the majority of treating practitioners. Instead of viewing the 'nerve doctors' as a coherent body of practitioners, this chapter examines and compares the academic credentials and quality of publications that they produced. In doing so, it reveals significant tensions and discrepancies between what it defines as the 'first tier' (academic physicians), the 'second tier' (social climbers and social reformers) and the 'third tier' (quacks) treating nervous disease. It focuses heavily on the first-tier leaders of the medical profession, who were the most respected, frequently consulted, and professionally influential body of practitioners. This chapter suggests that the relative absence of these 'serious' doctors from so many histories on the subject has contributed to the faulty image of nervous disease as a phenomenon more culturally contrived than clinically significant.

In a similar fashion, Chapter 3 highlights the shallow nature of stereotyped depictions of nervous sufferers. Indeed, patient correspondence, consultation letters and professional descriptions of nervous invalids by medical practitioners reveal a striking contrast between popular perceptions about, and the reality of, nervous patients. Despite the general reputation of eighteenth-century nervous disease as the exclusive preserve of the rich, this chapter underscores the presence of sufferers in the middle and lower classes. Whereas the period's popular discourse frequently portrayed nervous patients as eager sufferers secretly rejoicing in the modish implications of their maladies, this study further suggests that most patients seeking medical assistance were in genuine misery. Likewise, whereas nervous disease was commonly considered a pathological manifestation of fashionable sensibility and delicacy, patient consultation letters reveal that the symptoms of nervous disease were far from flattering. Unlike the vague swoons and nervous flutterings felt by fictional heroines in the mid-century's novels of sensibility, real nervous sufferers littered their disease descriptions with remarkably indelicate complaints of gas, painful indigestion and emotional instability.

My discussion of treatment in Chapter 4 also provides surprising revelations about the nervous experience. It explains the medical theory behind seemingly indulgent prescriptions like travel and trips to the spa, investigates the most common diet and exercise regimes for nervous sufferers, and provides details of the medications most commonly prescribed in such cases. In addition to explaining the theory behind these remedies, this chapter illustrates what it was like for nervous patients to undergo treatment; it explores the tastes, smells and side effects of the most popular medicines, as well as the methods behind more aggressive remedies like blisters, issues and electric shock therapy. Through actual patient accounts, this chapter shows how patients from all classes endured surprisingly objectionable and aggressive treatments in hopes of curing their very real, and often very painful symptoms.

The final chapter of this study further addresses the disparities between the discourse and reality of nervous disease. It demonstrates how popular portrayals of nervous patients as selfish malingerers in the late eighteenth century reflected serious national anxiety over Britain's ability to cope in a modern world. It explores how concern over a perceived increase in nervous sufferers diminished its fashionable exclusivity and heightened alarm over the perceived danger of depraved modern living. The late eighteenth century witnessed a significant moral backlash against sufferers who, by living loosely, had prompted their own nervous conditions and were consequently endangering the physical, moral and political health of the nation.

The fact that nervous complaints persisted throughout the century, even amidst mounting social condemnation of nervous weakness, proves that the experienced symptoms of nervous disease were far more lasting than their flattering social implications. Whereas the modern historiography frequently illustrates the ways in which the eighteenth-century medical world was influenced by culture, this study highlights the equal power of medicine to belie social prescription and to affect the period's cultural climate. By grounding our understanding of the cultural contexts of nervous disease with a better understanding of its clinical importance and lived experience, this study reveals that nervous disease in eighteenth-century Britain was as diagnostically significant as it was socially charged.

1 DEFINING NERVOUS DISEASE IN EIGHTEENTH-CENTURY BRITAIN

By the eighteenth century the disorders 'commonly called nervous' already had a long history, stretching back to the Hippocratic writings in the fourth century BC.[1] For hundreds of years doctors and natural philosophers debated the significance of a mind–body connection, the origins of hypochondria and hysteria, and the precise physiology allowing for what was widely acknowledged to be a confusing and inconstant set of symptoms. By the time the eminent nerve doctor Robert Whytt wrote his *Observations on the Nature, Causes, and Cure of those Disorders which have been Commonly Called Nervous, Hypochondriac, or Hysteric* (1764) in an effort to provide an updated and comprehensive medical text on these matters, the definition of nervous disease was as loaded as its history was long. Cultural implications of suffering from disordered nerves proliferated alongside clinical explanations for nervous disease. Hypochondria, hysteria and general nervous weakness encompassed a befuddling mixture of physical and emotional causes and consequences including emotional superiority, relaxed nervous fibres, wealth, dangerously strong passions, delicate physiology, genius and extreme sympathy between the mind and the malfunctioning body. Opinions regarding the verity and severity of nervous disease were as mixed as these explanations, with sceptics regarding it as an invention of overly sentimental novel readers and obsequious physicians, and believers insisting that anyone who doubted the pain and distress of nervous sufferers was simply 'ignorant and cruel'.[2] The confused history of this malady prior to the mid-eighteenth century illuminates the reasons behind these disparate opinions.[3] This history also elucidates the struggle of physicians to define the complicated set of disorders denominated 'nervous', and highlights the simple elegance and lasting significance of Whytt's 1764 definition of nervous disease as an ailment 'owing to an uncommon delicacy or unnatural sensibility of the nerves'.[4]

Historians have long acknowledged the vague nature of the definition of nervous disease and its cultural implications.[5] This chapter examines the reasons behind this ambiguity and explores the inevitable clash between cultural and pathological definitions of nervous disease in the eighteenth century.[6] By addressing these issues it clarifies the reasons behind scepticism about nervous ailments on the part of many medical practitioners and members of the public.[7] This chapter begins with an overview of the medical faculty's variety of opinions regarding the causes of nervous disease from the seventeenth to the early eighteenth century. It then explores the ways in which these professional debates prompted an increasingly medically informed public to devise their own opinions regarding nervous ailments. Ultimately it reveals how, fuelled by the popularity of Scottish philosophy and sentimental literature, public definitions replete with flattering social implications of nervous disease predominated over starkly pathological definitions from the 1730s to the middle of the century. As this chapter will show, it was only with Whytt's publication in 1764 that the medical world asserted its presumed dominion over nervous disease, and that the nerves, in turn, came to dominate the medical world.

Debates over the Structure and Function of the Nerves

For Hippocrates, hypochondriasis was an actual physical disorder in the spleen, or, more generally, the *hypochondrium*, an abdominal area located under the rib cage.[8] Despite this physical cause, the symptoms of a disordered hypochondrium identified by the ancient Greeks were largely psychological, including strong emotional turmoil and melancholia. Greek medicine acknowledged the presence of mind–body connection, with Hippocratic writings noting common sense examples of the phenomenon including the way in which fear could make a man turn pale, and anger could cause his face to redden. Galen called similar attention to how the pulse was easily 'altered by quarrels and alarms which suddenly disturb the mind'.[9] Consequently, it was not surprising to the ancients that in addition to the physical effects of a deranged *hypochondrium* like painful digestion and flatulence, patients also experienced emotional symptoms such as fear and sorrow.

According to the Hippocratic texts, hysteria was closely related to hypochondria, although it was most common in unmarried or widowed women. With the exception of emotional or physical fits whereby women would convulse or laugh and cry uncontrollably, hysteria exhibited the same symptomology as the male-dominated diagnosis of hypochondria: difficulty breathing, an irregular pulse, vomiting, belching, headaches and anxiety. Hysteria was commonly attributed to a 'wandering womb', in which the offending uterus would float upward, place pressure on the liver, and encumber the patient's breathing.[10] The simplest cure for hysteric patients was marriage and quick pregnancy, as a baby in the womb would supposedly help to weigh it down. Practitioners such as the respected Bath physician Robert Peirce subscribed to this notion well into second half of the seventeenth century. Among Pierce's published cases is one of a nineteen-year-old female who was 'more than ordinarily troubled with Vapours, and strange Fits (doubtless Hysterical)'. Although Pierce noted that his patient was cured by a course of the Bath waters, he prescribed marriage as the most reliable preventative of future fits. As he reflected in his published notes, 'I hope my Lady, her Mother, (by giving her to a good Husband) prevented a Relapse'.[11]

Medical theory changed little from ancient times to the seventeenth century. The celebrated seventeenth-century scholar Robert Burton's *Anatomy of Melancholy* (1621) still relied heavily on Hippocratic humoural theories, identifying the four humours as the root cause of all distempers. Consequently, Burton very traditionally associated the melancholic and depressive state with an excess of black bile.[12] Although he composed 1,392 pages on melancholy, Burton did little to clearly define the disorder, claiming instead that 'whether it be a cause or an effect, a Disease, or Symptome ... I will not contende about it'.[13] Among the symptoms of melancholy he listed feelings of fear and sorrow, disordered imagination and a loss of reason. Like his ancient predecessors, Burton believed strongly in a reciprocal relationship between mind and body:

> For as the Body workes upon the minde, by his bad humours, troubling the Spirits, sending grosse fumes into the Braine; and so *per consequens* disturbing the Soule, and all the faculties of it with feare, sorrow, &c. which are ordinary symptoms of this Disease: so on the other side, the minde most effectually workes upon the Body, producing by his passions and perturbations, miraculous alterations; as Melancholy, despaire, cruell diseases, and sometimes death it selfe.[14]

Like Hippocrates, Burton noted that emotional turmoil could result in hypochondria and hysteria. Further blurring the already vague distinction between melancholia, hysteria and hypochondria, Burton identified a particular type of melancholy as 'hypochondriacal melancholy'. The symptoms of hypochondriacal melancholy were twofold: those that affected the body, and those that affected the mind. Physical symptoms included 'winde, rumbling in the guts, belly ake, heat in the bowels, convulsions, crudities, short winde, sowre & sharpe belchings, cold sweat, paine in the left side, suffocation, palpitation, heavinesse of the heart, singing in the eares, much spittle and moist, &c'. Psychological symptoms included a tendency to be 'fearefull, sad, [and] suspitious' while experiencing 'discontent, anxiety &c'.[15]

Burton also acknowledged a strong connection between hypochondriacal melancholy and mental genius, insisting that most poets and academics were sufferers; *The Anatomy* included a lengthy chapter specifically devoted to the 'Misery of Schollers'.[16] Burton was hardly the first to suggest a connection between melancholia and creative genius. Hundreds of years earlier Aristotle even pondered why 'all men who have become outstanding in philosophy, statesmanship, poetry or the arts are melancholic'.[17] While Burton believed strongly in the ability of a superior mind to affect the body, he also believed that hypochon-driacal melancholy could have an 'inward' physical cause. The physical source of hypochondriacal melancholy remained a mystery, although the spleen, a 'cold stomach' and an 'over-hot liver' were the primary culprits.[18] Burton explained the difficulty of determining a physical cause, claiming that 'in this hypochon-driacal or flatuous melancholy, the symptoms are so ambiguous that the most well-trained physicians cannot identify the part involved'.[19] Thus, Burton left his readers with a blurred distinction between melancholy, hysteria and hypochon-dria, as well as significant ambiguity regarding their physical causes.

In 1667 the renowned London physician and member of the Royal Soci-ety, Thomas Willis, lent some clarity to this vague picture with his publication on the *Pathology of the Brain*. As G. S. Rousseau has argued, Willis's *Pathology* marked the beginning of a gradual shift from an understanding of the human body as a system of humours and hydraulics to the eighteenth-century's notion of the body ruled by the nervous system. Willis argued that the human soul/mind was located in the brain, and that the nerves, running from the brain to the rest of the body were responsible for all of the body's functions including sensa-tion, movement and thought.[20] Because melancholy, hysteria and hypochondria involved problems with both an overly passionate mind and a malfunctioning body, the nerves were the most likely source behind these troubles. '[T]hose distempers,' Willis proclaimed, 'are for the greatest part convulsions and con-tractions of the nervous parts'.[21] He explained,

> Sometimes the Melancholy, being disturb'd in the spleen, conveys thence the pas-sion to the Brain, whence disorderly and Hypochondriacal fancies happen: And on the contrary, when a violent Passion of the mind, occasionally rais'd within the brain troubles the Spirits residing in it, the impression given the fancy, is convey'd to the spleen by the course and successive affect of the spirits, lying within the nerves.[22]

This 'discovery' made Willis a pivotal figure in the history of the nerves and nervous disease. As the presumed link between the brain and body, interest in the nerves skyrocketed after Willis, becoming the most significant topic in phys-iology until the nineteenth century.[23] In addition to identifying hypochondria and hysteria as specifically 'nervous' disorders, Willis also expanded the group of symptoms traditionally associated with these ailments to include 'wander-ing pains', 'flushing of blood', 'a danger of swooning' and a tendency to imagine themselves 'being affected with diseases of which they are free'.[24]

While the nerves gained newfound importance in the seventeenth century with Willis's theory, they were not a new discovery; nerves were present even in the writings of Hippocrates and Galen, although they were often mistaken for sinews, ligaments and tendons. The ancients believed that the nerves were responsible for movement and sensation. The precise structure of the nerves was a matter of debate, with Aristotle arguing that the nerves emanated from the heart, and Galen rightly insisting centuries later that they stemmed from the brain. Galen further postulated that the nerves were hollow tubes, through which the body's animating fluid, described as 'pneuma psychikon' or 'animal spirits', flowed, carrying sensory impressions to the brain.[25] Fifteen centuries later, Willis agreed, contending that animal spirits were the method by which 'unseen messages' were sent from the brain to the rest of the body.[26]

Like, Willis, Thomas Sydenham, the 'English Hippocrates' of the late seventeenth century, also believed that nervous disease was the result of disordered animal spirits and convulsions or contractions of nervous parts. As Sydenham noted in his explanation of hysteria, 'From this very disorder of the spirits is born that disturbance, and the continually variable abnormalities of both mind and body which prevail in hysterics and hypochondriacs alike'.[27] Sydenham further maintained that hypochondria and hysteria were the same disease; female sufferers were simply hysterics, and male sufferers were hypochondriacs. His posthumously published *Compleat Method of Curing Almost All Diseases* (1693) noted of 'the disease called in women Hysterical; in men the Hypochondriacal Passion' that 'when the mind is disturb'd by some grievous accident, the animal spirits run into disorderly motions'.[28]

Whereas Sydenham acknowledged that a physical disorder or disorder of the animal spirits was the cause of hypochondriac and hysteric symptoms, he maintained that strong emotions typically initiated these ailments. Thus, hypochondria and hysteria were both mental and physical disorders. Sydenham warned practitioners of the consequent difficulty entailed in diagnosing nervous ailments; because these diseases were often instigated by 'disturbances of the mind', he argued that their symptoms could not 'be accounted for on the common principle of investigating diseases'. Instead, symptoms were varied and inconsistent, thereby frustrating physicians in search of a purely physical distemper.[29]

Two years after Sydenham's death, Sydenham's friend and Thomas Willis's prized pupil from Oxford, the medically educated philosopher John Locke, published his famous *Essay Concerning Human Understanding* (1690). In this essay, Locke discussed sensation at length, clearly adopting his tutor's ideas about the nerves. Just as Willis held the nerves responsible for sensory impressions, and consequently for knowledge, so too did Locke insist that the nerves were 'conduits', conveying sensations to a receptive mind.[30] Locke's work further cemented medical ideas about the connection between mind and body, showing how even a person's train of thought, association of ideas and state of mind could have 'considerable influence on the body'.[31] Eighteenth century philosophers like David Hume, who, as will be discussed, further shaped the evolution of nervous theory, were largely indebted to Locke's ideas about the association of ideas and the nerves. Of course, Locke's reasoning was not wholly owing to Willis's teachings;

Isaac Newton also greatly influenced his philosophy as is clear from the fact that Locke dedicated his *Essay*, in part, to him. Indeed, Newton's *Principia* (1687) had strong implications for the study of the nerves and sensation, suggesting that solid nerves conveyed sensation by vibration.[32] Newton's later *Opticks* (1704) discussed the nerves even more directly, explaining how they facilitated sight: 'do not the Rays of Light in falling upon the bottom of the Eye excite Vibrations ... Which, being propagated along the solid Fibres of the optick Nerves into the Brain, cause the sense of seeing?' Such vibrations, he continued, 'convey into the Brain the impressions made upon all the Organs of Sense'.[33] Newton's writings about the nerves also reveal a significant shift from traditional beliefs regarding nerve structure; whereas Willis and the ancient physicians believed in a hollow nerve, through which animal spirits or a 'nervous liquor' flowed, Newton instead envisioned a solid nervous fibre, whose actions depended upon the vibration of a weightless, invisible and stationary elastic aether. This aether, according to Newton, could capably transmit sensation, electricity and magnetic forces via the subtle vibration of its 'indivisible particles'.[34]

Newton's notion of a solid nerve and elastic aether were overshadowed by the significance that his mechanics held for late seventeenth and early eighteenth-century physiology. While Harvey's discovery of the circulation of the blood in 1628 prompted widespread adoption of vascular and hydrodynamic physiological theories, Newton's mechanics encouraged further emphasis on movement and interaction of matter within the body.[35] The resultant mechanical physiology depicted the human body as a composition of canals, funnelling vital fluids to every part. This mechanical model of the body gradually superseded ancient humoural medical theories in the early eighteenth century, with disease considered less the direct consequence of an imbalance of the four bodily humours than a defect in their movement as a result of clogged or malfunctioning moving parts. Thus, Archibald Pitcairne, the famed Newtonian physician and medical professor at the University of Leiden, attributed such symptoms as mental confusion and delirium to a malfunction in the hydrodynamics of the blood, which in turn disturbed the flow of animal spirits through the nerves.[36] Pitcairne's mechanistic view of the body also indicated his adoption of a Cartesian division between the soul and the physical body whereby the body functioned or malfunctioned independently, without reference to the immaterial soul.

Pitcairne's student, Hermaan Boerhaave, became the most famous mechanist physician of the eighteenth century. As the professor of medicine at the University of Leiden, the seat of medical learning in the seventeenth and early eighteenth centuries, Pitcairne enjoyed an unparalleled reputation as a master of medicine on the continent and in Britain.[37] Significantly, all four of the original faculty members at the University of Edinburgh's medical school in 1726 were educated by Boerhaave in Leiden. Not surprisingly, Boerhaave's mechanist ideas dominated the medical curriculum at Edinburgh for the first half of the eighteenth century.[38]

Like his mechanist predecessors, Boerhaave described the inner body as a complex configuration of tubes and vessels. The smallest of these tubes were the nerves, which connected directly to the body's muscle fibres, and through which animal spirits flowed. Like Willis, Boerhaave believed that animal spirits flowed from the brain; it was a surge of nervous juice flowing into the muscular fibres via the nerves that prompted muscular movement. Thus, as Hubert Steinke has explained, while the nerves were important to mechanist theory, they were regarded merely as 'passive transport structure[s], conveying impulses to and from the brain'.[39]

A quarter of a century after Newton published his *Opticks*, physicians became as interested in his ideas about nerve structure, as they were in his mechanical ideas at the beginning of the century.[40] From the 1740s onward, as physicians investigated the potential medical uses of electricity, discussion of Newton's elastic and electricity-transmitting aether consistently resurfaced.[41] Yet revived notions of Newton's aether as the communicative agent between body and soul irritated a number of physicians who opposed mechanistic and dualistic views of the human body. One such opponent, the founder of the Prussian medical school at Halle, Georg Ernst Stahl, defined the concept of animism, whereby arguments regarding the precise nature of nervous fluids, aether and spirits were rendered obsolete. According to animist theory, the soul (*anima*) directed all movement, sensation and emotion. The soul was the body's vital principle, independent of physical intermediaries like animal spirits.[42] Whereas mechanists like Boerhaave viewed the body as a healthy functioning or diseased and malfunctioning machine, separate from the immaterial soul, a growing number of animist physicians from the 1730s onward insisted that the soul had a place within the body, and that it played a dominant pathological role. Not surprisingly, discussion of the soul acting upon the body according to unknowable spiritual principles did little to solidify a uniform physiological understanding among medical professionals. Debate raged on regarding how the immaterial soul acted upon material matter, and the precise role of the nerves.[43]

Boerhaave's student, Albrecht von Haller, lent his own voice to the discussion in the early eighteenth century. Unlike Stahl, Haller rejected the notion of tubular nerves and animal spirits, arguing instead, like Newton, that the nerves were solid fibres. More significantly, Haller distinguished between animal motion and sensual perception, which, he claimed, corresponded with notions of 'irritability' and 'sensibility'. 'Irritability', Haller explained, referred to the contraction of a muscle as a result of a stimulus. Alternatively, 'sensibility' denoted the ability of the nerves to feel this stimulation, and to convey it to the brain.

Like Haller, the eminent Edinburgh physician and medical professor Robert Whytt rejected the notions of nervous spirits or a Newtonian aether flowing through the nerves. Like the animists, Whytt also insisted on the presence of the soul in the physical body, believing that the soul, which he termed the 'sentient principle', governed both the movement of the muscles and the workings of the mind.[44] Yet Whytt significantly differed from animists in his insistence that the sentient principle operated via the brain and nerves. According to Whytt, sense, reason and motion were due to the cooperative workings of the brain, nerves and soul.[45] Whereas animists believed that disease was the soul's attempt to rid the body of noxious agents by prompting physical symptoms, Whytt argued that the soul was unaffected by illness, and that the brain and nerves monitored disease.[46]

In accordance with Whytt, other professors at the University of Edinburgh medical school also placed the soul within the physical body and emphasized the significance of the nervous system.[47] However by the middle of the century, these professors referred more often to the state of a patient's 'sensibility' than they did to Whytt's elusive 'sentient principle' or state of the patient's soul.[48] Unlike the animists or Whytt, these new 'vitalist physicians' argued, as Roger French has explained, that the 'ultimate principle of life was no longer the immortal soul of Christian tradition, but some separate vital principle, and aether was less an agent of communication and more a vital principle itself'.[49] Whether the matter within the nerves was referred to as 'aether', 'animal spirits', or a 'nervous fluid' was of little consequence to most vitalist physicians, who preferred the less visual term of 'vital principle'. As one of Whytt's vitalist colleagues noted in a medical lecture later in the century,

> Whether [the nerves] are solid strings, which vibrate from one extremity to another; or along which a fine elastic Aether moves; or if they are canals transmitting a fluid; hath long been, and still is a dispute which it is perhaps of little consequence to determine.[50]

More important was the vital principle's role as a life sustaining nervous energy, responsible for muscle movement.[51] The level of nervous energy experienced by an individual was dependent upon sympathetic, mental and external forces. These emphases on sensibility and on the role of the nerves as agents of the 'vital principle' invited a strongly holistic view of disease whereby external impressions, emotions and environment could physically affect the body through nervous sensation.[52] Vitalists believed that factors as disparate as grief, joy, climate and topography, could prompt a response by the sensible nerves and result in a somatic disorder.[53]

By 1750 the nerves were of paramount importance to medical theory. The shift from the late seventeenth and early eighteenth-century's emphasis on the vascular system to an emphasis on the nervous system by the middle of the eighteenth century was further facilitated by the new generation of physicians joining the faculty of the Edinburgh medical school. No longer educated by Boerhaave or loyal to his mechanist theories, these physicians, sensitive to the connection between mind and body and the power of nervous sensation, took centre stage in the medical world.

Consequences of Medical Debate on the Status of Nervous Disease in the Early Eighteenth Century

The wealth of debate over the structure of the nerves, and the pathology of hysteria and hypochondria over the course of the seventeenth century did little to clarify the definition of nervous disease. Rather, as nervous diseases were attributed to patients' disordered minds *and* bodies, their origins became more difficult to pinpoint, their symptoms became more difficult to isolate, and their legitimacy was increasingly questioned by an ever more dubious public. Sir Richard Blackmore, author of *A Treatise of the Spleen and Vapours: or, Hypochondriacal and Hysterical Affections* (1725), noted that hypochondriac and hysteric patients were often 'unwilling their Disease should go by its right name' due to popular perceptions that their symptoms were 'imaginary and fantastick Sickness of the Brain, filled with odd and irregular ideas'. Consequently, Blackmore explained, many people treated nervous patients with 'derision and contempt'.[54]

The psychological dimension of nervous disease was not the only factor leading to public incredulity regarding its physical reality. Disagreement within the medical profession also shook the faith of British laymen. Without question, the published literature on nervous disease by medical practitioners from antiquity to the late seventeenth century revealed a significant amount of professional discord and revised theory. Debate over the function and structure of the nerves – their hollow or solid natures, their accordance with humoural theory, their use of animal spirits, or their tendency to vibrate when 'plucked' like the strings of an instrument – continued well into the eighteenth century and beyond. In his *Treatise of the Hypochondriack and Hysterick Diseases* (1730) the physician-philosopher and social critic Bernard Mandeville reviewed with frustration the contradictory history of these disorders, exploring the 'several Causes to which the Hypochondriack Passion has been believed to owe its Rise'.[55] The reason for such varied accounts, Mandeville insisted, was the tendency of physicians to engage in empty speculation. Instead, he insisted, physicians should be honest about their ignorance and openly recognize the limits of human reason. Medical knowledge should be based on experimental evidence, rather than the narcissistic rantings of philosophizing physicians. In the introduction to his *Treatise* Mandeville wrote,

'Tis Pride that makes the Physician abandon the solid Observation of never-erring Nature, to take up with the loose Conjectures of his own wandering Invention; that the World may admire the Fertility of his Brain ... But if the Reasons that are often given by the one ... were to be strictly examin'd into; it would almost induce a Man of Sense to disown his kind, and make him blush, when he is called a Rational Creature.[56]

Beyond undermining faith in the integrity of physicians, Mandeville's comment also raised doubt about the lasting truth of medical explanations. In 'looking back,' Mandeville argued, 'you may all along observe a fashion in Philosophizing as much as in wearing of Cloaths'.[57]

While physiological theories continued to rise and fall like fashions even after Mandeville's time, some experienced occasional revivals. For instance, although Newton's notion of solid nerves and vibrating aether dominated theories of hollow nerves and animal spirits from the late seventeenth century onwards, its new reign was not uncontested. Medical publications relating accounts of unhealthy 'clogged' or 'drained' tubular nerves surfaced well into the eighteenth century. As late as 1751, the Scottish physiologist Malcolm Flemyng argued with Newtonian thinkers, providing an 'easy' argument in defence of his more traditional beliefs:

I wonder that an easy and obvious manner of reasoning did not come into their minds, to this purpose; as the animal spirits are the finest and most subtle of all the liquids in the animal body, the nerves must be nourished solely by these.[58]

Flemyng dismissed the 'cloud of arguments' surrounding the question of whether or not animal spirits actually flowed through the nerves, preferring instead to devote his attention to the precise composition of this spirit which he amusingly determined to be a mixture of 'phlegm or water, oil, animal, salt, and earth, all highly attenuated ... and intimately mixed and incorporated together'.[59]

It was because the nerves were too small to have their tubular or fibrous structure incontrovertibly proven with a microscope that nervous theories were dependent upon the philosophical reasoning which Mandeville found so objectionable. Critics of the medical profession also objected to this philosophical reasoning, accusing practitioners of concealing the limits of their medical knowledge with imaginative theories. Many physicians staunchly defended their profession against this criticism. As Flemyng claimed, 'it is, I think, much more to be wondered at, that, in so abtruse an enquiry, human penetration should have been able to proceed so far, than that it hath made no farther advances'.[60] Other physicians passively acknowledged the limits of experimentation and human reason in discovering the structure and inner workings of the nerves. For instance, in his *New Essay on the Nerves and the Doctrine of the Animal Spirits* (1737), the physician David Kinneir expressed content with even a vague understanding of the role that animal spirits played in causing health or sickness. After insisting that 'good animal spirits' meant health and 'harmony between soul and body', he noted, 'but how that comes about is, and probably will always be, a mystery to human reason'.[61] In light of the ever changing nature of medical theories and the mysteriously vague pathological explanations of the professional community, nerves and nervous diseases were increasingly viewed as fair game for investigation and speculation by an ever more medically informed public.

Public Definitions of Nervous Disease in the Early Eighteenth Century

Medical knowledge was not the exclusive domain of medical professionals in the eighteenth century. Costly professional medical advice was beyond the means of most. Furthermore, in an age when most citizens self treated with trusty household remedies inherited from earlier generations or in accordance with medical advice offered in comprehensive self-help guides, formal medical consultations often seemed an unnecessary if not useless expense. Britons of every class owned inexpensive medical manuals like John Wesley's *Primitive Physic* (1747) and William Buchan's *Domestic Medicine* (1769).[62] Comprehensive in nature, these manuals addressed every imaginable disorder, including nervous disease. More specialized texts, like George Cheyne's *English Malady* were, realistically, only within the means of the wealthier classes. Ownership of specialized medical volumes implied that a person had the money to purchase them and the leisure time to study them. In this way, detailed medical knowledge became the mark of a gentleman. [63] The fashion for dabbling in amateur medical studies encouraged the further proliferation of popularly accessible medical publications.

Medical treatises once exclusively published in Latin for a scientifically learned audience now expanded their readership with the release of new editions and publications in English. Likewise, doctors who once published purely for the edification of, and recognition from, their fellow physicians, now wrote highly accessible health manuals and treatises for the edification of, and recognition from, an interested purchasing public. Along with laymen's growing interest in specialized medical matters like nervous disease came heightened self confidence in their ability to discuss and judge the theories behind these ailments, their symptomologies, their treatments, and perhaps most significantly, their status in the hierarchy of bodily distempers. The physician Robert John Thornton bitterly acknowledged this fact in the first edition of his *Philosophy of Medicine*:

> there are three things which almost every person gives himself credit for understanding, whether he has taken any pains to make himself master of them or not. These are: 1. *The art of mending a dull fire*; 2. *Politics; and,* 3. PHYSIC.[64]

Whereas the medico-philosophical community at the close of the seventeenth century largely embraced the works of Locke and Newton, the publication of these works in English meant that they also received an enthusiastic reception from the public. Following these vernacular publications, Lockean and Newtonian ideas regarding sensation and nervous physiology were disseminated quickly in the public realm. Locke and Newton's discussions of the nerves were often quoted and discussed in the popular London publication *The Spectator*. Likewise, John Wynne's 1696 abridgement of Locke's *Essay* was in its eleventh edition by 1774, and Jeffrey Gilbert's easy to read *Abstract of Locke's Essay Concerning Human Understanding* (1709) ran through at least four editions during its first four decades in print. Newton's work was frequently diluted for its ever-increasing audience, leading to such publications as James Thomson's 'Poem to the memory of Sir Isaac Newton' (1731), which praised the significance of his works in verse, and Francesco Algarotti's *Sir Isaac Newton's Philosophy Explain'd for the Use of Ladies* (1739). [65] Given the wide propagation of Newton's and Locke's theories, it was generally accepted early in the eighteenth century among physicians, philosophers and even ladies 'with not the least Notion of Physics', that nerves were the all-important link between mind and body. [66]

The respected names of 'Locke' and 'Newton' became so well known that a mere citation from one of their books could lend credibility to the work of any aspiring medical author. As the fictional physician Philopirio in Mandeville's *Treatise of the Hypochondriack* sarcastically noted, 'A Man of Wit and good Parts, that has a little smatt'ring of the *Newtonian* Philosophy, is seldom at a Loss now, to solve almost any Phoenomena'. [67] Cheyne was quick to lay claim to his Newtonian roots, repeatedly noting his indebtedness to the 'late *sagacious and learned* Sir Isaac Newton' in *The English Malady*. [68] As a student of the famed Newtonian Archibald Pitcairne, there is little doubt that Cheyne's Newtonianism was sincere. Nonetheless, there is also little doubt that he hoped to profit by flaunting his respectable and increasingly fashionable intellectual heritage. Cheyne was eager to impress the public; unlike the majority of previous treatises written on the nerves and nervous disease, his *English Malady* was intended for a lay audience. His appeal to a popular audience was highly successful, with the *English Malady* going through six official and one pirated edition in its first two years in print. [69]

Like Newton, Cheyne envisioned solid nerve fibres which, when unhealthy, would become 'lax, feeble, and *unelastik*'. [70] Whereas the vibration of moderately taut and healthily elastic nerves would convey the appropriate senses and perceptions to the brain, loosely strung nerves would distort this sensibility, causing a sharp excess of feeling. Unlike many of his seventeenth-century predecessors, Cheyne stressed the somatic nature of nervous disease, arguing that physically weak nerves were the cause of the depressed spirits so common among hypochondriacs, hysterics and melancholics. By emphasizing the physical origin of nervous disease, Cheyne sought to rescue it from its reputation among the general population as a purely mental malady. Explaining the ill repute of nervous disorders in the non-medical world he wrote,

> Nervous *Distempers* especially, *are under some Kind of* Disgrace *and* Imputation, *in the Opinion of the* Vulgar *and* Unlearned; *they pass among the Multitude, for a lower Degree of* Lunacy, *and the first Step towards a* distemper'd Brain; *and the best Construction is* Whim, Ill-Humour, Peevishness *or* Particularity ...[71]

In reality, Cheyne argued, nervous diseases were exclusive physical ailments, afflicting only the most sensitive and hence, refined members of society:

> *The Truth is, it* [nervous disease] *seldom, and I think never happens or can happen, to any but those of the liveliest and quickest natural Parts, whose Faculties are the brightest and most spiritual, and whose Genius is most keen and penetrating, and primarily where there is the most delicate Sensation and Pain.*[72]

Cheyne flattered nervous sufferers by insisting that their ailments were the result of refinement and over-civilization. Nervous patients, Cheyne contended, were most often city dwellers who anguished over business concerns during the day, then played hard at night with banquets, spirituous liquors, card playing and dancing; their nervous bodies were mentally exhausted and physically weak. Long days of sitting at an office desk, or for people of leisure, endless hours of polite inactivity, sipping tea, writing letters and reading books, was a far cry from the hearty activity of the lower classes who engaged in daily manual labour. Hearty living meant healthy nerves. Alternatively, the luxurious and physically lazy lifestyles of the upper classes meant weak and overly-elastic nerves, with all of their consequent symptoms: a weak pulse, fainting fits, shortness of breath, headaches, cold extremities,

> all *Lowness of Spirits, Swelling of the Stomach, frequent Eructation, Noise in the Bowels or Ears, frequent Yawning ... Restlessness, Inquietude, Fidgeting, Anxiety, Peevishness, Discontent, Melancholy, Grief, Vexation, Ill Humour, Inconstancy, lethargick or watchful Disorders,* in short, every Symptom, not already classed under some particular limited Distemper ... [73]

While distressing, these symptoms could appear alluring to a public believing Cheyne's claims regarding the superior class of nervous sufferers. Undoubtedly this appeal was only heightened by Cheyne's additional claim that that '*Fools, weak* or *stupid* Persons, *heavy* and *dull Souls,* are seldom much troubled with Vapours or Lowness of Spirits'.[74] Beyond afflicting people with the money to afford a luxurious or indulgent lifestyle, Cheyne argued that nervous disease also attacked people with superior intelligence and sensibility. Early in his *English*

Malady, Cheyne explained the way in which people of elevated rank and mental ability also had the greatest sensibility, and hence, the greatest susceptibility to disordered nerves:

> There are as many and as different Degrees of *Sensibility* or of *Feeling* as there are Degrees of *Intelligence* and Perception in *human* Creatures ... One shall suffer more from the Prick of a *Pin*, or *Needle*, from their extreme Sensibility, than others from being run thro' the Body; and the *first* sort, seem to be of the *Class* of these *Quick-Thinkers* I have formerly mentioned.[75]

Similar to Burton's claims about melancholy, Cheyne's association of nervous symptoms with 'quick thinkers' was also reminiscent of Bernard Mandeville's assertion three years before *The English Malady*, that hypochondria was often referred to as 'the Disease of the Learned; because they are more subject to it than other people'.[76] Cheyne's notion of a hugely powerful mind–body connection was also already widely accepted among his eighteenth-century readership and physicians. As Cheyne stated, 'It is well known to *Physicians* what wonderful Effects the *Passions* ... have on the Pulse, Circulation, Perspiration, and Secretions, and the other Animal Functions, in *Nervous* Cases especially, even to the restoring from Death, and destroying Life'.[77] This would not have surprised a public that was used to seeing 'grief' and 'fear' listed as official causes of death on the London Bills of Mortality.[78] The physician and poet Edward Baynard also displayed the general public's awareness of the connection between mind and body. His poem, *Health* reminded readers in the first verse of a forty-five-page rhyme of the importance of regulating their emotions:

> If twice Man's Age you would fulfil,
> Let Reason guide you, not your Will;
> Let all the Passions of the Soul
> Be subject unto her Controul[79]

Despite the many well-established themes discussed in the *English Malady*, Cheyne's spectrum of class-based nervous physiology was original. Whereas the wealthy and learned suffered most from nervous disease, Cheyne instituted a graded system wherein the '*indolent* and Thoughtless' suffered the least, and the '*Stupid* and Ideots *not at all*.[80] In this way, Cheyne classified all British citizens into orders based upon the intensity of their emotional responses and the composite strength or laxity of their nerves; no one was exempt from the taint or privilege of these meaningful fibres.

The publication of Cheyne's *English Malady* brought with it new meaning and a restored reputation for nervous disease. Suddenly these disorders were deserving of admiration rather than scorn. The importance of *The English Malady* to the history of nervous disease cannot be overlooked; the book was widely read, with 'Cheyne' becoming a household name from the time of its initial publication, through to the end of the eighteenth century.[81] Yet the fact that so many people were aware of Cheyne's book does not mean that everyone agreed with him, or his methods. In the first instance, many physicians strongly objected to his flagrant disregard for professional boundaries by writing for the public. Self-help guides only served to empower patients, giving them the tools to self diagnose and self treat. As a result, they could compromise the demand for lucrative private consultations and undermine the significance of trained medical professionals.

Professional distaste for self-help guides already had a long history before Cheyne. Even seventeenth-century books like John Archer's *Every Man His Own Doctor* (1671) exacerbated the angst felt by many physicians over their perceived lack of recognition for their specialized skills. Yet Cheyne's *English Malady* inflicted an additional wound on this already irritated profession. As many physicians feared, his insistence upon the flattering social significance of nervous disease could potentially encourage people eager for status to feign nervous sufferings. It was with this in mind that Doctor Samuel Johnson warned his friend James Boswell not to take Cheyne's message to heart: 'Do not let him teach you a foolish notion that melancholy is a proof of acuteness'.[82] The temptation for 'patients' to fake fashionable nervous sufferings would only cast additional doubt on the reality of an already pathologically vague disorder. Likewise, as many physicians believed, the very fact that nervous disorders were so clinically confusing meant that they could only be properly diagnosed by discerning medical professionals. Yet for a population already primed in the subjects of the nerves, sensation and perception by such authorities as Locke and Newton, diagnosing nervous disease with the help of Cheyne's *English Malady* seemed an appropriate and manageable task. As newspapers and journals began to discuss nervous disease, debating the physical or mental nature of its symptoms and advertising miraculous cures capable of curing any nervous ailment, popular interest in the nerves sharply escalated.

Novels and the Nerves

The rise of the sentimental novel in the 1740s further fuelled the popularization of nervous disease. Interestingly, Cheyne's influence was also strongly felt in the literary world. As the physician to the novelist and hypochondriac Samuel Richardson, Cheyne regularly advised the author on the causes and treatment of his nervous sufferings.[83] Throughout these letters, Cheyne conveyed his belief in the superiority of Richardson's condition, blaming his 'extremely frightful and lowering' 'vapourish and nervous' complaints on his situation as part of the 'Sedentary, Studious, and Thinking Part of Mankind'.[84] As is clear from their correspondence, Richardson's nervous symptoms were particularly violent after writing his novel, *Pamela*. Cheyne responded to his patient's complaints with a heavy dose of sympathy, writing, 'Now as to yourself I never wrote a Book in my Life but I had a Fit of Illness after'.[85]

In addition to advising Richardson of the threat that his literary endeavours posed to his health, Cheyne also advised him on the nervous sufferings of his fictional heroine in the novel, *Clarissa*. Upon the novel's release Clarissa quickly became an icon for glamorous female delicacy and suffering. Throughout the novel, her weak condition is identified with her overwhelming sensitivity thereby implicitly affirming her place among Cheyne's 'thinking and feeling' part of mankind. Clarissa's excessive sensibility is a symptom of her superiority. As a woman too sensitive for a harsh world, the novel concludes with her death as a result of her tremendously strong emotion. Prior to her demise, Clarissa explained her pathetic state in psychosomatic terms: 'My countenance ... is indeed an honest picture of my heart. But the mind will run away with the body at any time'.[86] This romantic portrayal of extreme emotional and nervous weakness was common to sentimental novels throughout the century; Clementina from Richardson's *Sir Charles Grandison* (1754) fell victim to 'hysterical disorders' as a result of her strong passions; Laurence Sterne's Yorick from *Tristram Shandy* (1759) was remarkably sensitive to his constant nervous sensations; Tobias Smollett's Matthew Bramble from the *Expedition of Humphry Clinker* (1771) suffered from 'nerves of uncommon sensibility', and Henry Mackenzie's *Man of Feeling* (1771) espoused the virtue inherent in a sensitive, delicate, nervous, though arguably effeminate character.[87] As several literary historians have described, 'heroines now fainted at the sight of distress compulsorily'; they were 'sick by their sensitivities', and 'became frail and pale, priding themselves on being able to swoon at length and weep at will'.[88] As a result of these popular novels, the public became even better acquainted with the notion of a fashionably debilitating nervous sensibility.[89]

Of course, the 'nervousness' to which the reading public was becoming accustomed was a far cry from the nervousness discussed by the majority of physicians. Doctors writing treatises for their fellow medical practitioners described nervous disease in a clinical context as a technical malfunctioning of nervous fibres, tubes, animal spirits, membranes, or bodily organs. Alternatively, avid novel readers in the eighteenth century perceived nervous disease as more of a cultural phenomenon than a pathological disorder. Hypochondria, hysteria, weak nerves, 'the vapours' and melancholia signified social superiority, good breeding, heightened sensibility and admirable feminine delicacy more than any physical distemper.[90] Even diagnostic explanations by fictional medics in novels like *Clarissa* were void of any technical language or serious medical theory. As Wayne Wild has noted, Clarissa's apothecary only offered a vague explanation of her poor health, stating that 'so much watching, so little nourishment, and so much grief ... is enough to impair the most vigorous health, and to wear out the strongest constitution'.[91] Also acknowledging the ambiguous explanation for nervous sensibility in *Clarissa*, the literary historian Raymond Stephanson has thoughtfully explained that

> For Richardson and his readers the physical implications of acute or excessive nervous sensibility are painfully clear, and although his dramatization of physiological 'realities' in *Clarissa* does not always repeat the technical jargon of Cheyne's more professional descriptions, the fact is that they do not *have* to be any more detailed than they already are since Richardson is touching on a common stock of truths that to a large extent exists at the level of unspoken assumption.[92]

This 'common stock' of ideas was able to form and perpetuate a 'cultural template' whereby the reading public could interpret the nervous sufferings of themselves and those around them.[93] The literary and medical worlds of the eighteenth century were, as Clark Lawlor has explained, 'in constant dialogue'.[94]

This dialogue was often disconnected. In addition to lacking technical theory, novels of sensibility also presented a highly sanitized view of nervous disease. Clarissa and Pamela were not free from all physical symptoms of their nervous sensibility; rather, they were simply free from any less-than-glamorous symptoms. Pamela was anxious and consistently swooned, while Clarissa remained lethargic, pale and weak from emotional distress. Yet other nervous symptoms regularly listed in health manuals such as excessive flatulence, moodiness and belching remain conspicuously absent in fictional accounts. The reason behind this sanitization of symptoms is easy to comprehend: it is hard to imagine that Richardson's novels would have met with such success had his romantic heroines been afflicted with flatulence rather than fainting fits. Still, the nervous symptoms exhibited in novels of sensibility served a rhetorical purpose. Because medical theory emphasized nervous disease as the consequence of extraordinary depth of feeling, the display of these symptoms offered novelists an alternative to a basic character description. Instead of stating the existence of a heroine's inner sensibility and extreme delicacy, nervous symptoms presented writers with a way to display their protagonist's emotional temperament.[95] In short, novelists employed nervous symptoms to diagnose their characters' temperament, not their disease.

Thus, eighteenth-century readers became accustomed to the sanitized and largely romanticized view of nervous disease presented in novels of sensibility. Some readers, carried away by the fashionable implications of a newly glamorized disease, complained of their own nervous sufferings in a fiction-inspired manner, somatizing their superior sensibility in what Mark Micale has referred to as 'nervous self fashioning'.[96] For instance, after completing the novel *Clarissa*, one reader wrote to Richardson,

> I verily believe I have shed a pint of tears, and my heart is still bursting, tho' they cease not to flow at this moment, nor will, I fear, for some time ... in agonies would I lay down the book, take it up again, walk about the room, let fall a flood of tears, wipe my eyes, read again, perhaps not three lines, throw away the book, crying out, excuse me, good Mr Richardson, I cannot go on.[97]

As John Mullan has explained, Richardson 'made it possible to believe that delicate feelings were morally admirable, and could be tested and enlivened by reading'. As many authors hoped, readers of their sentimental novels would be able to 'experience, in the very activity of reading, those 'refined and elevated feelings' associated with nervous sensibility.[98] Henry Mackenzie, the Scottish author of *The Man of Feeling* clearly considered himself a much a moralist as a novelist.[99] In a private letter to his cousin, Mackenzie insisted that novels were the best means by which to convey his ideas on 'men and manners' to a public audience given that they interested 'both the memory and the affections deeper than mere argument or moral reasoning'.[100] Mackenzie's sentimental novels were intended to encourage proper admiration for the refined feelings and actions of his delicate protagonists and to develop the public's capacity to feel for others. Inspired by the cultural implications and fictional caricatures of nervous sufferers, the reading public often held a very different view of nervous ailments than their more serious minded or, at times, professional counterparts.

The literary world was not unilaterally flattering of these seemingly sensitive characters; Henry Fielding responded to Richardson's *Pamela* with a satire titled *Shamela* (1741), in which he portrayed her less as a delicately swooning victim than as a manipulative and 'conniving tart'.[101] Like Fielding, other novelists also offered caricatures of nervous sufferers who were more calculating than emotionally moved. As will be discussed in the final chapter of this study, these negative stereotypes were more prevalent in the latter part of the eighteenth century, when nervous sufferings were associated less with admirable sensibility than a pathetic inability to cope in the real world. Yet for the majority of successful novels in the middle of the century, glamorous nervous sensibility remained the hallmark of a proper protagonist.

Philosophy and the Nerves

In the preface to his *Essay on Regimen* (1740), Cheyne described philosophy as 'the science of living'. 'Physic', he explained, was 'but one branch of this Philosophy'.[102] This relationship between philosophy and medicine was unquestioned by physicians and philosophers of the eighteenth century; both subjects offered rules for proper living, and the interdependence of the soul and body meant that medical and philosophical prescriptions were equally important.[103] In this vein, emotional and medical sensibility belonged as much to philosophers as it did to pathologists.[104]

Haller's physiological sensibility met its cultural counterpart in Scottish Enlightenment philosophy. In his explanation of the role of the nerves in the sensual perception of outward stimuli Haller noted, 'I call that a sensible part of the human body which upon being touched transmits the impression of it to the soul'.[105] As Van Sant has explained, the metaphor of 'touching the soul' was easily applied to emotional sensations and responses.[106] The Scottish philosopher David Hume observed in his *Treatise of Human Nature* (1739) how sensations could be transmitted from one person to another, declaring that there was 'No quality of human nature more remarkable, both in itself and its consequences, than that propensity we have to sympathize with others, and to receive by communication their inclinations and sentiments, however different from, or even contrary to, our own'.[107] The 'scientist of ethics' and friend of David Hume, Adam Smith, detailed a strong philosophical case for the power of sensibility to touch the soul and prompt virtuous behaviour.[108] As he argued in *The Theory of Moral Sentiments* (1759), the act of witnessing the suffering of one person could stir painful passions of a sensitive onlooker. Smith and his fellow Scottish moral philosophers contended that the nerves were the responsible physiological party for human compassion. Scottish intellectuals heralded the notion of 'sympathetic exchange' as the most effective path to societal improvement. Often equated with sociability, sympathetic sensibility was also the means by which Scotland could avoid the self-absorption, selfish emphasis on luxury, and other irritating qualities of their new English in-laws.[109] Whytt's concept of medical sympathy both infiltrated and borrowed from the philosophical writings of men like Smith and Hume. Just as Scottish enlightenment philosophers praised the power of sympathy and sensibility to form bonds among men, Whytt noted in his *Observations* that 'doleful or moving stories, horrible or unexpected sights, great grief, anger, terror and other passions, frequently occasion the most sudden and violent nervous symptoms'.[110] The relationship between observing suffering and feeling sympathy was as much an 'ethical commonplace' as it was a 'medical fact'.[111]

Consequences of Social Definitions of Nervous Disease in the Early Eighteenth Century

The fashionable implications of nervous disease meant that some patients eager for status might feign, or at least over indulge their nervous complaints. As Tom Lutz has joked, while nervousness supposedly denoted the superiority of its sufferers, 'the signs of such uncommonness were surprisingly common'.[112] Such instances only encouraged sceptics to insist that nervous disease was imaginary, and that nervous sufferers were deluded by romantic ideas about sensibility. Together with the absence of a clear-cut pathological definition for nervous disorders, their imprecise symptomology also prompted significant incredulity towards their reality.

Nervous symptoms were undeniably vague. Buchan's *Domestic Medicine* even described their symptoms as 'Proteus-like, they are continually changing shape; and upon every fresh attack, the patient thinks he feels symptoms which he never experienced before'. Further elucidating their amorphous nature Buchan wrote, 'a volume would not be sufficient to point out their various symptoms. They imitate almost every disease; and are seldom alike in two different persons, or even in the same person at different times'.[113] Among these symptoms were bodily weakness, poor digestion, headaches, fainting fits, hiccups, loss of voice, lowness of spirits, flatulence, frequent urination, wandering thoughts, disturbed sleep and heart palpitations, to name but a few. It was widely acknowledged among the medical faculty that beyond the display of singular symptoms, nervous patients could also exhibit an infinite combination of complaints.

In addition to the muddled group of symptoms associated with nervous disease, writings intended for the public very rarely distinguished between different types of nervous complaints. Rather, hypochondria, hysteria and melancholia were most frequently lumped together under the term 'nervous'. Attempts to separate the disorders were generally in vain, as evidenced by the definition of 'Hypochondriack' in Johnson's *Dictionary* as 'Melancholy', and the definition of 'Melancholick' as 'hypochondriacal'.[114] Cheyne acknowledged the haphazard nature of these diagnoses in a letter to Samuel Richardson in 1742:

> we [doctors] call the *hyp* every distemper attended with lowness of spirits, whether it be from indigestion, head pains, or an universal relaxed state of the nerves, with numbness, weakness, startings, tremblings, &c.! So that the *hyp* is only a short expression for any kind of nervous disorder, with whatever symptoms, (which are various, nay infinite,) or from whatever cause.[115]

Academic definitions of nervous disease during the first half of the eighteenth century were in equal disarray. In addition to the difficulty of classifying nervous disorders, treatises intended for medical professionals also reported varying and frequently discrepant descriptions of disease aetiologies. These contradictions were particularly due to the fact that the formal educations of learned physicians were classical in nature, relying heavily upon the ancients. Given the ever-changing explanations of conditions like hysteria and hypochondria from Hippocrates to the seventeenth century, it is easy to see how this appeal to history would result in a confused mix of out-dated theory and continued argument over basic nerve structure.

Adding to this ambiguity, many doctors writing for the public focused heavily on the cultural definition of nervous disease, more concerned with the suave implications of nervous sufferings than any technical theory. As will be discussed in the following chapter, physicians who published on the subject purely for medical students or their peers in the medical faculty frequently accused practitioners writing for a lay audience and stressing the cultural implications of the disorder of compromising the purity of medical inquiry. Already by the 1740s medical men and laymen alike suspected that the fashionable nature of nervous disease had prompted false suffering on the part of some patients eager for elegance. This, in turn, raised suspicion among many conservative members of the medical faculty that popularly publishing physicians were greedily shaping their discussions of nervous disease into forms that were most palatable to potentially lucrative patients. Indeed, struggling medical practitioners like the naval surgeon Adam Neale blatantly over emphasized the way in which wealth and class instigated nervous ailments. Sympathizing with his readership and potential clientele Neale wrote,

> although their [nervous sufferers'] circumstances are in the most flourishing condition, their tables spread with all the most delicate dainties that art and nature can provide; yet that great *blessing content* is absent from their dwellings, so that they *eat* their bread with greater carefulness and anxiety, than those that beg it from door to door. Thus far has it pleased the Divine Providence to level the greatest lord upon a square with the meanest beggar.[116]

Alternatively, most academic physicians publishing for their professional peers focused only on the physiological aspects of nervous disease, ignoring their flattering implications of money and social station.

The Clinical Response to Fashionable and Literary Definitions of Nervous Disease

Even among physicians supposedly delivering strictly theory-based treatises on the nerves, nervous disease remained difficult to define. Simple discussions regarding what types of disorders were nervous was a contentious issue, with some doctors limiting nervous disease to the traditional array of hysteria, hypochondria and melancholia, while others extended this list to include more serious convulsive or paralytic diseases like epilepsy and palsy.[117] This nebulous definition was severely damaging to the credibility of nervous ailments. Desperate to rescue what he believed was a serious medical condition from diagnostic disarray, the Edinburgh Professor of Physic Robert Whytt composed his *Observations* in 1764. In the introduction to this treatise, Whytt complained of the flippant way that so many practitioners diagnosed their patients as nervous: 'physicians have bestowed the character of *nervous*, on all those disorders whose nature and causes they were ignorant of'.[118] Potential misdiagnoses, therefore, could further threaten the integrity of nervous disorders as a legitimate illness. In an effort to relieve nervous disorders of this role as a catchall diagnosis, Whytt's *Observations* offered an exhaustively comprehensive record of the 'most common and remarkable' symptoms of nervous diseases.[119] The fruit of this labour was a six-page catalogue of potential nervous symptoms. Despite this seemingly complete list, Whytt still had to admit that nervous disorders were difficult to diagnose. Because symptoms could appear in an infinite number of combinations, Whytt openly acknowledged the 'impossibility of fixing a certain *criterion*, by which nervous disorders may be distinguished from all others'.[120] Adding to the problem of properly identifying the root cause of ambiguous symptoms was the notion of 'sympathy'. In a vicious cycle of circular symptomology, the nerves were vulnerable to weakness not only on their own, but also by acting in sympathy with other diseased parts of the body. Thus, nerves could become weak through sympathy with other diseased organs, and other organs could suffer as a consequence of a body's diseased nerves.

Struggling to find order amidst this symptomological chaos, Whytt also sought to distinguish between the various types of nervous ailments. Again, he faced difficulty in defining manageable parameters for his discussion. For as Whytt explained, nearly all disorders were nervous in some way.

> The nerves must not only suffer, when they themselves, or the brain and spinal marrow are primarily affected, but also when the other parts are diseased: and hence the difficulty, perhaps the impossibility, of fixing a certain *criterion*, by which nervous disorders may be distinguished from all others.[121]

The closest Whytt could come to creating the desired criterion was his claim that nervous diseases were chronic ailments, caused by an 'uncommon delicacy or unnatural sensibility' of the nervous system.[122] Toothaches, for example, while clearly causing great pain to the nerves of the teeth, were not 'nervous' unless 'convulsions or faintings are added'. Only then, Whytt noted, 'being the effects of an uncommon delicacy of the nervous system, [they] may be justly called *nervous*'.[123]

Whytt acknowledged to his medical students in his clinical lectures in the early 1760s that 'many speak of this [nervous] disease as a Proteus of no determined shape'. Of course, Whytt continued, 'such an account of it to you would be vague and useless'. Consequently, despite instances of irregular or unusually convoluted nervous cases, Whytt believed that in order to provide a useful definition for his medical students and future diagnosticians, he needed to isolate the most 'general & diagnostic description of the disease'.[124] Whytt's *Observations* boldly created this much needed general definition. Dividing nervous disease into three categories, the 'simply nervous', the 'hysteric (women)', and the 'hypochondriac (men)', Whytt delineated their most basic characteristics. Patients that were 'simply nervous' were, he explained,

> such as, tho' usually in good health, are yet, on account of an uncommon delicacy of their nervous system, apt to be often affected with violent tremors, palpitations, faintings, and convulsive fits, from fear, grief, surprise, or other passions; and from whatever greatly irritates or disagreeably affects any of the more sensible parts of the body.[125]

Hysterics, Whytt claimed, generally exhibited all of the aforementioned symptoms in addition to 'indigestion, flatulence in the stomach and bowels, a lump in the throat ... giddiness, flying pains in the head ... frequent sighings, palpitations, inquietude, fits of salivation, or pale urine, &c'.[126] Hypochondriacs did not necessarily exhibit all of the traditional nervous symptoms. As Whytt noted, hypochondriacs 'from a less delicate feeling, or mobility of their nervous system in general, are scarce ever affected with violent palpitations, faintings, or convulsive motions, from fear, grief, surprise, or other passions'. Still, hypochondria came with a few bothersome and unattractive symptoms of its own, including 'indigestion, belching, flatulence, want of appetite, or too great craving, costiveness, or looseness, flushings, giddiness, oppression or faintness about the *praecordia*, low spirits, disagreeable thoughts, watching or disturbed sleep, &c'.[127] The primary difference between hysteria and hypochondria lay in the sex of the sufferer. Quite simply, hysterics were female, and hypochondriacs were male. According to Whytt, hysteria was more prevalent than hypochondria given that women's nervous systems were 'generally more moveable than in men'.[128]

Whytt's treatise met with quick success, going through three editions in its first two years in print. As a highly respected member of the faculty at the most prestigious medical school in Europe, his words carried immediate weight. Whytt's *Observations* comprised part of the curriculum for medical students at Edinburgh, thereby asserting a strong influence over a generation of physicians during the second half of the century. Not surprisingly, his name littered the footnotes of treatises on the nerves long after his death in 1766. In his attempt to cast a net over the increasingly nebulous definition of nervous disease, Whytt reined in what was becoming an unwieldy culturally charged diagnosis. By attempting to define and assign a comprehensive list of symptoms to nervous disease, Whytt was, in a sense, reclaiming it from the public sphere for the medical profession. His book did not mention the social distinction, wealth, or superior class of nervous sufferers. Rather, he simply discussed, in the most precise terms he could, the physiology of nervous disease. Nor did Whytt offer his book to the public. Although written in English instead of Latin, his book was technically dense and clearly intended for members of the medical profession who were capable of correctly recognizing a nervous disorder, with all of its stubbornly perplexing symptoms. Indeed, symptoms remained confusing. Despite his best efforts, Whytt could not help but justify his inability to define precisely the causes, symptoms and root of nervous disease by citing the 'sagacious Sydenham's' observation that 'the colours of the *chameleon* are not more numerous and inconstant, than the variations of the hypochondriac and hysteric disease'.[129] Given the persistent aura of imprecision surrounding nervous disease, the nerves remained a significant topic of discussion well after Whytt's publication, in both the public and professional spheres.

Definitions of Nervous Disease after Whytt

William Cullen, Whytt's colleague and professional successor as the chair in the theory of medicine at the University of Edinburgh, adopted Whytt's definition of nervous disease, making only a few adjustments regarding the relationship between the muscles and the nerves. Whereas Whytt believed that the nerves and muscles were separate entities, Cullen argued that the muscular fibres were merely a continuation of the nerves. In his *Nosology* (1769), an extensive 240-paged taxonomy of diseases, Cullen coined the term 'neuroses', identifying them as all disorders relating to the nervous system that occurred without any sort of physical structural change, lesions, or inflammations. Among Cullen's neuroses was a 'smorgasbord of conditions' including hysteria, hypochondria, melancholia, migraines, epilepsy, diabetes and even mania.[130] The reason for this seemingly odd grouping was Cullen's insistence on the connection between the muscles and the nerves; any disorder exhibiting a disturbance of sensation or muscular motion, such as a seizure or convulsion, was considered nervous.[131]

The *Nosology* officially identified the nervous system as the nexus of all physiological processes influencing health and disease.[132] Consequently, maintaining a clean boundary between the neuroses and other diseases was not easy. Echoing Whytt, Cullen openly acknowledged this fact, later claiming that 'in a certain view, almost the whole of the diseases of the human body might be called NERVOUS'.[133] This conviction was reflected in his private consultations. In a letter regarding a patient who suffered from a seemingly disconnected array of symptoms Cullen wrote,

> I own it would be difficult to account for the various appearances and resolutions which have happened in his constitution. But upon the whole I am of [the] opinion, that the foundation of all his complaints ... is a weakness and mobility of his nervous system which is liable to every variety of derangement.[134]

Surviving professional correspondence reveals doctors and patients alike, linking the nervous system to a wide range of diseases and ailments. For instance, one physician writing to Cullen in 1780 regarding a patient suffering from a 'violent

cough' began his four page letter with a short paragraph intended to familiar-
ize the doctor with the patient's constitution. The fifty-year-old patient was, he
wrote,

> of a fair complection, & rather delicate thin robust frame ... below the middle stature,
> not given to much excess in his way of living, past threw a great part of his life with-
> out great ailment, yet sometimes troubled with nervous complaints, as indigestions,
> flatulence in his stomach, sleepless nights now & then, always accompanied with pale
> urine & a pulse scarce perceptible.[135]

In this way, the weak state of the patient's nervous system was synonymous with
his weak constitution. It was a common belief that nervous weakness could
increase a patient's vulnerability to other diseases. One father writing to a physician on behalf of his ailing daughter suggested that her debilitating cough was
the result of the fact that her nerves had 'been too much relaxed & debilitated'.[136]
Conversely, other diseases could also dangerously weaken the nervous system;
another patient writing to his doctor in 1778 indicated how his 'unlucky' venereal infection resulted in a nervous disorder seven weeks later.[137]

While in practical terms Cullen's efforts to demarcate the definition of nervous disease met with little success, his *Nosology* represented a sincere attempt to
relieve the profession of at least some of its frustrating theoretical ambiguity. His
efforts were well received by professionals and medical students. With the publication of his *Nosology,* the first volumes of the *Institutions of Medicine* (1772),
and the *First Lines of the Practice of Physic* (1777), Cullen earned an international reputation as a leading physician, professor and nerve expert. One medical
student delivering a paper on hypochondriasis at the University of Edinburgh
even praised his professor for 'illustrating this distemper, as distinct from others,
and rescuing it from the rubbish with which it had been involv'd by more antient
authors'.[138]

Despite such praise, popular understanding of nervous disease by laymen
and most medical practitioners remained, in practice, more indebted to Whytt's
three categories of 'simply nervous', hysteric and hypochondriac than to Cullen's
Nosology. Very few medical publications on nervous disease in the second half of
the century mentioned any other than these three very traditional 'neuroses'. For
example, in his *Enquiry into the Nature, Causes, and Method of Cure, of Nervous
Disorders* (1781), the physician Alexander Thompson acknowledged the fact
that the term 'nervous' included a wide range of disorders including 'apoplexy,
epilepsy, and convulsions'. Nevertheless, Thompson declared in his introduction
that his book would 'be restricted to those complaints more particularly denominated nervous' including hysteria, hypochondria and general nervous disorders
depending 'upon extreme sensibility of constitution'.[139]

Even for physicians who rejected Cullen's precise taxonomy of disease, like the American physician Benjamin Rush, Cullen was still considered the gem of the medical profession, credited with formally situating the nervous system in its rightful place at the centre of medical theory. Reflecting on the contribution of his Edinburgh professor to the medical field, Rush wrote:

> Many ... of the operations of nature in the nervous system have been explained by him; and no candid man will ever explain the whole of them, without acknowledging that the foundation of his successful inquiries was laid by the discoveries of Dr Cullen.[140]

Rush further declared that 'While astronomy claims a Newton, and Electricity a Franklin, Medicine has been equally honoured by having employed the genius of a Cullen'.[141]

Despite such predictions, Cullen's classificatory system came under increasing attack at the end of the century by several less starry-eyed members of the medical profession. The most famous opponent of Cullen and his system was his previously prized student, John Brown.[142] Hatefully rejecting Cullen's formal disease classification, Brown referred to Cullen's *Nosology* as a 'brat, [a] feeble, half-vital, semi-production of phrenzy, the starveling of strained systematic dullness'.[143] Instead, Brown offered a rival system of disease classification. According to Brown, all diseases were of two types: sthenic diseases, defined as diseases induced by excess nervous excitability, and asthenic diseases, or diseases of deficient nervous excitability. Summarizing Brown's theory, one anonymous medical student noted 'diversity of symptoms implies no diversity of cause'.[144] Rather, variations in symptoms were due simply to the degree of sthenia or asthenia attained. Eager to lend what he perceived was some much needed simplicity and precision to the medical world, Brown designed a numbered scale by which doctors could measure their patients' level of over or under stimulation. Sthenic diseases like smallpox and dysentery were, according to Brown, caused by increased bodily excitement and cured by techniques designed to relax the nervous system such as lying in bed, bleeding and eating a spare diet. Alternatively, hypochondria and hysteria were asthenic disorders 'marked out by symptoms of dyspepsia, Flatus [and] sluggishness' and requiring 'powerful stimulants' in order to regain the proper level of excitement.[145] Health, Brown maintained, consisted of a perfect balance between sthenia and asthenia.

Followers of Brown, known late in the century as 'Brunonians', also rejected the designation of Cullen's 'neuroses', regarding it as a meaningless category guilty of complicating a truer and simpler disease nomenclature. The ardent Brunonian Robert Thornton remarked on the confusing nature of Cullen's precise system of classification, exclaiming, 'how different this arrangement from the simple method we have adopted, and how confounding must it be to the medical writer, who is obliged to treat separately of each disease!'[146] Likewise, Thomas Beddoes, who, in 1795 wrote a biographical preface to Brown's *Elements of Medicine*, mocked Cullen's *Nosology* in his commonplace book claiming that 'Cullen laid diseases upon the Procrustes bed of his nosology, and tugged at this, and hacked at that, but all in vain. They could not be made to fit, as all who compare his frame with nature must acknowledge'.[147]

Brown conducted several lectures in Edinburgh from 1778 to 1786, drawing his audience primarily from members of the University's Royal Medical Society. While it is impossible to tell how many members of the medical profession actually adopted Brunonianism, it is clear from the Royal Medical Society's dissertations that it was a frequent topic of discussion. Debates between society supporters of Cullen and Brown became so heated as to require a ruling that any members who duelled over the credibility of Brown's system would be expelled.[148] After making many enemies among Cullen's loyal colleagues and failing to secure any sort of formal employment at the Edinburgh medical school, neither Brown nor his system achieved the same renown as Cullen and his *Nosology*. Nevertheless, aspects of Brown's system were widely adopted with notions of excitability unwittingly infiltrating the medical lexicons of Brunonians and Cullen supporters alike. Indeed, *The Edinburgh Medical and Physical Dictionary* of 1807 noted in its entry on 'Brunonianism' that 'the remarkable thing is that the majority of persons who ... become converts to the doctrine, are totally unable to recollect, when or how they were converted'.[149] Discussions by medical professionals about nervous excitement continued well through the Victorian period, with physicians believing that the nerves possessed only a limited capacity for nervous excitement, which, if surpassed, would lead to nervous exhaustion and disease.

Ironically, although Brown created his theory in direct opposition to Cullen's supposedly complicated and confusing system, his own system also harboured significant ambiguities. The very premise of Brown's system, 'excitability', remained sadly undefined. Brown even admitted this fact in his *Elements of Medicine* (1788), claiming, 'we know not what excitability is, or in what manner it is affected by the exciting powers'.[150] Furthermore, the theory behind Brunonianism did not depart from previous systems as much as Brown wanted to claim; Cullen spoke of the 'excitement of the nervous system' long before Brown.[151] Likewise, although Brown's system defined nervous disease, not as 'neuroses', but as mere degrees of asthenia, the recommended treatments for these conditions via stimulation or relaxation was identical.[152]

Conclusion

Although divergent medical ideas between supporters of Cullen and Brown resulted in heated debates, duels and personal slander, it is clear from the majority of publications on nervous disease in the second half of the century that most doctors simply agreed to disagree on the specifics of nerve theory and the precise definition of nervous disease. Most publishing physicians openly acknowledged the variance of opinions before offering their own explanation of disordered nerves in their introductions. Other medical authors, like the London physician Sayer Walker, preferred simply to acknowledge their ignorance of the physiology. As Walker claimed, 'the precise mode in which these organs [the nerves] perform their office still remains among those arcana of nature which we are not permitted fully to discover'.[153] Others happily embraced this ambiguity. Thomas Trotter's *View of the Nervous Temperament* (1807) welcomed vague definitions of the nerves and their disorders, believing that they best facilitated an easy understanding of an otherwise technically impenetrable phenomenon:

> nervous feelings, nervous affections, or weak nerves, though scarcely to be resolved into technical language, or reduced to a generic definition, are in the present day, terms much employed by medical people, as well as patients; because the expression is known to comprehend what cannot be so well explained.[154]

Yet even among publications that complacently professed the superfluous nature of a precise definition of the nerves, Whytt's contribution was quietly visible. For as much as doctors disagreed on the specifics of nervous disease, Whytt's insistence that they were chronic ailments caused by an 'uncommon delicacy or unnatural sensibility' of the nervous system was virtually unquestioned by 1764, and either implicitly or explicitly discussed in every eighteenth-century publication on the nerves thereafter.[155] Most importantly, Whytt's heavily academic treatise on the nerves encouraged further academic investigation into the subject, prompting educated leaders of the medical profession to adopt a more technical understanding of nervous disease, based more on objective observation than subjective expectations gleaned from literary sources and popular discourse.[156]

Of course, the newfound lustre of technical and pathological discussions of the nerves did not entirely eclipse or separate from more cultural understandings of the nerves. As will be discussed in the final chapter of this study, as the medical profession took nervous disease more seriously as a legitimate threat to the human frame late in the century, both they and the general public also took it more seriously as a potential threat to the societal framework. By the final third of the century, the once-flattering connotations of nervous disease took a more sinister turn, becoming less an object of praise than of moral censure. Thus, while Whytt's treatise on the nerves failed to silence all sceptics of nervous sufferers, it did establish a permanent space for hysteric, hypochondriac and 'simply nervous' cases within medical academia and the national consciousness for the remainder of the century. Far from becoming a mere footnote in the literary history of the 1740s, nervous disease breathed new life after 1764 as a medically significant disorder, as worthy of serious discussion as it was of social discourse.

2 QUACKS, SOCIAL CLIMBERS, SOCIAL CRITICS AND GENTLEMEN PHYSICIANS: THE NERVE DOCTORS OF LATE EIGHTEENTH-CENTURY BRITAIN

In the introduction to John Brown's *Elements of Medicine* (1795), the Bristol physician Thomas Beddoes categorized the medical faculty into genus and species.[1] The first genus, 'doctors as desirous, at least, of doing good and extending knowledge, as of amassing wealth' included such species as the 'philanthropic doctor' who was 'equally sensible of the importance and imperfection of medicine', the 'shy philanthropist' who 'keeps too closely retired from public notice', and the 'renegado philanthropist' who, fed up with the 'helpless state' of the medical art, applied instead 'his talents to literature or science'.[2] The second genus, 'mere collectors of fees, regardless of medical science' included such species as the 'bullying Doctor' who 'looks big, struts, swaggers, [and] swears', the 'solemn doctor with garb, voice, gestures, and equipage, contrived to overawe weak imaginations', the 'club hunting doctor' usually found 'talking much and loud', the 'burr doctor' eager to fasten 'himself upon you as tenaciously as the heads of the noisome weed', and the 'Adonis *wheedling* doctor with a handsome face' that 'flourishes at watering places'.[3] While mostly written in jest, Beddoes's satirical classification of doctors highlights the disjointed nature of the medical profession in the late eighteenth century. Although broad differences between barber-surgeons, apothecaries and physicians are well documented in the historiography, Beddoes's categorization reminds historians of the further diversity of practitioners within these groups.[4] This study argues the importance of additional classificatory refinement with regard to Britain's late eighteenth-century nerve doctors.[5] Whereas such doctors were most commonly portrayed in popular discourse as the 'Adonis *wheedling*' type, this chapter demonstrates the inaccurate and wildly over-stretched nature of this blanket stereotype. It reveals that far from providing any sort of unified front against nervous disease, the confused nature of the disorder significantly divided the medical profession. By analysing the similarities and differences of social backgrounds, treatment regimens and professional writings of practitioners diagnosing nervous diseases, this chapter divides the nerve doctors into quacks, social climbers, social critics and gentlemen physicians, revealing a striking hierarchy even within this narrow species of medical professionals.[6]

The categorization of nerve doctors into separate tiers is based upon prosopographical research of thirty medical practitioners publishing on the nerves.[7] Practitioners were divided based upon the level and quality of their education, career credentials (including honours awarded and prestigious hospital appointments), participation in academic societies, and the number and innovative nature of their publications on the nerves. The sphere of influence of various doctors was also taken into account through an examination of the number of editions of their publications, their appearance in the footnotes of publications of fellow medical practitioners, and their inclusion or omission in collections of medical biographies during the period. Of the thirty practitioners included in this study, thirteen are identified as 'gentlemen physicians', or, members of the medical elite, with the most thorough medical educations, most heavily academic publications, most traditional methods of treatment, and the most respected reputations among all medical practitioners.

The next group of practitioners consists of ten 'second-tier' social climbers or social critics, who, while generally advising the same methods of treatment as their first-tier superiors, lacked the same social and professional connections. The style of second-tier nerve doctors' publications was less academic than those of the first tier, as they were intended for a public audience. In writing for the public, second-tier physicians had ulterior motives; social climbers sought to boost their second-rate status by boasting publicly about their supposedly superior healing abilities, and social critics used their discussions of nervous disease as forums for discussions of social and political reform. The final group of practitioners consists of seven quack doctors. Unlike first- and second-tier nerve doctors, the third-tier quack doctors were less concerned with the format of their publications or with fostering long-term professional connections than with their desire to sell patent medications. The defining characteristics of each of these tiers, as well as specific examples of practitioners belonging to these groups will be discussed in detail below.

Historians have successfully established the presence of a group of 'nerve doctors' in the late eighteenth century.[8] The role of these practitioners' participation in a larger competitive 'medical marketplace' has also been effectively discussed, with particular attention paid to the most outspoken men of the profession, including James Graham, James Adair, Thomas Trotter and Thomas Beddoes.[9] This study analyses the professional lives and medical theories of a much wider group of late eighteenth-century nerve doctors. Instead of placing these practitioners in the context of the rest of the medical profession, it evaluates them in the context of other nerve specialists. Through a detailed examination of clinical and medical lecture notes and publications on nervous disease, as well as surviving case records, consultation letters and personal papers of various nerve specialists, this chapter details the professional hierarchy of Britain's late eighteenth-century nerve doctors. It demonstrates the way in which the practitioners' status within the profession significantly shaped the format and style of their publications on nervous disorders and influenced their methods of treatment.

This chapter also reveals how the status of publishing physicians helped mould popular opinion regarding the validity of these much discussed and frequently debated ailments. Quack doctors were, as will be explained, the most ostentatious and visible group of medical practitioners treating the nerves. Consequently, it is easy to understand why nerve doctors were so often stereotyped as a group of mercenary and theoretically unsound practitioners. Nevertheless, the physicians actually driving the medical theory behind nervous disease, and the practitioners most sought after for treatment from the middle of the eighteenth to the turn of the nineteenth century were, in fact, the educated elite of the medical profession. Nervous disease was far more the preserve of respected physicians than of the quacks.

In addition to subscribing to critical stereotypes regarding the nerve doctors, the public, along with many members of the medical profession, frequently questioned the validity of nervous diseases altogether. As discussed in the previous chapter, debate concerning the authenticity of nervous disease was largely prompted by its vague definition and formless symptomology. The military physician Adam Neale defensively claimed in his *Dissertations on Nervous Complaints* (1796) that it was practitioners unable to make sense of these complicated diseases who were likely to condemn them as imaginary: 'some gentlemen, when they cannot reasonably account for those surprising phenomena that often arise in nervous diseases, are so ready to resolve all into whim, or a wrong turn of the fancy'.[10] Alternatively, critics of the medical profession insisted that nervous disease was simply a catchall diagnosis, or a formal name that doctors could attach to a disease when they were unable to make sense of their patients' symptoms. For while the causes of nervous disorders, such as excess in eating or drinking, a sedentary lifestyle, strong passions, or over-sensibility of the nervous system, were generally finite and agreed upon by doctors, their concurrent symptoms were far more complex. As discussed in the previous chapter, the most widely recognized symptoms among medical practitioners included such problems as bodily weakness, poor digestion, headaches, fainting fits, loss of voice, lowness of spirits, flatulence, frequent urination, wandering thoughts, disturbed sleep and heart palpitations, to name but a few. Yet physicians consistently observed additional or unique groupings of symptoms. For instance, William Buchan added symptoms like cramps, flushing, night sweats, hiccups and nightmares in his popular self-help guide, *Domestic Medicine*; others like William Heberden noted how in some patients 'tears flow from the eyes without grief; the nose and ears are filled with ideal odours and sounds: and a mist will seem to obscure the sight. A giddiness, confusion, stupidity, inattention, forgetfulness and irresolution' could also torment these sufferers.[11]

In addition to their multiple symptoms, nervous disorders were notoriously difficult to diagnose and treat due to the fact that they were chronic rather than acute ailments. In his personal casebook, Robert Whytt discussed the inherent difficulty in dealing with chronic disorders, claiming,

> chronick diseases are much more irregular[,] anomalous and unlike one other than acute ones, and therefore their nature & causes, are not only more difficult to be traced, but also the method of cure is much less similar than in acute diseases, which all require the same general treatment ... [E]very Physician who has practiced for any considerable time, will readily confess that he has been much more puzzl'd and disappointed in the treatment of chronical than of acute diseases.[12]

Given the difficulty that a diagnosis of nervous diseases posed to even such a qualified and well-respected physician as Whytt, it was clear to most eighteenth-century citizens that these disorders were well beyond the league of lesser medical practitioners like surgeons or apothecaries; obscure internal disorders and constitutional problems were typically considered the physician's domain. Unlike surgeons who supposedly dealt with obvious outward contusions, setting broken bones and pulling teeth, the physician's role was presumed to be far more cognitive. R. Campbell's *The London Tradesman* (1747) identified the necessary attributes for becoming a physician:

> the particular genius cut out by Nature for a Physician may be easily deducted... He must have a natural Turn of mind to the Healing Art... He must be possessed of a solid judgment and a quick apprehension... He must at once take in the whole Process of the disease, and conceive instantly both Cause and Effect.[13]

Lesser medical practitioners including surgeons and apothecaries, who, at least according to contemporary stereotypes worked more with their hands than with their heads, would not necessarily require or possess this sagacity. Campbell put it quite bluntly with his claim that the 'mere apothecary... requires very little Brains'.[14] Nervous disorders, as complex and chronic ailments with a visibly undetectable origin (most doctors argued that they could not even be detected through autopsy), were something to be explained through theory, intuition and reason – all considered the special capabilities of the physicians. In particular, nervous diseases were widely acknowledged among late eighteenth-century citizens to belong to the domain of the most elite and genteel medical practitioners. It was with this understanding that one doctor deferentially wrote to Cullen after asking for advice on a hypochondriac case, 'I shall be proud to make you my own telling oracle in all difficult chronic cases, where my patients case afford such advice.'[15]

Satirists of the medical profession insisted that it was primarily wealthy money-minded physicians that diagnosed nervous disorders, in hopes of flattering their patients with a diagnosis suggestive of high living and a fashionable excess of sensibility. While physicians treating nervous patients vehemently denied these mercenary motives, they did not reject the image of themselves as a socially elite and professionally superior group of practitioners. Neither did they deny that the definition of nervous disorders was confused and complicated. Rather, by acknowledging the difficulty of correctly detecting these ailments, doctors treating and publishing on nervous disorders could reinforce their reputations as a privileged and elite few; only they were shrewd enough to detect nervous disease amidst the mass of jumbled symptoms, and only they possessed the upper-class sensibilities necessary to properly sympathize with and relate to what was commonly perceived to be a largely upper-class group of sufferers.

First-Tier Nerve Doctors: Gentlemen Physicians

A large proportion of the authors publishing on nervous disorders in the late eighteenth century were, in fact, genteel members of the medical elite.[16] The vast majority of these gentlemen practitioners were wealthy, well-connected, well-respected and well-educated MDs, frequently holding competitive and prestigious positions at voluntary hospitals and memberships in the Royal Medical Society and Royal College of Physicians of London or Edinburgh.[17] Even the fact that these physicians had regular medical degrees set them apart from the bulk of medical practitioners. Given the lack of any effective professional regulation or medical licensing in the eighteenth century, most practitioners simply learned through apprenticeships. If they did receive more formal medical training, they generally enrolled in a haphazard smattering of classes at a medical school.[18] Students paid for formal medical educations by the lecture, and the majority took only the classes that they could afford and which interested them the most. Alternatively, students studying for a formal medical degree were expected to have taken courses in 'all branches of Medical teaching' including Chemistry, Anatomy and Surgery, Botany, Materia Medica, Medical Theory, Pharmacy, and to have attended clinical lectures. While only approximately 33 per cent of medical students attending the University of Edinburgh (the leading medical school of the period) actually enrolled in clinical lectures, graduates from the University never totalled more than 20 per cent of the student body.[19] These graduates composed the elite of the profession, and their active membership in exclusive medical societies such as the Royal Medical Society or Royal College of Physicians added further sheen to their already illustrious credentials. While the Royal College faced a flagging membership and internal strife among its licentiates and fellows during the eighteenth century, membership still conveyed prestige, and the simple letters 'FRCP' or 'LRCP' consistently adorned the title pages of members' publications. Among this privileged group of elite nerve doctors are such well-known names as Robert Whytt, William Cullen, John Gregory, Ebenezer Gilchrist, Sayer Walker, John Cooke and Andrew Wilson.

Complicating this group of elite nerve doctors of the period are the names of several other eminent physicians for whom nervous diseases were only peripherally discussed in their publications, yet for whom nervous disorders made a small, but decidedly consistent portion of their surviving case counts or personal writings. Included among this group are John Coakley Lettsom, Caleb Hillier Parry, William Falconer, William Heberden, William Oliver and Henry Halford. While these doctors did not publish on nervous diseases at such length as the other elite physicians, the format of their writings and their recommended treatments were practically identical. Generally intended for their fellow medical practitioners or, in the case of Whytt and Cullen, for medical students at the University of Edinburgh, the writings of the elite physicians were replete with heavily academic and strongly theory-based discussions of nervous diseases.[20] Cullen, for example, described diseases of the nervous system, or 'neuroses' as 'preternatural affection[s] of sense and motion, without idiopathic or primary pyrexia, and without local disease'.[21] It was precisely this technical language that separated the cream of the profession from the curds. As Penelope Corfield has explained, a 'mastery of tongues' was common to the elite in every profession, who wished to set themselves apart from other less well-educated members of the profession and to encourage the public's need for 'professional' assistance.[22]

These elite or 'first-tier' physicians repeatedly reinforced their status as 'the' doctors diagnosing nervous diseases by referring to and footnoting one another's treatises. For example, Whytt's *Observations* recommended Gilchrist's treatise on *The Use of Sea Voyages in Medicine* (1756), Falconer's *Remarks on the Influence of Climate* (1781) referred readers to Lettsom's 'ingenious' essay on the dangers of drinking tea, and Walker's *Treatise on Nervous Disease* (1796) quoted several times from the 'celebrated' Dr Cullen.[23] These citations reveal strong professional connections among the medical elite. In addition to being acquainted with one another's work, the elite nerve doctors were also well-connected to other learned members of society and powerful figures through memberships in other local and national clubs like literary and philosophical societies, musical societies and agricultural societies.[24] These professional connections extended beyond national borders. Cullen, for example, was an absentee member of Philadelphia's prestigious American Philosophical Society, founded by Benjamin Franklin. The correspondence of several of the Philosophical Society's American members also reveals that they read and regularly recommended books such as 'Whyte on nervous disorders', 'Lettsom on tea', and all of Cullen and Gregory's works.[25]

The first-tier nerve doctors were highly regarded by other members of the public for their wide range of knowledge, polite manners and charitable endeavours. For instance, Forbes Winslow's *Medical Sketch Book, Exhibiting the Public and Private Life of the Most Celebrated Medical Men of Former Days* (1839) noted that in addition to Cullen's well-cultivated professional knowledge, he also possessed 'more than the average information of the fine arts'.[26] Another medical author noted shortly after Cullen's death that 'in his intercourse with the world he exhibited the manners of a well-bred gentleman. He exercised upon all occasions the agreeable art, in which true politeness is said to consist, of speaking with civility, and listening with attention to every body'.[27] Gregory was praised in similar terms, with Winslow claiming that Gregory combined

> in a degree seldom equalled, the studies and acquirements of a man of science, with the taste and honourable feeling of a high-born gentleman. His society was sought after by the first persons of rank and eminence in this country.[28]

Heberden's polite manners and charitable nature were discussed even more directly when he received a letter of appreciation for donating a set of astronomical instruments to his former college in 1767 stating, 'your removal into the Polite world and uncommon eminence in your profession have not induced you to forget the place of your former residence'.[29] First-tier nerve doctors also commonly held positions as hospital physicians. Although voluntary, these positions were highly competitive and conveyed much prestige upon the possessor.[30]

In addition to their similar methods of social and professional networking, first-tier physicians' treatments for nervous sufferers were also highly traditional, encouraging moderate and medically sound lifestyle changes like diet and regular exercise. Heavy and rich foods and sauces were commonly blamed for nervous complaints. Consequently, these physicians generally advised the consumption of simple and plainly dressed foods that were easy on the stomach. Exercise was unanimously regarded as the most effective way to strengthen weakened nerves, and was also valued for its ability to distract the minds of sufferers from their complaints. While medicines were certainly prescribed by the elite physicians to treat nervous disorders, they were usually recommended in conjunction with changes in regimen, or as a last resort. As will be discussed in Chapter 4, bitters, emetics and spa waters were the most frequently prescribed medications, although there was never much consensus regarding the benefits of these remedies. There was consensus, however, on the fact that medicines were likely to be the most ineffectual remedy for nervous disorders. In his *Treatise on Nervous Disease* (1796), Walker expressed a common frustration among the elite physicians, complaining that patients were too eager to fly to drugs as 'quick fixes' instead of taking the more proactive, albeit arduous preventative step of regulating their diets and getting more exercise; 'it is too common', Walker argued, 'for patients vainly to expect to be cured, without making any sacrifice on their part'.[31]

The patent similarities between the writings of the elite doctors can be largely explained by the fact that their recommendations were traditional in nature, harkening back to Hippocratic and Galenic notions of balance and moderation. Thus, while hardly cutting-edge, the treatments recommended by the elite physicians at the end of the eighteenth century appeared moderate and medically sound. The traditional nature of these physicians' treatments is also indicative of their formal educations; several of the elite physicians treating nervous disorders, including Lettsom, Falconer and even practitioners abroad like Rush, were educated at Edinburgh by 'the great' nerve doctors, Whytt, Cullen and Gregory.[32] The fact that so many of the period's nerve doctors sprang from this University is hardly surprising; aside from being one of the most internationally renowned medical schools in the eighteenth century, it was also one of the largest.[33] Even within Britain, Edinburgh produced 2,594 medical graduates from 1751 to 1800 as opposed to only 246 from Oxford and Cambridge combined.[34] Falconer's notebook from his days as a medical student in the 1760s includes notes from Cullen and Whytt's clinical lectures, which clearly recommend horseback riding, dietary changes and chalybeate waters as the primary methods of treatment for hypochondria.[35] Given the way in which knowledge was formally passed on through lectures, it is not surprising to see the younger practitioners espousing the medical dictums of their predecessors. Beyond illustrating this intellectual inheritance, Falconer's notebook also reveals the significance placed on nervous diseases in the University of Edinburgh's prestigious medical curriculum. Whereas Falconer's notebook opens with a very basic introductory lecture explaining the importance and value of clinical lectures for allowing students to study diseases first hand, by page fifteen, hysteria and hypochondria had already been discussed at length. Of 314 pages, twenty-five were dedicated to a discussion of nervous diseases including hysteria, hypochondria and melancholia. While the difficulties of diagnosing nervous disorders and other chronic diseases were repeatedly mentioned in Falconer's notes, the fact that these disorders were consistently discussed – especially so early in the course – implies that the privileged students attending the lectures, and receiving such a strong regular education, would ultimately be the ones capable of making these diagnoses. Cullen strengthened this notion when on the first day of class in 1772 he advised his students that the nervous system was the most important topic they would learn.[36] His sincerity is evidenced by the fact that two thirds of his physiology lectures were on the nervous system.[37]

Nervous disorders were not only discussed in the clinical or classroom setting at Edinburgh Medical School. Student members of the exclusive Royal

Medical Society, described by Guenter Risse as a 'finishing school for budding medical gentlemen', also grappled with the subject of nervous diseases.[38] The weekly dissertations presented to the society from 1751 through to the end of the eighteenth century include a slow but significantly steady stream of presentations on the subject, with such titles as, 'Have Nervous Diseases Increased Since the Introduction of Tea and Coffee?', 'What are the Diseases Induced by a Sedentary and Literary Life?', and several case reviews on hypochondriac and hysteric patients observed in the clinical wards of the Royal Infirmary.[39] Like Falconer's notes, these dissertations commonly emphasized the difficulties of dealing with nervous diseases. Francis Claxton, the disgruntled society member assigned the complicated question regarding the relationship between coffee, tea and nervous disorders, could not help but express his discomfort with the subject, whining that 'the term nervous is too vague to admit of the precision which we would attempt in the discussion'. Hence his disclaimer early on in the essay, that it is 'with the greatest diffidence we enter on the discussion of a question so intricate ... Numerous are the subtleties which it involves and numberless the disadvantages with which we set about the enquiry'.[40] Although nervous disease was a frustratingly complicated topic, the fact that it was consistently discussed in the prestigious society's meetings implies that it was considered worthy of the members' attention. The confusion expressed by society members also reinforced the notion that nervous disorders were the property of the learned. If even the University's most privileged and elite students holding memberships in the Royal Medical Society had difficulty describing and discussing nervous ailments, certainly they could be considered well beyond the comprehension of students acquiring less formal educations.

Some first-tier nerve doctors like Lettsom explicitly accused 'lowly' practitioners of being unable to detect nervous ailments accurately. As part of his campaign to expose the quacks of the medical profession, Lettsom published several pieces attacking the German-born uroscopist and supposed quack Dr Theodor Myersbach in 1776.[41] In one such piece designed to display Dr Myersbach's ineptitude, Lettsom reviewed several cases in which Myersbach's patients – including many nervous patients – had been misdiagnosed. In the case of one Elizabeth Nottingham, Myersbach diagnosed a disorder of the womb, recommending his own mysterious green drops and pills for a cure. When these remedies did not relieve her symptoms, Elizabeth sought a second opinion. 'When she applied to me,' Lettsom disdainfully gloated, 'she suffered a variety of nervous complaints: her strength, her appetite, her spirits were totally impaired'.[42] Likewise, a male patient diagnosed by Myersbach as suffering from '*slime in his blood*' also sought a second opinion from Lettsom after months of unsuccessful treatments with Myersbach's medications. Lettsom again proceeded to make a corrected diagnosis: 'I found he was a hypochondriac, and laboured under many nervous symptoms; but with the use of the usual nervous remedies, and gentle exercise upon horseback, he recovered his former health in the space of a few weeks'.[43]

In response to Lettsom's revelations came the anonymously penned *Impostor Detected; or, the physician the greater cheat* (1776). In this pamphlet, the author, presumably hired by Myersbach due to his own difficulty with the English language, criticized physicians with formal medical educations and memberships in the Royal College of Physicians.[44] 'It is nothing but the pride and arrogance of education', the author snarled, that 'impresses the *learned* with a belief, that it is impossible the unlearned should know what *they* are not qualified to understand'.[45] Such a statement undoubtedly smacks of bitterness towards the elite of the medical profession. Yet there is little doubt that Lettsom fully intended this snub, firm in his belief that only a learned practitioner could correctly detect and diagnose such an elusive disorder.

The elite status of the physicians teaching about and diagnosing nervous disorders was further reinforced by their recognition from outsiders. For instance, one patient writing to Cullen regarding his 'troublesome & unpleasant' nervous disorder indicated that he sought Cullen's particular assistance given the 'general voice' of praise for his 'judgment & abilities'.[46] Likewise, in a letter home to his brother in Philadelphia, the Edinburgh medical student George Logan wrote that

> The World is so acquainted with Dr Cullen's abilities that it is unnecessary to say anything with respect to them. You know he has established a new theory of Medicine... As the Boerhaavians accounted for every disease of the body from... the fluids, so on the other Dr Cullen refers them to... the nervous system.[47]

At times, less qualified practitioners would, when faced with the necessity of dealing with a nervous case, formally defer to their 'superiors' for help. Among the thousands of surviving consultation letters written to Cullen are numerous letters from physicians, surgeons and apothecaries asking for advice on treating nervous disorders and other, usually chronic, complaints. For instance, 'Dr Turner' from Warrington consulted Cullen regarding his persistently nauseous nervous patient 'Miss Woodcocks'.[48] Likewise, the apothecary Edward Watson from Sunderland wrote to Cullen on behalf of one nervous patient, listing several drugs that his patient had unsuccessfully tried, and politely requesting, 'if a remedy can be found, that will take off this agitation of the nervous system, please do send it to me'.[49] Several physicians with difficult cases, including one Doctor Stark from London, encouraged their problem patients to consult Cullen directly by letter. Such practitioners maintained their authority over their patients by providing Cullen with their own 'professional' account of their patients' histories. For example, as Stark wrote to Cullen in 1774,

It gives me great pleasure to know that my Patient has, at length consulted you on his very obstinate Disorder, for which he has had the advice of many Physicians, to very little purpose. I have had the pleasure, more than once, of mentioning to him your eminent ability, and am persuaded that you will, if possible, reinstate him.

In such cases, the recommending physicians would convey as much information as they thought might help Cullen in his diagnosis. For instance, Stark wrote,

It may be proper to inform you that, on enquiry, I learned that his Mother had been always subject to a bad stomach, and a variety of complaints call'd Nervous: and that I have lately seen a Brother of his, on my return from Paris, who consulted me for a similar disorder, tho' not so complicated.

There was no shame in these secondary consultations. Rather, sharing news of patients and asking for advice would only bolster the practitioner's place in the professional arena. Prompting even a professional correspondence with a physician so eminent as Cullen could help forge a valuable connection for otherwise less-connected or less-established medical practitioners.

Although asking for second opinions could reveal a humble and good-natured professionalism on the part of the writer, it was also important for him not to appear lazy or incompetent. For this reason, in addition to making the standard remarks regarding the patient's past treatments, Stark was careful to inform Cullen of the uncooperative nature of his patient – something which undoubtedly would have been left out of the patient's self-history, and which might excuse his own inability to treat his patient with success:

I hope it will appear to you that every probable mean has been tried, tho', I acknowledge, with very little advantage, save that of procuring a more regular habit of Body, and, at times, longer intervals of ease. There was indeed a Period, when I began to flatter myself with a prospect of success: But, his aversion to exercise; his indulgence in Bed, late hours, and frequent trespasses in point of Diet, deprived us [Stark and all other consulted physicians] of our capital resources.[50]

These letters, usually addressed simply to 'Dr Cullen, Edinburgh', or even more simply, to 'Dr Cullen' came from all over the United Kingdom, Europe and even as far away as America. Although not nearly the authority that Cullen was on nervous diseases, Lettsom also received letters from abroad acknowledging his expertise in the area. One letter from an American physician, James Jay, in 1812 expressed deep regard for Lettsom's character and opinion, detailing Jay's wish that he could receive feedback from Lettsom regarding his upcoming publication: 'such is the critic and such the friend, a man would wish to consult who is preparing a work for the Public, especially on such subjects as Gout and Nervous Disease'.[51]

At times, eminent physicians received requests for aid regarding nervous cases even without ever having written on the subject, suggesting that status alone was frequently sufficient to qualify a practitioner to treat nervous diseases. For instance, the famed London physician Matthew Baillie received a letter from one 'Mr Collyns', a surgeon near Exeter, providing details of a nervous patient and asking for his advice on treatment.[52] This letter is particularly interesting for two reasons; not only does it reveal a surgeon feeling out of his depth with a nervous case, but it also raises the question of why Mr Collyns wrote to Baillie for help. Baillie's response is professional, concise and void of any extraneous niceties, suggesting that the two were not acquainted on a personal level. Yet Baillie did not publish, or specialize in nervous diseases in any way that would have promulgated his reputation as an authority in the area. Thus it appears that his privileged status as a physician to the royal family, Fellow of both the Royal College of Physicians and the Royal Society and physician to St. George's Hospital, was enough to qualify him, in the surgeon's eyes, as a nerve expert.[53]

Second-Tier Nerve Doctors: Social Critics and Social Climbers

If high status could qualify someone as a nerve specialist, many less-esteemed, less well-connected and frequently less-informed practitioners hoped that by presenting themselves as experts on nervous disorders, they could in turn advance their professional reputations. The late eighteenth century witnessed a large proportion of status-hungry practitioners – surgeons and physicians – trying to stake a claim in this supposedly elite medical terrain by publishing on nervous diseases. The primary difference between these 'social climbers' and the elite physicians was in their motivation for writing. The elite physicians wrote about nervous diseases as a consequence of their station; as well-educated doctors, patients and other medical practitioners expected them to be well versed in the subject. Alternatively, the doctors whom I define as social climbers, including James Makittrick Adair, James Rymer, Adam Neale, William Perfect, Alexander Thomson, John Hill, Hugh Smith and John Scot specifically wrote about nervous diseases as a means of attracting attention, in hopes of somehow 'duping' the public into believing that they were part of, or, in some cases, better than, the elite and exclusive sphere of nerve doctors.

Closely related to this group of social climbers is another group of practitioners, whom I define as 'social critics'. Like the social climbers, the social critics had fewer illustrious credentials, and were generally less esteemed than the elite physicians. Although not in itself a reason for their secondary status, the social critics also wrote about nervous diseases in order to attract wider public attention. Yet unlike the climbers who sought personal recognition through their writings on nervous diseases, social critics hoped instead to use a discussion of nervous ailments to highlight their larger concerns regarding Britain's supposed national and moral decline. Together with the social climbers, the social critics Thomas Beddoes and Thomas Trotter compose what I refer to as the 'second tier' of nerve doctors.[54]

In addition to adopting the subject of nervous diseases in an effort to attract attention, second-tier practitioners had a tendency to quote heavily from, and adopt the structure and arguments of the first-tier nerve doctors. The majority of these authors were not shy about citing the 'major' authorities as the inspiration behind their work. For example, in his *Cases of Insanity, the Epilepsy... and Nervous Disorders, Successfully Treated* (1785), William Perfect announced that he would 'take the liberty of giving the common, and most remarkable symptoms [of nervous disorders], in the words of the ingenious Dr Whytt' before proceeding to quote the doctor's five-paged list of symptoms.[55] In this way, it appears that the use of names or quotations from prominent nerve doctors could help lend a veneer of respectability to practitioners eager for such a sheen. Quotations from 'the authorities' could also be indicative of a practitioner's education; the Edinburgh physicians also educated many of these 'second-tier' nerve doctors, including Adair, Beddoes, Rymer and Trotter. By openly paying homage to their professors, these doctors could reveal their well-respected connections, and in turn, boost their own credibility.

The importance of publishing and forging professional connections was discussed overtly in a letter to Cullen from a former student, Dr De La Roche. Writing to Cullen in 1772, De La Roche admitted his difficulty in establishing a successful private practice. Since leaving school, he confided, he had enjoyed 'little practice... at least of such as can give any reputation & lead a man to fortune; there is no wonder in that as I am so young; but what is worse I see but little prospect'. The reason for his pessimism, he explained, was that 'no body has so few connections as myself'. To compensate for this disadvantage De La Roche proposed a plan:

> Among other means of making myself known in the public as a Physician I have pitched upon one which will be an arduous task, it is writing a book – I see what credit some Physicians have acquir'd by publishing... I have therefore thought on a subject & the one that I find to suit best my intention is that of Nervous disorders...

The problem with this strategy, he acknowledged to Cullen, was that

> I cannot give any thing interesting upon that matter but what I have learn'd from you & as it is not my opinions but yours that I wish to offer to the public I will not undertake any thing towards it 'till I have your leave of doing it.

While promising Cullen that he would be sure to 'inform my readers of the source whence I have taken my ideas on the subject', De La Roche's boldness did not end there. He complained to Cullen that there were many aspects of nervous disease 'which I don't well understand'. He then included a list of questions for Cullen to answer about nervous disease, while asking the doctor to also advise him regarding a 'general plan' for his book, as 'I have none well form'd as yet'. For whatever reason, it does not appear that De La Roche ever published his treatise. Yet like the publishing second-tier physicians, De La Roche hoped to boost his career by writing for the public and allying himself with the elite of his profession, regardless of his apparent intellectual inferiority.[56]

Whereas academic first-tier physicians were the driving force behind the evolution of eighteenth-century nerve theory, second-tier physicians were far less innovative. Like De La Roche, second-tier nerve doctors often aimed to regurgitate the original writings of their teachers and other elite practitioners into a form more easily digested by readers. These efforts were not always well received; one critic of Trotter's *View of the Nervous Temperament* complained that Trotter's work was verging on plagiarism of Whytt's *Observations*, claiming that it was 'but an old song to a new tune'. 'We cannot,' the critic argued, 'be deceived by the author's pretensions to novelty, while it is in our power to confront him with Dr Whytt'.[57]

Despite their apparent similarities, there remained several distinct differences between the treatises written by the second-tier practitioners and those composed by the medical elite. Unlike the genteel nerve doctors who primarily wrote their treatises for their fellow practitioners and medical students, the social climbers and critics specifically addressed the public in their writings. Lacking the professional connections that could help boost an otherwise overlooked practitioner into public notice, these practitioners were forced to take a more direct route. Most announced their intention to write for the public in the introductions to their treatises, with Adair even going so far as to claim of his book, *Medical Cautions* (1785), 'I flatter myself that this morceau will become a very fashionable *powdering book*; insomuch that every fine lady and gentleman will consider it as necessary an article of *toilette* furniture...'[58] Five years later, Adair further unabashedly acknowledged the plagiaristic trend in popular medical writing:

> It has become very much the Fashion of the present Day to catch the Eel of *Science* by the Tail; and though she is apt to slip through our Fingers, somewhat of the Flavour adhering to the exrementitious *Mucus*, which besmears the Surface, still remains. From *this delectable Source*, many ingenious and useful Labours are ushered to the Public.[59]

Whether slimy or simply diluted, treatises intended for the public also differed from those written by the first-tier nerve doctors in their tendency to pair discussions of nervous disorders with social commentary. Whereas books like

Cullen's strict *Nosology* (1769) and Walker's straightforward *Treatise on Nervous Disease* (1796) withheld judgment on nervous sufferers and an increasingly nervous society, the social critics Beddoes and Trotter freely vented their social and political concerns in their medical publications on the nerves, accusing effeminate hypochondriacs and weakly valetudinarians of sacrificing the nation's morals and strength.

The fact that these men wrote for the public and invoked social and political commentary in their publications is not in itself indicative of their secondary status. As will be discussed in the Epilogue, doctors at the turn of the nineteenth century were increasingly expanding their professional role as medical practitioners into that of moral guardians. Convinced of an interdependent relationship between social, moral and physical health, these new medical and moral guardians appealed directly to the public to live virtuous and disciplined lives for the sake of their personal well-being and the health of the nation.[60] Likewise, although the emphasis on medico-moral writing increased in the late eighteenth and early nineteenth century, this trend does not imply that the second-tier nerve doctors were necessarily of a younger generation than the first-tier doctors. While the average date of the first publication on the nerves by second-tier nerve doctors included in this study was 1781, the average date of the first publication on the nerves by first-tier nerve doctors was only five years earlier, in 1776. Furthermore, many first-tier doctors embraced their new professional role as moral guardians. Yet unlike the second-tier nerve doctors, these younger first-tier physicians still published innovative and academic treatises on the nerves that were significant to the development of eighteenth and nineteenth-century nerve theory.

It is certain that the social critics' popular and non-academic treatises on the nerves did not boost their reputations within the medical profession in the same way that publishing innovative treatises for a professional audience did for members of the first tier. Many elite members of the medical profession at the turn of the century still viewed writing for the public as an opportunistic and mercenary endeavour. Even Beddoes acknowledged the supposed superiority of medical publications written for a purely professional audience. In the introduction to his book *Hygeia*, published for a popular audience in eleven monthly instalments from 1802 to 1803, Beddoes wrote:

> I believe it is an unquestionable fact that medical writings for the profession have at all times been infinitely superior in their kind to those for the public. No wonder therefore that I should feel too proud to be gratified by a comparison, however to my advantage, with certain predecessors. But there does exist a model to which I am truly humble at the idea of being referred. It is *that*, which daily contemplation of domestic sufferings must have created in the breast of every experienced and discerning physician, whose feelings are not bound up in the profits of his craft.[61]

Thus, it was out of a humane desire for the public good that Beddoes claimed to sweep aside any inhibitions about popular writing. Convinced that poor health was quickly becoming a matter of national concern, Beddoes believed that the public had as much need to be informed of medical matters as medical professionals. Ultimately the result of his popular writing was to warn Britons of the dangers posed by modern luxuries and material comforts. Such luxuries, he claimed, were hardly worth the cost of consequent ill health: 'the encouragement of manufactures, that is, the creation of a miserable and sickly population is a paltry excuse for lying... in the stew-pan of luxury, till we become miserable and sickly ourselves'.[62]

Beddoes laboured to make his writing accessible to the public, even prefacing his discussion of the 'most desirable state of the nerves' with a statement declaring his belief that his readers would prefer to learn by example rather than by technical theory. As he explained, 'I choose an example, as thinking my lady and lady-minded male readers who hate metaphysics, will prefer an example to description'. He then added a footnote to this statement noting, 'I hate metaphysics too'.[63] While such an admission may have boosted his appeal as an honest, entertaining and accessible medical writer among the public, it did little to impress the rest of the profession, which valued theoretical innovation as the mark of an eminent nerve doctor.

Trotter's *View of the Nervous Temperament* (1807) also valued examples over complex theories. As Trotter claimed,

> On the whole there will be found little of what is called theory in this discussion: unshackled by any attachment to system, and unseduced by the love of novelty, I have endeavoured to delineate the NERVOUS TEMPERAMENT, as I have seen it in actual practice, and in a large intercourse with mankind.[64]

By writing such an accessible treatise, Trotter hoped to appeal to as wide a public as possible. Written during the Napoleonic wars, Trotter believed his message was immediately necessary for a public which was fast becoming weak-nerved and self-absorbed. In the *View*, Trotter expressed his fears that Britain would never retain her ascendancy among 'rival states' unless citizens reduced their nation's number of nervous sufferers by resisting the temptation to over eat, drink too much tea, dress in fashions impeding proper exercise, and otherwise indulge themselves in the growing consumer society. Trotter warned that exotic products from England's colonies only served to 'weaken her [Britannia's] manly character, and overwhelm her with nervous infirmities' which would in turn make her more susceptible to potential French invaders.[65]

Medical critics believed the overtly political agendas of these medical writings were only intended to boost sales. Reviewers at the *Edinburgh Medical and Surgical Journal* in 1805 dismissed Trotter's discussion of 'the influence of nervous diseases on the character of nations, and on domestic happiness' as 'a sort of politico-economical rhapsody, intended, we suppose, for Dr Trotter's general readers, and dished up to their taste'.[66] The fact that these doctors' medical discussions had social, political and possible mercenary motivations does not necessarily imply a lack of sincere concern on their part regarding nervous diseases. Beddoes's personal correspondence expressing his fears over issues like modern sedentary lifestyles, excessive sensibility and the consequent degeneration of British citizens, proves that his published writings were not all for show.[67] Likewise, Trotter's involvement in military and medical reform at the time of England's struggle with France can easily explain the political bent of his writing, stressing the debilitating effect of unhealthy nerves on the nation's military manpower.[68] Nevertheless, as with Beddoes, the non-academic style of his publications together with his intention to avoid any technical discussion of nerve theory clearly set him apart from the innovative nerve doctors of the first tier.

Second-tier nerve doctors also inadvertently distanced themselves from the first-tier physicians by frequently insisting upon the exclusively upper-class nature of nervous sufferers. Echoing Cheyne's claim from earlier in the century, practitioners like the naval surgeon James Rymer still insisted that it was a malady of the learned.[69] In terms similar to those of his professional predecessors, Rymer insisted that hypochondria belonged more to 'men of learning, genius, and property, whose minds are constantly upon the rack of thought, than among the illiterate, the stupid, and the indigent'.[70] Even more dramatic was Rymer's insistence that people

> possessed of fine sensibility, and irritability, of great vivacity, spirits, and ready wit, are more liable to these diseases than those who appear on all occasions easy, careless and unconcerned; who have no humane and tender feelings, and upon whose hardened hearts the distresses and calamities of human nature make no impressions.[71]

Rymer's message was clear: to be nervous was to be superior.

Rymer provides a contrast with elite nerve doctors of the late eighteenth century who, while still sympathetic to nervous sufferers and often associating disordered nerves with an exquisite civilization-induced sensibility, no longer vehemently stressed nervous disease as a strictly upper-class malady.[72] As will be discussed in Chapter 5, from the 1760s onwards, academic nerve theories stressed the universal threat which nervous disease posed to people of all classes. For instance, Whytt's clinical lectures alerted students to the fact that while 'the idle, voluptuous & luxurious are the most subject' to hysteria, 'it sometimes attacks labouring women'.[73] Likewise, Walker argued in his *Treatise on Nervous Disease* that 'whilst luxury and inactivity may introduce the malady into the circles of the rich and studious, so hard labour, with a slender diet, joined to great anxiety respecting a comfortable provision, may produce it amongst those of a different class'.[74] Records from clinical lectures given by elite doctors like Cullen and Gregory at the Edinburgh Royal Infirmary in the 1760s and 70s also reveal that first-tier physicians were comfortable diagnosing pauper patients with nervous diseases.[75]

Certainly by the time Rymer wrote his treatise in 1785, the notion of nervous disease as an exclusively upper-class ailment was, at least in terms of medical theory, already out dated. Yet when paired with his unusual and underprivileged status as a surgeon treating nervous diseases, Rymer's old-fashioned medical view takes on new meaning as a likely ploy intended to attract a wealthy clientele. By insisting that nervous diseases were a plague of the upper class, Rymer could at once flatter his patients regarding the exclusive nature of their sufferings, and flatter himself by advertising his ability to treat these maladies.

Not all second-tier doctors insisted on the elite nature of nervous diseases. For example, Trotter expressed fears at the universal threat which nervous disorders posed to British citizens, anxiously arguing in the *View* that 'nervous ailments are no longer confined to the better ranks in life, but [are] rapidly extending to the poorer classes'.[76] In one particularly bold passage, he claimed that 'in the present day, this class of diseases, forms by far the largest proportion of the whole, which come under the treatment of the physician'.[77] While the views of these second-tier doctors were very different, they were both extreme, and both were designed to boost the practitioners' popular appeal. For Rymer, insisting on the exclusivity of nervous disease would appeal to an upper-class group of potential sufferers who rejoiced in the implication of heightened upper-class sensibility that nervous disorders could convey. For Trotter, alerting the public to this supposed threat to national health allowed him to highlight his role as a selfless moral crusader. As he claimed in his introduction, 'mankind have seldom been delighted with a picture of their infirmities... But... it must be the duty of some person to sound the alarm, and to announce the danger, however unprofitable the talk'.[78] Given Trotter's role as a naval physician as well as the fact that at the time of publication he was just settling into his first private practice, it is certain that any publicity gained through the apocalyptic style of his writings could help boost his career. In his *Medicina Nautica* (1797) Trotter specifically discussed the difficulty of entering private practice after a naval career:

> The sea-life assuredly begets a disposition of mind, that unfits him [a naval physician] for the exercise of his profession in private practice. He is, therefore, in the decline of his days, frequently left in a state of precarious dependence: his naval servitude, in the prime of youth, had prevented him from making friends and forming connections, that would have been favourable to his future prospects in medical rank and reputation.[79]

By stressing his professional popularity in his publications, Trotter could compensate for this occupational disadvantage. His preface to the second edition of the *View* acknowledges the way in which the publication promulgated his professional reputation: 'since the publication of this book, I have been consulted by letter[s], from different parts of England, by a numerous list of nervous patients, who seem to have been much gratified by the explanation which is here given of these diseases'.[80] Even in other publications, such as his *Essay Medical, Philosophical, and Chemical on Drunkenness and its Effects on the Human Body* (1804), Trotter stressed his connection with those whom he referred to as the 'men at the summit of the Medical profession', emphasizing the warm reception of his work from men like Cullen, who, he claimed, had 'commended the design, execution, and importance' of his work.[81] By going to such lengths to highlight publicly his connection with these men at the 'summit' of the medical profession, Trotter inadvertently set himself apart.

Another characteristic distinguishing the second-tier doctors from the established nerve doctors was their self-conscious tendency to justify their ability to treat nervous diseases. Second-tier physicians consistently emphasized their sympathy for nervous sufferers. Of course, sympathy for nervous patients was the hallmark of all nerve doctors; sympathy towards patients was also indicative of the practitioner's own sensibility – his ability to relate to his patients, and to feel or understand their pain. Scottish Enlightenment philosophers like David Hume and Adam Smith insisted that sensibility was greatest among the most civilized members of society. Not surprisingly, elite physicians treating nervous disorders (many of whom where also Scottish) expressed appropriately civilized sympathy for their nervous patients. Gregory noted that physicians should exhibit 'particular tenderness', when dealing with nervous patients, as their sufferings 'are of all distresses the greatest, and demand the most tender sympathy...'[82] Cullen also exhibited the appropriate sympathies for his station, prompting one passionate admirer to send him a two-page poem praising the his 'superior lustre' and sensibility:

> For in thy breast the softer graces dwell...
>   Thine is the breath sincere of Friendship, thine the Compassion of unaffected ardour, thine the husband's & the father's tender love, and warm benevolence incircling all.[83]

Following Cullen's death in 1790, Rush composed a eulogy praising his 'quick' and 'exquisite' sensibility, remarking that when Cullen dealt with patients, 'so gentle and sympathizing was [his] manner, that pain and distress seemed to be suspended in his presence'.[84] Similarly, a eulogy for Lettsom after his death in 1815 noted how

> It is part... of the medical function to apply the balm to the troubles that alarm the
> imagination, the pangs that agonize the senses, the sensibility that bleeds at the heart,
> and the nerves that tremble to the sickness of the soul![85]

This capacity for strong sensibility set the elite of the medical profession apart
from the rest. Not surprisingly then, the doctors most eager for prestige and
social recognition were the ones to write about nervous sufferers in the most
consciously sympathetic terms. For instance, in his treatise on hypochondria,
John Hill represented patients suffering from the disease due to prolonged study
as having made a noble sacrifice of their health for the good of civilization. As he
dramatically claimed, study 'sinks the body to the grave, even while it carries up
the mind to heaven'.[86] By conspicuously exhibiting their own sensitivity, doctors
eager for prestige attempted to display a specifically upper-class sensibility.

Justification for treating nervous disorders also came in the form of extreme
self-promotion, with treatises like that of the surgeon William Perfect claiming
an ability to treat difficult nervous disorders where other 'eminent', 'experienced
and approved' physicians including a 'Gentleman in London celebrated for his
peculiar attention to disorders of this kind' had failed.[87] Perfect was also eager to
inform his readership that he had been consulted by other members of the medical faculty for his expertise on nervous disease. As he claimed in his published
book of cases,

> A man, near fifty years of age, applied to me... with a letter from a Gentleman of the
> Faculty, in the village where he lived, describing his case... that it was nervous, and
> wishing, that I would endeavour to assist him.

According to Perfect, this 'Gentleman of the Faculty' carefully followed his
advice when treating the patient, later writing him a letter to inform him that 'he
had punctually, and without variation, adhered to my plan, and, had the pleasure
to inform me, the patient was amazingly amended for the better'.[88]

The surgeon Adam Neale also ranked his supposedly vast experience with nervous diseases above that of some well-respected physicians. Neale's *Dissertations
on Nervous Complaints* (1796) detailed the story of a physician of 'considerable
fame', who, upon failing to sympathize with his patient's nervous symptoms, coldly
insisted that they were imaginary, and would be gone by the next day. As a consequence of this gentleman physician's cruel disbelief, the patient, Neale gleefully
informed his readership, 'expired before that period; so that, if he was well, according to this gentleman's prognostication, it was in the other world'.[89]

Despite such stories, none of the well-established nerve doctors felt a need
to respond with similar self-promotion. Revealing intra-professional contention
was considered poor professional conduct. As Thomas Percival maintained in
his *Medical Ethics*, written in 1792, and published nine years later, 'opposition of

interest' in the medical profession should never be 'communicated to the public; as they may be personally injurious to the individuals concerned, and can hardly fail to hurt the general credit of the faculty'.[90]

Another reason for the lack of retaliation or blatant published self-promotion on the part of elite practitioners was that others did it for them. In his journal, Rush wrote of Cullen that 'it is scarcely possible to do justice to this great Man's character, either as a scholar – a physician – or a Man'.[91] More public promotion of the elite practitioners could be found in local newspapers, particularly in the area around Edinburgh medical school. For instance, on 24 September 1771 the *Edinburgh Advertiser* proudly proclaimed that

> It is with pleasure we inform the public that the University here daily increases in its reputation for medical knowledge; and indeed, what university has been able to boast of having at the same time, four such great professors as Cullen, Monro, Gregory and Black?[92]

It is clear that such complimentary news of first-tier physicians like Cullen spread successfully, with many patients like one in 1774 writing to the physician, 'Sir, having heard of your famed knowledge of Physick &c. [I] thought [it] proper thus to consult you of a Lingering Disorder I've been afflicted with near two years'.[93]

At times, the self-promotion of second-tier practitioners reeked of quackery. Even William Rowley, a Licentiate of London's Royal College of Physicians from 1784, was ultimately rejected by the College following a number of publications, including a treatise on nervous diseases in which he tirelessly footnoted himself and criticized other authors publishing on hysteric and nervous complaints.[94] Even worse was Rowley's tendency to include under his list of qualifications on the title page of his publications that he was a member of Oxford University. For this, the *London Medical and Physical Journal* remarked disgustedly that 'his modesty has induced him to take a title, which any term-trotter may assume, almost as soon as matriculated'.[95] The manuscript inscription on the first page of the Wellcome Library's copy of Rowley's *Treatise on Female, Nervous, Hysterical, Hypochondriacal, Bilious, Convulsive Diseases &c* reads, 'in a conversation with the Earl of Oxford about Dr Rowley – he observed that he knew him, and that he was a great fop, and a great quack, an observation which this book fully confirms'.[96] Likewise, Rowley's entry in the usually bland and encyclopaedic Munk's Roll leaves no doubt of the damage such writings did to his reputation:

> his writings, which were numerous, are most of them popular in style, addressed to the public rather than to the profession; and were calculated to promote his own private interests rather than to advance the science and art which it was his province to cultivate and practise... They have long fallen into complete and deserved oblivion. Neither his character nor career were of a kind we delight to dwell on.[97]

Third-Tier Nerve Doctors: the Quacks

While some practitioners occasionally displayed quackish behaviour, there was no shortage of 'real' quacks also trying to diagnose nervous disorders.[98] In addition to the pretension and lack of respect for the rest of the medical profession which some of the social climbers revealed, 'real' quack doctors belonging to the third tier of nerve doctors were brazen self-promoters who profited primarily through the sale of their own secret remedies.[99] Most quacks either dealt with their clients once (while making a sale), or else sold their remedies through a third person whereby they did not come into contact with their 'patients' at all. Unlike the social climbers, the quack doctors' treatment of nervous diseases differed greatly from that of the established nerve doctors. Whereas the great Edinburgh physicians like Whytt, Cullen and Gregory always emphasized the importance of regimen over medications in treating nervous diseases, men such as James Graham, William Brodum, Samuel Solomon and the more elusive W. D. Knight, Joshua Webster and William Lowther shamelessly sang the praises of their nervous tinctures, pills, drops and balsams.

These medicines were frowned upon by the elite physicians treating nervous diseases, who were constantly forced to wean stubborn patients away from the promise of a quick and easy cure. The men creating these medicines were respected even less by the medical faculty than the supposedly bogus remedies that they sold. In 1793 the *Medical Spectator* claimed, 'he must be a poor creature indeed, that cannot invent a vegetable syrup or an antiscorbutic drop, a nervous powder, or a pectoral lozenge, a cordial tincture, or a justly famous pill'.[100] Despite such harsh words, recent historians have revealed that quack doctors' proprietary medications were almost identical in composition to medicinal remedies sometimes prescribed by first- and second-tier physicians; many simply included a higher dosage of palliative ingredients like opium and alcohol.[101] This fact did not go completely unnoticed by regular practitioners in the eighteenth century. Yet as most such doctors insisted, it was not simply the composition of the drug that made it effective; it was, more importantly, the individualized care with which the drug was prescribed and applied. As one physician remarked early in the nineteenth century, 'the mischievous tendency of a quack medicine does not depend upon its composition, but upon its application'.[102] Most first and second-tier nerve doctors complained, quack doctors encouraged an inappropriate and indiscriminate use of their patent medications for all patients with the money to purchase their drugs.

Ever eager to make a sale, the shameless James Graham no doubt piqued other members of the profession with his advertisement for a Nervous Aetherial Balsam. Graham's salesmanship crescendoed in this pamphlet with his comment that 'many fanciful, rich, and luxurious people, who are in fact in good health, and who ought by no means to take this precious aetherial balsam' would be in no danger should they still decide to indulge in a few unnecessary doses. 'With such people,' he noted, his medication would

> produce no other operation or sensation, than a more genial and brisker flow of the blood and animal spirits, – and that species of contentment, thankfulness, and benevolent gladness of heart, which makes us happy in ourselves, and agreeable to all about us.[103]

With so many doctors like Beddoes, Trotter and Lettsom decrying the propensity of nervous patients to become addicted to alcohol and drugs, Graham's strong recommendation of his balsam, tempting the nervous and curious alike to indulge in medication, was strikingly irresponsible.

The writings of quack doctors were designed, not to inform their readership about nervous diseases, but to make a sale. This difference is further reflected in the distinctive format of quack publications. Whereas the other nerve specialists composed formal treatises, quacks published in pamphlet form, or, more commonly, in short newspaper advertisements. Void of any complex theoretical discussion of nervous disorders as espoused by the elite practitioners, quack publications unproblematically employed vague definitions and confused symptomology. Unlike publications by first- and second-tier practitioners, quack doctors did not footnote or reference any authorities on the subject other than themselves. Of course, as independent salesmen frequently living an itinerant lifestyle and without a steady or regular clientele, third-tier quack doctors had little need for networking.[104] Their singular status and lack of theory did not necessarily mean that they were socially or intellectually inferior to other tiers of medical practitioners. Lettsom's enemy, Myersbach, was rumoured to have collected up to £1,000 per month in fees, and even Graham studied in Edinburgh under Cullen and Whytt's expert tutelage, though he did not earn a formal degree.[105] Likewise, quack doctors did not cater exclusively to poorer patients unable to afford physicians' fees. Rather, they appealed to patients of all classes.[106] Whereas some quacks appealed even to illiterate customers, verbally advertising their wares on street-corners and attracting attention with bright costumes and theatrical performances, others appealed to a more exclusive and educated clientele by holding formal lectures in which they discussed the unparalleled benefits of their remedies. P. S. Brown's study of the prices of patent medicines advertised in eighteenth-century Bath newspapers also points to the wide appeal of quack remedies, showing how they ranged in price from as little as one shilling, to more exclusively priced remedies costing up to twenty-six shillings.[107]

Because quack doctors so frequently sold their medications through advertisements and without personal consultations, their remedies were necessarily less individualized than those of their professional superiors. Whereas first- and second-tier physicians composed personalized regimens of diet and exercise for their patients, quack doctors instead advertised their medications' universal appeal. Thus, quack doctors confidently assured the purchasing public of their medication's ability to treat any and all nervous symptoms, from headaches to horrific feelings of 'dejection and despair'.[108] For instance, W. D. Knight's *Hint to Valetudinarians* (1796) recommended a fourteen day course of 'DR FOTHER-GILL'S DROPS' for the cure of nervous complaints, citing the successful cure of a nervous tradesman's wife who suffered from low spiritedness, oppression, a weak stomach, a loss of appetite, giddiness and 'fear and trembling on hearing an unknown noise'.[109] Similarly, Dr Lowther's Nervous Powders and Drops, advertised in a January 1766 edition of *Pope's Bath Chronicle*, promised 'extraordinary Efficacy and Success in the Cure of the Fits and all nervous Disorders', and claimed to

> restore the Memory, and prevent confused and wandering ideas; remove Anxieties, Tremors, Horrors, Startings, restore an Appetite, dispel Flatulencies, Vapours and Flushings. They wonderfully exhilarate and invigorate the Constitution, so as to overcome all Faintness and Lowness of Spirits, and radically cure every Species of Convulsion and Weakness, arising from the nervous system.[110]

The *Chronicle* also advertised 'the Genuine British HERT TOBACCO and SNUFF' promising to strengthen the nerves and stomach while preserving the sight, and Vandour's Nervous Pills, assuring readers that they would 'give a serene Chearfulness of Disposition, in the Place of those Horrors which so dreadfully oppress the People of weak Nerves'.[111]

The number of quack advertisements for nervous medications printed in eighteenth-century newspapers was considerable. Brown's study examined the Bath papers from 1744 to 1800, counting 302 advertisements for patent and proprietary medications among the 636 issues reviewed. Among this sample, he found nineteen medications for mental symptoms and diseases of the nervous system, appearing in no less than 597 separate advertisements.[112] Although the scope of his study was limited to Bath, Brown's results shed light on the role that newspapers played in shaping public opinion of nervous disorders. Given this constant publicity, there is little doubt that the quacks were the most publicly visible practitioners treating nervous complaints.

Conclusion

Given the high visibility of quack doctors, the frequent stereotyping of the nerve doctors in public discourse as a group of mercenary and theoretically unsound practitioners is not surprising. This reputation is not wholly deserved. The physicians driving the medical theory behind the phenomenon were the elite of the medical profession who composed detailed treatises on the nerves void of any flattering or fashionable notions of nervous weakness. As is clear from their professional and personal writings, these doctors believed wholeheartedly in the medical significance of the nerves, even establishing nerve theory as the basis of a medical education at the University of Edinburgh. The writings of elite first-tier physicians were intended for an exclusive professional audience, whereas publications by second- and third-tier physicians appealed to progressively larger audiences. Consequently, it is not surprising that public opinion regarding nerve doctors was generally based upon the most visible lower orders of nerve specialists whose diagnoses were frequently fuelled by a desire for money, fame, or a fashionable clientele. Yet although some of the most public nerve doctors comfortably fit such stereotypes, private contributions from less visible and arguably, more professional medical practitioners tell a different story.

The nerve doctors were not a coherent group; practitioners' methods of treatment and attitudes towards nervous disorders varied greatly with respect to their level of prestige, education and career ambitions. These factors could vary significantly even within each tier; no one would doubt that Cullen was a more elite and better-known gentleman physician than Falconer; Beddoes was undoubtedly a higher calibre 'second-tier' physician than Perfect, and Rowley was less of a quack than Graham. Following his own classification of the species of medical practitioners Beddoes remarked that individuals are 'apt, like hybrid plants, or mule animals, to exhibit the marks of two species, wholly or in part'.[113] As a specialized group of medical practitioners, the nerve doctors were equally subject to these hybrid tendencies. Such complexity further highlights the inappropriate nature of stereotyping eighteenth-century nerve doctors as a homogeneous group of obsequious and mercenary practitioners. This popular image of nerve doctors does not do justice to the diversity or sincerity of so many treating physicians, or the status which nervous disease held in the period as a legitimate subject of medical inquiry.

3 'FESTER'D WITH NONSENSE': NERVOUS PATIENTS IN LATE EIGHTEENTH-CENTURY BRITAIN

To date, historians writing on nervous disease have focused largely on celebrities and fictional sufferers for evidence of nervous patients. Hence, the hypochondriac and melancholic sufferings of James Boswell and Samuel Johnson are well documented, as are the constant sniffles of Henry MacKenzie's overly sensitive man of feeling and the nervous swoons of Richardson's Pamela and Clarissa. While such sources reveal much about the public face of, and contemporary response to nervous sufferers, they leave us with very little sense of how the majority of nervous patients experienced their illness. The first part of this chapter seeks answers to this question, examining the symptoms, feelings and concerns of nervous sufferers as revealed by their diaries, letters written to friends and family and letters written to their physicians. The bulk of the material for this section comes from the surviving professional correspondence of the eminent Edinburgh nerve specialist, William Cullen. Housed in the Royal College of Physicians Library in Edinburgh, the several thousand patient letters written to Cullen provide a rare glimpse into the lives and sufferings of numerous nervous, melancholic, hysteric and hypochondriac patients.

The second part of this chapter complements this qualitative material with a more quantitative approach. Through a statistical analysis of surviving hospital records, private case notes, published disease reports and notes and papers written by medical students 'walking the wards', this section illuminates important basic details about the presence of nervous sufferers in eighteenth-century Britain, including their average age, sex, class and number. Ultimately, through both qualitative personal accounts and institutional statistics, this chapter reveals the seriousness with which nervous disease was taken by patients and their practitioners in the late eighteenth century, and proves that the experience of nervous suffering was far from fiction.

Patient Accounts of Nervous Disease

Patient diaries, publications and personal correspondence all provide windows into the experience of suffering from a nervous disease in the late eighteenth century.[1] Yet the best systematic evidence of nervous sufferers comes from surviving postal consultations. Postal consultations were common in the eighteenth century. Involved physical medical exams were not a normal part of doctor-patient relations until the late nineteenth century with the invention of the stethoscope.[2] Even if a patient did see a doctor, the physician's professional diagnosis was informed primarily from the patient's own case history. The patient would explain to the physician when and why they thought the complaint began, and provide a description of their symptoms. Patients typically informed their physicians of their daily regimen, including diet, exercise and sleep patterns. In turn, the doctor would contextualize the patient's disease history within his knowledge of the patient's past ailments and general constitution. Based upon this, as well as a basic visual examination, noting the colour of the patient's tongue, complexion and the taking of the pulse, the physician would usually offer a diagnosis. He would then suggest changes in regimen, and potentially prescribe medication to be mixed by the patient at home, or by a local apothecary.[3]

Given the rather cursory and superficial nature of medical examinations in the eighteenth century, together with physicians' overwhelming reliance on their patients' own histories, the prevalence of postal consultations is easy to understand. Furthermore, given the relative lack of diagnostic technology in the eighteenth century, a postal consultation could be just as effective as one conducted in person. Cullen conducted a significant amount of his private practice by post. The value of his surviving letters extends far beyond their ability to provide basic evidence of the quantity and sex of nervous sufferers in the period; for in the patients' attempt to convey the depth of their physical and emotional pain, their letters allow historians a window into their lives at their most vulnerable and unguarded moments.

Detailed descriptions of a patient's disorder were crucial to a doctor's ability to provide reliable and useful medical advice. The importance placed upon a meticulous case description is evident from a letter written to Cullen by the hypochondriac 'G. Watts' in 1784. Accused by his wife of previously submitting an inaccurate account of his symptoms to the doctor, Watts was coerced into sending a follow-up letter. He wrote,

> I am almost ashamed to trouble you with another [letter], and so soon too: but the truth of the matter is, Mrs Watts has, ever since I told her what I had written to you, been displeased & said I had deceived you & insists my writing you a letter to undeceive you, by giving you a more full & a more just representation of my case. She says

my appetite is good & that I eat three quarters of a pound of flesh meat ever day at dinner. I think she is mistaken, but she is positive.

After elaborating upon the details provided in his first letter to the physician, Mr Watts reiterated the depth of his distress:

I have suffered so much for about 32 years, from faintness ... gnawing, & weakness of stomach, that my spirits & resolution are in a manner quite exhausted, & had I not a family, who, I thank God, are grown up, I should wish to die, rather than live as I now do, for the above complaints have been worse than usual for above a twelvemonth.[4]

As will be discussed later in this chapter, Cullen received many such letters from distraught nervous patients. The more severe the patients' complaints, the more urgently they requested his advice. For instance, the frantic patient 'J. Nicholson' wrote to Cullen in 1785 expressing intense frustration with the doctor's apparent failure to respond immediately to his letter.[5] Nicholson wrote,

I am unfortunate in not being favor'd with an answer to my last in which I related the unhappy state of my nerves ... I am under apprehension you have not received it or you wou'd not surely tamper with me. I am now at Doncaster – write immediately and direct to the post office.[6]

Yet for most nervous patients, a response from Cullen was not so pressing. Given the chronic nature of nervous disease, the majority were long-time sufferers who had tried countless remedies, and were already under the care of a local practitioner. These patients frequently contacted Cullen for a second opinion. For example, one Lieutenant Colonel Clark wrote to Cullen from his station in New York that he was 'very nervous', suffering from cramps in his legs and feet, fever, poor sleep, a fast pulse, headaches and 'heaviness & anxiety after eating'. While already under the care of a 'very sensible clever young man' who had studied in Edinburgh and worked as a physician to the General Hospital, he expressed his 'wishes to have the opinion of Doctor Cullen', specifically regarding 'the effect of different climates for me'.[7]

Another patient, Mr Rae, wrote to Cullen in 1777 of his complaint 'call'd Nervous' which, he claimed, 'has harass'd me exceedingly' with poor sleep, gas and a 'vast and undescribab[le] uneasiness which I so frequently feel in my mind'. He informed Cullen that he had already 'consulted Dr. Fothergill who is reckoned skillfull'. Yet whereas Fothergill recommended sea bathing for his complaint, Mr Rae informed Cullen that another physician had told him that 'bathing in salt water would be no way serviceable'. Lamenting the way in which 'drs. will differ in judgment', Mr Rae confessed, 'I am at a loss what to do'. Expressing the depth of his sufferings and his faith in Cullen's discerning faculties he concluded,

> I hope you will be able to hit upon the cause of my sufferings and by the favour of
> God be likeways able to prescribe something that may afford relief – my utmost
> endeavours is altogether ineffectual in raising the spirits to that height which would
> make life desireable.[8]

Acknowledged as an expert in nervous disease by his professional brethren, Cullen was also approached directly by physicians eager for a second opinion. This was particularly common in cases where a patient's disorder was not responding to treatment. In one such typical instance a physician wrote to Cullen explaining all that he had done for his nervous patient, admitting that none of it had proven successful. He concluded, 'Having laboured so long under this obstinate Indisposition, and tried so many Remedies without Success, he [the patient] is anxious about himself, and wants to be advised of the most probable means of removing all his Complaints and recovering his Health'.[9]

It was also common for physicians like Cullen to receive letters from self-diagnosed patients who had begun treatment regimens of their own devising. This was particularly the case in the eighteenth century, when disease was regarded as a highly individual phenomenon owing to a patient's personal constitution and lifestyle choices.[10] It was common sense that patients knew their bodies best and would be most acutely aware of any changes in their bodily functions and physical or mental states. The proliferation of self-help guides during the period also helped patients become acquainted with medical matters and terminology. The inexclusivity of medical knowledge made self-treating a practical and economical choice for many patients, especially those without the money for private consultations.[11]

The tradition of self-help was strong even as early as the 1500s. Paul Slack's review of vernacular medical books from the *Short Title Catalogue* has estimated that approximately 153 such books were published between 1486 and 1604. Slack also suggests that by 1604, at least one of these books would have been in use for every twenty people. Yet as Ginnie Smith has discussed in her study of self-help advice in the eighteenth century, the market for self-help guides reached new heights in the eighteenth century with books like John Wesley's *Primitive Physic* running through no less than twenty-four editions from its first publication in 1747 to 1800, and thirty-five editions by 1842.[12]

Well versed in such sources, patients were acutely aware of both the causes, and the generic prescriptive artillery used by physicians to combat nervous disease, including gastronomic overindulgence, general inactivity and depression. Consequently, nervous patients often wrote to their physicians merely for confirmation of conclusions they had already reached and treatments they had already undertaken. For instance, when Lady Hester Newdigate wrote to her husband in 1792 regarding what she perceived was a nervous disease affecting their daughter, she mentioned that the consulting physician 'confirms my opinion of it [the child's complaint] being nervous', and that his 'opinion so perfectly coincides with my own that it satisfys me'.[13] Similarly, Ann Ormston, one of Cullen's more frequent correspondents, expressed her satisfaction with the doctor's initial assessment of her self-described 'tedious & lingering' condition including weak nerves, sweatings, headaches, oppression of spirits and poor sleep:[14]

> I have the greatest reason to join the general voice in praise of Doctor Cullen's judgments, since no person that has yet been consulted has seemed to understand my case at all, & his sentiments exactly coincide with my own opinion & Feelings, as I had frequently said from the beginning of my Illness, that there was a weakness in my Constitution that would require much Time & Care to remedy.[15]

Thus, it was with much confidence that she began a course of daily bathing and gentle exercise.

In a letter to Cullen, one Mr Surteer went even further, concluding his letter with the suggestion that sea bathing 'might be proper' for his complaint, only asking Cullen at the very end of his letter, 'What is your opinion?'[16] Likewise, Mr Nicholson, who consulted Cullen about a nervous disorder in 1785, informed him that 'I have been drinking hard', and concluded his letter by saying, 'My profession does not [expose] me to hard labour and I have time for exercise'.[17] There is little doubt that Mr Nicholson was aware that exercise and moderation in eating and drinking were crucial to combating nervous disease. Accordingly, it is likely that Mr Nicholson anticipated a letter from Cullen recommending moderation in drinking and increased exercise. It appears that he requested professional affirmation of the fact to calm his mind and possibly strengthen his personal resolve to make such lifestyle improvements.

Patients anticipating a prescription for travel were often so bold as to suggest specific destinations. For instance, one nervous patient wrote to Cullen in 1773 claiming that he believed England's climate was largely to blame for his condition. As a result, he wrote to Cullen of his plans for a sea voyage to Bermuda: 'Bermuda is situated in 32 degrees of North Latitude, and enjoys by all accounts, a most serene, equal and temperate Air its not being so hot there, as on the American Continents and on the same degree of Latitude'.[18] In this case, the patient never even asked Cullen for advice; he simply offered Cullen the opportunity to object to his plans. James Burnett, writing to Cullen in 1782 was slightly more flexible with his suggestions, asking the physician 'what town or County in England you think most proper to spend the winter in – or should I be ordered abroad, what place in France, which I would prefer greatly to any other foreign country'.[19]

In addition to informing patients of the common causes and treatments for nervous disease such as travel, self-help guides and popular medical literature could also inform patients of the intricate physiological details of their disorder. A few nervous patients writing to Cullen proudly displayed their technical understanding of the nervous system. One such patient wrote to Cullen in an effort to share 'a few of my Thoughts relative to the Nature of my Indisposition'. He acknowledged the mysterious nature of nervous disease, describing it as 'full of dark, intricate and perplexing paths, where one may wander for evermore, without being able to attain a distinct and satisfactory Idea of it'. Because of its confusing nature he wrote,

> I must take care therefore not to penetrate too far into it, which would be labour in vain – and besides, a long and painful Search, would neither suit with your time nor mine, neither have I strength of Spirits sufficient for it – I shall therefore be as short as I can.[20]

Nineteen pages of his 'short' letter survive.[21] Much of what survives is, in fact, a lecture upon the working of the nervous system. The author wrote to Cullen, 'There are certain parts of a Human Body which Physicians call the Nerves, and to which they attribute Sensation, or the power of feeling'. Such an elementary introduction would hardly have been necessary for the founding father of 'Neuroses'. Nevertheless, the patient's discussion quickly became more complex, as when he described his most bothersome symptom as

> an extra-unnatural degree of Sensibility – an high degree of an irrasable and Spasmodick disposition in the Stomach and Bowels – whether in these Organs, or in the Membranious Muscular and Nervous Parts, external from them, I am not able with precision to say … [22]

Interestingly, much of this patient's technical description of his nervous disease seems borrowed from Whytt's *Observations* which spoke of the 'unnatural sensibility' of disordered nerves which in turn could affect the 'stomach, liver and bowels', and produce a 'spasmodick contraction' of the muscles.[23] While some such patients attempted to present professional descriptions of nervous disease as their own, others were perfectly willing to reveal their familiarity with medical literature. In an effort to forgo the trouble of listing his extensive nervous sufferings, one patient, Mr Bradley Smith wrote to Cullen, 'I find most of my symptoms enumerated by Dr. Withers in his treatise on chronic weakness'.[24] Regardless of their familiarity with nervous disease, many patients (and their physicians) wrote to Cullen simply to take comfort in the fact that they had pursued the best medical advice possible.

    It is difficult to tell precisely how many of the patients writing to Cullen were actually nervous; Cullen's responses are stored separately from these consultation letters and it is difficult to pair the two.[25] Adding to this complication, Cullen very rarely offered a definite diagnosis in his letters. Most often, he simply provided some discussion of the presumed causes of a patient's disorder such as indigestion, or a weakness of the constitution or nervous system, along with his recommended treatment. Likewise, many patients merely provided Cullen with lists of symptoms that were typically described as nervous according to self-help guides and medical texts. Others specifically complained of their 'nervous', 'hypochondriac', or 'hysteric' disorders. It is not surprising that so many of the patients writing to Cullen were nervous; as a leading proponent of nerve theory at Edinburgh Medical School with a string of publications heavily focused on the nervous system, his reputation in the field was paramount. His academic fame naturally fuelled his private practice, resulting in a steady stream of new clients. As the nervous Reverend Charles Charleton wrote in the introduction to his first letter to Cullen, 'Sir, I am induced to submit my case to your judgment from the merit you have deservedly acquired both in the medical and literary world'.[26]

Symptoms and Sensibility

Roy Porter and G. S. Rousseau have examined the popular discourse surrounding nervous disease, effectively emphasizing the fashionable and upper class implications of nervous suffering.[27] Their work has revealed how exhibiting extreme sensibility or melancholy was frequently considered during this period as a 'badge of identity' or a 'mark of refinement in the man of feeling'.[28] Certainly in the first half of the century in the context of Cheyne's *English Malady* and the publication of the first novels of sensibility, the notion of superior nervous sufferings was commonplace. Moreover, unlike other contagious or disfiguring diseases, nervous disease was, as Porter has described, 'mercifully free of disgusting visual and distasteful cultural associations'.[29] Thus, confident in the glamour of their fashionable malady, well to do Britons spoke and wrote openly of their strained nerves. The correspondence of the illustrious socialite and litterateur, Lady Elizabeth Montagu, reveals some such pride in her supposedly strained nerves. In 1765 she received a poem from her correspondent George Lyttleton, titled 'A Dialogue between Mrs Montague's Soul and Body'. Referencing the toll that fine feeling took on her nerves, Lyttleton wrote,

> T'other night as they lay together in Bed
> Mrs Montagu's soul to her Body thus said,
> I could sleep very well, if it was not for you –
> With your nerves and your spasms there's so much to do
> That, though I am ever so calm and serene
> I can take no more rest than if I were a Queen!
> ... Her Body was piqued to hear alma so chide –
> Good Madam, said she, when our cause shall be tried,
> I am confident, it will appear very plain
> That I have most reason by far to complain ...

> If a Friend, or Friend's Friend, is sorry or sick, my poor Heart is
>   immediately pierced to the quick.
> You fret all its fibres, disturb all its Pulses,
> And make Business enough for ten Dr. Hulses.[30]

Apparently pleased with this portrayal of her physical sensibility, Montagu forwarded this poem to her good friend, the physician John Gregory.[31] Yet this poem, as with Lady Montagu's own references to her strong sensibility in her letters, were intended more as a flattering commentary on her character than an actual medical complaint. Not surprisingly, these descriptions of her nervousness were, as Porter describes, free from disgusting visual symptoms.

Lady Maxwell, the elite Edinburgh resident famed for her extreme piety and generous philanthropy, also took pride in her nervous condition. Eager to share her private pains with a public audience, her writings about her disordered nerves also bore greater resemblance to a description of her strong character than a pathological complaint. Born in 1742, Lady Maxwell married in 1760 at the young age of seventeen, only to have her husband and first young child die by 1762. As a result of this tragedy she experienced a deep religious conversion, becoming a staunch Methodist and personal friend to John Wesley.[32] Over the course of her life, Lady Maxwell saved her correspondence and personal writings (including over 300 letters and a 2,300 paged diary covering forty-two years), with the intent that they should 'be transmitted to one of the Wesleyan Ministers' upon her death.[33] While not publishing her writings herself, she made clear to her friends her 'sanguine' hope that after her death, her diary and letters 'would soon be given to the religious world'.[34] In this context, Lady Maxwell's regular references to her nervous disease in her writings from 1770 until her death in 1810 are particularly interesting; her 'private' discussions of her disorder within her diary and personal correspondence were clearly intended for a very public audience. Predictably, detailed accounts of precise nervous symptoms are nowhere to be found in her writings. Rather, she speaks only vaguely of her 'exquisite' sensibility, including general sweeping comments claiming that '*Weakness of nerves* and *spirits*, subjects me to painful feelings' while often remarking upon 'how amazingly ... the whole frame [is] unhinged, when the nerves and spirits are affected!'[35] Lady Maxwell depicts her experience with nervous disease as a divine challenge, or test of faith. She describes this point of view to her friend and fellow nervous sufferer, Lady Hope, in a letter in which she commiserates with her friend's sufferings and offers her own experienced advice:

> Your tears are caused by the weak state of your spirits and nerves, and also your bad dreams. I am no stranger to either ... An increase of faith and love is the best receipt. Keep your mind easy; be not too rigorous in your exactions from either mind or body at present. Your path of duty, just now, is to *suffer* the will of God ...

Three years later, in 1783, Lady Maxwell was still prompting her friend to rise to the challenge of proving her faith and overcoming her nervous symptoms:

> There is nothing so hurtful to the nervous system, as anxiety; it preys upon the vitals, and weakens the whole frame; and, what is worse than all, it grieves the Holy Spirit. But I hope you will be made conqueror over that, and ... prove God's utmost salvation and fullness of love: then you will find, 'where the spirit of the Lord is, there is liberty'.[36]

This didactic tone is equally visible in Lady Maxwell's diary entries. Referring to a particularly difficult month in 1779 in which her nerves and spirits were acutely agitated, Lady Maxwell wrote:

> I have been severely and unexpectedly tried; but my God has been good, supported me, and brought me through. From *weakness of spirit and nerves*, the animal frame was more agitated than was needful ... My severe distresses in early life, with a firm belief of the Christian religion, which quickly followed, and a comfortable persuasion of my interest in the glad tidings of the gospel, produced a serenity and solemnity of mind, with a sobriety of manners, which have, more or less, abode with me ever since.[37]

Thus, Lady Maxwell's bout with nervous disease was an ongoing test of faith, which, as she reveals through her writings, she ably passed. Far from being a punishment for an overly-luxurious lifestyle, Lady Maxwell believed that her nervous disease was heaven-sent, providing her the opportunity to set an example and prove her faith to the world.[38] As Porter has explained, public accounts and autobiographies of nervous sufferers often 'reek[ed] of literary convention, the stilted clichés of role players'.[39] Given the consciousness with which such 'private' writings were intended for emulation by, and edification of the public, there is little doubt that Lady Maxwell practiced some degree of 'nervous self fashioning', crafting her virtually symptom-less descriptions of her disorder to exhibit her 'superior sensibility'.[40]

Lady Montagu and Lady Maxwell wrote about their nerves in the same manner that so many eighteenth-century novelists wrote about the nerves of their fashionably delicate heroines: less as a medical condition than as a description of their inner character. The symptoms discussed in such cases are entirely inoffensive, consisting of extreme emotional sensibility, social sensitivity and polite physical delicacy. It would be unfair to impugn the reality of Lady Montagu and Lady Maxwell's perceived nervous disorders on the basis of these fashionable descriptions. Nevertheless, it appears that their intended audience significantly shaped, and potentially filtered, their descriptions of their nervous experience. In search of flattery, faith, or fame, their public writings served a very different purpose than a private consultation letter to a physician.

Despite his emphasis on the flattering and often insincere disease narratives of public sufferers, Porter's work on Samuel Johnson's melancholy rejects the automatic assumption that public personalities feigned their nervous complaints. Porter argues that Johnson's celebrity status did not mean that his disorder was an 'artificial construct' or that he used his illness 'as a public act towards his own career advancement.'[41] As an example, Porter shows how Johnson's personal 'reflective writings' offer historians a sincere and 'private view of a soul in turmoil.'[42] To prove that Johnson's melancholy was 'no mere literary caprice', Porter cites entries in Johnson's private diary, such as one from 1777 in which Johnson described his life as 'nothing but a barren waste of time with some disorders of body and disturbance of the mind, very near to madness.'[43] John Wiltshire has also mined Johnson's writings, providing evidence of his sincere concern over his many health conditions, which, in addition to his debilitating hypochondria and melancholia included poor sight and hearing, insomnia, asthma, strange tics and gout.[44] Wiltshire also investigates the writings of Johnson's correspondents and his biographer, James Boswell, who likewise documented Johnson's nervous condition. Indeed, in the *Life of Johnson* Boswell described his subject as

> overwhelmed with an horrible hypochondria, with perpetual irritation, fretfulness and impatience; and with a dejection, gloom, and despair, which made existence misery. From this dismal malady he never afterwards was perfectly relieved ... '[45]

As in other studies detailing the nervous sufferings of Samuel Johnson, the work of Porter and Wiltshire reveal his heartfelt self-disdain and very real pain, further undermining the temptation to doubt the sincerity of a patient's suffering based upon their public personality.

While this study in no way denies the reality of celebrity sufferers, its focus remains on medical case notes and consultation records from more 'ordinary' patients for dependable evidence of the nervous experience. Uncomplicated by celebrity or the presumption or possibility of a hugely public readership, the symptoms and consequences of nervous disease described by treating practitioners and patients seeking private professional medical advice were typically far more candid and serious than those described in novels, autobiographies, or open correspondence. For instance, writing to her husband relating the details of a medical consultation for her nervous adopted daughter, Sally Shilton, Lady Newdigate described how after the doctor left Sally's room, she

> follow'd him out of y[e] Room to know his real opinion & he has frighten'd me sadly. He says her nerves seem to be very delicate & that she has a Scorbutic irritability about her, that must be prevented fixing there taking care to keep her in an even tranquil state of Mind; that he has known Girls at her Age with y[e] Like delicate sensations lose all power of voice, even of speech, have a Paralytic Stroke or become stupify'd from great exertion of Spirits.[46]

Such a grim prognosis was particularly disturbing to Lady Newdigate, who was priming her daughter for a career as an opera singer.[47] James Lucas, a surgeon from Yorkshire related an even more grievous case from 1773 in which a twenty-five year old clergyman's wife was diagnosed with a nervous disorder after the unexpected death of two of her children. Among her dramatic symptoms Lucas listed headaches, stomach aches, vomiting, loss of sleep, great anxiety, large quantities of pale urine and coughing up blood. Her course of treatment was equally severe, with Lucas bleeding her sixty times and prescribing her three hundred grains of opium over the course of five months before she was finally cured.[48] While most nervous cases were not so life threatening, the symptoms discussed in medical contexts and cases were far more serious and pathologically grounded than the vague symptoms of nervous sensibility typically discussed in novels and sources intended for public consumption.

Indeed, most nervous patients experienced an impressive assortment of unflattering symptoms. The nervous patient Mrs Wynn exhibited a 'profuse perspiration' in the night, 'requiring a change of linen every 3 or 4 hours'.[49] Alternatively, the Edinburgh physician John Mitchell's response to his nervous patient 'Mr James' early in the nineteenth century reveals that one of Mr James' most bothersome symptoms was a collection 'of phlegm about the throat, with a troublesome and frequent husking up of it'.[50] The most common, and arguably the least flattering symptoms discussed by nervous patients in these letters are burping and flatulence. While these symptoms were commonly discussed in physician's publications on nervous disease, the detail with which patients describe their experiences is still surprising. For instance, the hypochondriac Mr Watts informed Cullen that

> When my food begins to digest, the air let loose from my food begins to distend the membranes of my stomach, merely because they are too weak to resist its expansive power. Wind never flies off my stomach easily & involuntarily, by the contraction of its membranes: but I force it off ... with difficulty; I suppose, by pressing my stomach between the diaphragm & abdominal muscles.[51]

Mr Shields, a nervous patient in Bristol, also complained of his dramatically debilitating wind: 'I am ready to die every instant, the wind is so powerful in my stomach, & when I can't bring it up, it suffocates me, & am panting for Breath & in danger of expiring momently'.[52] Troubled on the other end, a German patient wrote to Cullen in 1789 informing him that as a result of his 'hypocondriacal sickness' and 'irritability of the nerves' he suffered from a 'continual rumbling of wind in my stomach, and belching upwards which lasts for hours together.'[53]

Cullen's patient Ralph Ogle described in 1785 the benefits of sea bathing and horseback riding for his condition, although he complained of ongoing flatulence. He wrote, 'At intervals during the day, by means of exerting [and] straining myself a good deal, I can produce violent Eructions; & also in the mornings before I rise, the wind passes both upwards and downwards'. He went on to explain unabashedly to Cullen how 'immediately upon coming out of the [spa] water, I perceive a great tightness (as it were) across my stomach, both above & below the navel, for a short time; but am often relieved by several loud belchings, before I get my cloaths on'.[54] It is clear from this letter that Ogle intended the description of his symptoms to serve a very functional purpose; there is no evidence of him trying to display fashionable symptoms or glamorous sensibilities. Instead Ogle tells Cullen about his symptoms in a factual, honest and incredibly open way. Female sufferers were not exempt from unflattering flatulence or such candid descriptions. One physician writing on behalf of the nervous Miss Betty Ogilvie in 1782 informed Cullen that 'she complains much of being troubled with wind, is distressed with flatulent Rumblings in her Belly and has her stomach often oppressed with a sensation of fullness, and belches up wind from the stomach at these times'.[55] Although Miss Ogilvie did not write this description, it is clear that she originally voiced the complaint. Moreover, it is clear that she was little concerned with the supposed prerogative of nervous females to flatter themselves with symptoms indicative of delicacy and refinement.[56]

Fashionable Patients

Professional medical correspondence was not entirely void of fashionable or flattering interpretations of nervous sufferings. Although few in number, Cullen's private consultations do include some patients who contextualized their nervous ailments in the framework of high status or superior mental sensibility. In one such anomalous case, the nervous patient Robert Ligertwood wrote to Cullen from Aberdeen in 1781 offering a highly self-congratulatory view of his ailment. After telling Cullen of how his nerves and stomach were causing bile and costiveness, Ligertwood haughtily noted how 'when the Bile is thrown off, my mind is so distinct & clear that I can almost discern into the very Heavens'. Advising Cullen to be straightforward with him regarding the potentially mental causes of his nervous disease, he wrote,

> For I am persuaded that what is stored up in my mind is too exquisite for sense, so that I have often thought, Providence has thrown many things on my Person to Bear down the Aspiring & growing powers of my mind; yet I know it is my duty to Combat & nobly resist the Human Impulses, which many of the bravest & worthiest men have sunk under.

Such a heavily stylized letter, loading nervous sufferings with an abundance of cultural meaning, does not fit well with the other generally straightforward and candid patient letters written to Cullen. Moreover, Ligertwood's letter lacks any sort of graphic discussion of his symptoms or vital signs. Interestingly, Ligertwood notes in the post-script of his letter, 'My thoughts on reading have been so much employed & Delighted with the Nervous System that I could not restrain my self from committing what occurred to me to paper & publishing a small Treatise on the subject.'[57] Four months later, Ligertwood sent Cullen another letter, together with a copy of his book, which he stated had been published at the 'earnest request' of some of his 'particular friends'.[58] Ligertwood's desire to publish on the subject of his nervous disorder further suggests that it was the patients most eager to 'go public' with their nervous ailments that were the ones most likely to frame their sufferings in the context of mental or emotional superiority.

Interestingly, it appears that Ligertwood's own understanding of his illness changed over time. The flattering way that he described his disease in 1781 is significantly different from the way that he contextualized his disorder just five years earlier, when he first wrote to Cullen at the age of twenty-two. In this letter, rather than attributing his disorder to deep philosophical thought, Ligertwood admitted his belief that his distemper originated with an excess of 'venereal pleasures'. As a consequence, he suffered from 'frightfull appearances as if I was to be seized with a delirium or a fitt of the eppilipses'. He also complained of 'much trouble with the wind on my stomach which oppresses my Lungs and causes my breathing to be much affected'.[59] His embarrassment in his condition was clear from the postscript of his letter which stated, 'I begg youl not mention to any person that I have wrote you'.[60]

Writing again in 1778, Ligertwood complained of the continuation of his nervous symptoms, reiterating that he had lived a life of venereal intemperance so despicable that 'it would be impossible for me to paint out in proper colours, in so glaring a manner as it deserves'. As a result of his 'constant Devoir to the Ladies', Ligertwood noted that he suffered from a 'vertigo & giddiness in my head', 'a difficulty of breathing' and a 'horror and gloominess of mind'. In the mornings following his excesses, Ligertwood disclosed that he typically endured 'a calcaneous saliva attended with a deal of wind in the stomach'. He concluded his letter by relating to Cullen what he had read about the 'bad consequences that are produced by too great a discharge of the semen'. According to these sources, Ligertwood informed Cullen that offending young people

> Have the air and appearance of old age[.] [T]hey become pale[,] effeminate[,] benumbed[,] lazy[,] stupid and even imbecile. They have an utter distaste for every thing. That too great an abuse of amorous pleasures occasions disorders of the brain and of the nerves and destroys the Intellectual powers and that frequent emissions of the seed relax[,] dry up, weaken[,] enervate and produce a crowd of evils, the brain itself in this case appears consumed[;] the person in fact grows stupid and becomes so rigid that he is almost deprived of motion ... No wonder for the strength being gone impoverishes the Nervous system to such a degree that the mind seems at times in a state of delirium by being overcome with hypochondriacal complaints'.[61]

It is clear from this letter that Ligertwood's suffering and fear was very real. Plagued by guilt and anxiety over his condition, his letter reads like a private confession. Interestingly, by the time he decided to offer a public account of his nervous disorder three years later, his expressions of embarrassment and remorse were replaced by self-congratulation, and the description of his disorder was remarkably clear of any moral blemish or unsavoury symptoms.

In another seemingly stylized case, the Scottish judge and well-known philanthropist, Lord Gardenstone, wrote to Cullen in the summer of 1777 providing a detailed account of the nervous disorder by which he was 'horribly afflicted'. His letter began,

> I was born in the year 1722. I have from my earliest youth suffered the various complaints and infirmitys which arise from a Delicate or weak state of nerves – otherwise my constitution has been good and even vigorous – I can not deny that as long as I was able my life has been very irregular – pursuing every course of Fashionable pleasure with little reserve and suffering the usual consequences.[62]

The mere mention of his disorder in the context of a 'fashionable' lifestyle distinguishes Gardenstone's letter from the majority of Cullen's nervous patients. Although Gardenstone discussed specific symptoms in his letter, including nightmares which caused him to wake 'hastily in Horrors', 'imaginations very strong of immediat death', and convulsive fits followed by a sensation of feeling 'very languid & distress'd', it lacks the typical physical detail found in other letters regarding such mundanities as his daily bowel movements, rate of pulse, or even diet.

Like Ligertwood, Gardenstone also composed a public account of his trial with nervous disease, publishing a multi-volume set detailing his extensive travels in pursuit of health titled, *Travelling Memorandums*. In this memoir he wrote openly of his ailing nerves, even quoting the opinions of his many doctors that 'my nervous complaints are not curable, but may be mitigated and relived, - not by medicines, but by proper regimen, moderate exercise, and change of air'.[63] The obvious pride that Gardenstone had in his delicate valetudinary state (and his ability to spend so much time and money nursing his health) was evident from his description of his extreme efforts to procure the particular French water prescribed by his physician during his visit to Plombières. After being told by an 'esteemed' physician that the local mineral waters were too hot for his constitution, Gardenstone wrote,

> His counsel was cautious and candid – It suited my own opinion perfectly, and I adopted it ... He advised me to drink the cold chalybeate water, which is brought here from a village at the distance of about eight leagues; and to use a barh compounded from different fountains here.

As Gardenstone subtly bragged, the local hot waters might be serviceable to people of robust constitutions, 'but I am sure they are hurtful, or at least very dangerous to delicate constitutions, and relaxed nerves'.[64] Gardenstone's prideful description of his 'delicate' condition and his willingness to publicize his poor health is unlike the majority of nervous patients in Cullen's practice.

In very rare instances, romantic accounts of nervous disease can be found among unpublished letters of patients who have no intention of 'going public'. Yet in such cases the patients' flattering discussions of the instigating causes of their nervous disorders are paired with very personal details of physical symptoms and bodily functions. For instance, in one 1774 letter, a Genevan husband wrote to Cullen describing his wife's nervous symptoms, alluding to the way in which her extreme sensibility was the root cause of her ailment. As he explained, 'about 4 or 5 years ago, after much excess in dancing, she became extremely weak'. Following this weakness, she then 'played a tragedy which moved her much, the consequence of which was the disease for which I consulted you, namely fits of tension in the neck with great excitement of the imagination, followed by a general relaxation & languor both of the body & mind'. Together with her tendency to tax herself physically by singing too much, her dancing and emotional sympathy were, according to her husband, the causes of her 'evidently nervous' maladies.[65] Although this unpublished letter reveals a flattering and arguably fashionable depiction of feminine weakness and nervous sensibility, it still contains details not to be found in published accounts. Her husband provides information to Cullen regarding the time of her menses, as well as a record of her pulse. While minor, these details prove that although he discussed nervousness in a somewhat flattering way, the perception of the fashionable causes of her ailment did not come at the expense of his sincere concern or its role as a serious medical condition.

Again, it would be unfair to dismiss all patients who revelled in the fashionable implications of their sensibility-induced disorders as mere actors. In her discussion of the modishly delicate health of so many French enlightenment philosophers, Anne Vila has thoughtfully remarked that their tendency to conflate physical ailments like indigestion and dyspepsia with their superior mental and sentimental powers did not necessarily come at the expense of their sincerity. Rather, Vila argues, their tendency to dwell upon and publicly discuss their ill health

> was rooted in motivations that were jointly somatic, philosophical, and social: *philosophes* fretted over their stomachs partly because they were truly suffering, partly because they were fascinated with the body's mechanisms, and partly because having chronic digestive problems facilitated conversation with their high-born benefactors, who tended to complain loudly of their own "flighty" digestion.[66]

Voltaire, Vila explains, 'interwove his dyspepsia with his celebrity, exploiting both to advance his relations with high-born patrons'. Nevertheless, she explained, 'Voltaire truly believed that he had been cursed by nature with a horribly frail stomach that was liable to carry him to the grave at any moment'.[67]

British philosophers often exhibited the same pride over their nervous sufferings. For instance, in 1734 the renowned Scottish Enlightenment philosopher David Hume wrote to his physician George Cheyne that he was suffering from the 'Disease of the Learned' after spending too much time in solitude reading 'books of Morality, such as Cicero, Seneca & Plutarch'. Ultimately Hume's study served only 'to waste the Spirits, the Force of the Mind meeting with no Resistance'. In an effort to treat his nervous disorder, Hume took several courses of anti-hysteric pills, undertook a gruelling exercise regimen, and, most importantly, made sure to study more 'moderately, & only when I found my Spirits at their highest Pitch, leaving off before I was weary'.[68] Here Hume was clearly proud of his irritated nerves. Yet again, this pride did not necessarily come at the expense of the legitimacy of his sufferings; in another letter composed for a medical professional but never sent, Hume expressed earnest concern over his fate as a sufferer from the 'Disease of the Learned'. He ended his letter with a set of questions for the doctor:

> Whether among all those Scholars you have been acquainted with you have ever known any affected in this manner? Whether I can ever hope for a Recovery? Whether I must long wait for it? Whether my Recovery will ever be perfect, and my Spirits regain their former Spring and Vigour, so as to endure the fatigue of deep and abstruse thinking?[69]

While every patient contextualized their disorder in their own way, each sufferers' narrative of their illness 'reflected their lived reality'.[70] Thus, a particular emphasis on fashion, wealth, celebrity, sympathy, or intelligence was not necessarily exclusive of a patient's candor. Rather, patients could employ these contexts in an effort to make sense of their symptoms, and to find meaning in their misery.

Typical Patient Accounts

Of course, even the slightest notion of superior or romantic suffering was vastly different from the opinion held by the majority of nervous patients writing privately to Cullen. Whereas patients writing publicly about their symptoms often dwelled on their superior feelings and supremely sensitive natures, patients like John Warrandice, writing to Cullen in 1785, complained instead of a lack of feeling and a numb sensibility as a result of his disorder. Reflecting on the period in which his symptoms were most severe, he wrote, 'Sometimes I was in a state of stupefaction – indifferent to every thing around – I knew myself to exist and that was all - & Neither grief, joy, love, fear, or any passions of the mind seemed to have the same influence as formerly'.[71] Other anxious patients writing privately to Cullen displayed fears that their nervous complaints would not be taken seriously. This fear was not entirely unfounded. Satirical prints and written caricatures of nervous patients tirelessly presented them as self-obsessed sufferers likely to exaggerate, or even fake, the physical symptoms of disease. The public audiences for these caricatures were meant to laugh at the absurdity of hypochondriacs' physical complaints, knowing all the while that their symptoms, if real at all, were only in their minds.

Not surprisingly, nervous and hypochondriac patients often responded to this stereotyping by insisting on the physical reality of their complaints. For instance, in a postal consultation with Cullen in the summer of 1776 the patient John Henderson asserted that 'some weeks ago I imagined I was in a way to regain my ordinary degree of health, but of late my complaints seem to have caught a faster hold on me, & tho' they may still be of the nervous kind I am confident they are not imaginary'.[72] Likewise, after a lengthy consultation letter expanding upon the minutia of his 'flatulency, want of appetite', 'violent perspiration' and other nervous symptoms, Thomas Christie apologized for his potentially irritating level of detail, declaring:

> I did not mean ... to ... bias your judgment by any thing which I have said, but only to shew you that my opinion of my own case is not altogether founded in whim and Fancy, which are generally thought to govern entirely those who are afflicted with Nervous Complaints'.[73]

While this seems an obvious response for a sufferer whose diagnosis was so frequently called into question, most nervous sufferers had little trouble acknowledging the mental and imaginary dimension of their disease.[74] As the famed hypochondriac James Boswell explained to readers of his column, 'The Hypochondriac', a nervous sufferer's awareness of the imaginary nature of some of his complaints did little to lessen the reality of his pain. For, he wrote, while the sufferer 'knows that his mind is sick, his gloomy imagination is so powerful that he cannot disentangle himself from its influence, and he is in effect persuaded that its hideous representations of life are true'.[75]

Many nervous patients from Cullen's practice also discussed the role that imagination played in their disease. For example, after listing the symptoms and potential reasons for his nervous condition one patient wrote to Cullen, 'some of the Circumstances I have mention'd are trivial if not impertinent – but it is generally accounted one of the Symptoms of this Disease, to be more or less Whimsical – and it is proper this should appear in my case also'.[76] Similarly, the nervous Mr Sandilands wrote to Cullen in 1789 openly acknowledging the mental aspect of his malady:

> I am persuaded that these uneasinesses are, if I may be allowed the expression, in
> some measure mechanical, that is to say arising not so much from bodily infirmity
> as from perturbation of mind produced by indulging extravagant but very harassing
> thoughts.[77]

Likewise, the hypochondriac William Stewart confided in Cullen his understanding that 'distress of mind ... must affect the body' while listing such physical
symptoms as stomach aches, heartburn and an irregular heartbeat, together with
emotional symptoms including low spirits, 'gloomy' and 'absurd' ideas ('because
they are absurd, Nervous they must be'), as well as a 'shyness & diffidence about
me with too great an anxiety to please which often [makes] me feel uneasy'.[78]

Particularly pained by distressing thoughts, the nervous George Walide
wrote to Cullen in 1780 that his extreme sorrow upon the recent death of his
father had 'introduced a train of complaints which I have for some time past
been subject to'. He informed the doctor that he first experienced 'this severe
disorder' when he 'received the account of the death of a younger & much loved
Brother, which had so powerful an effect upon my spirits & so much agitated my
Mind, that it produced a Complaint which till that afflicting stroke I had been
totally unacquainted with.' He then listed his nervous symptoms, including
headaches, stomach cramps, heart palpitations and 'a trembling which affected
my whole body, & was preceded & attended by great chillness'. Yet his mental and emotional symptoms were the worst of all. As Walide explained, 'The
depression of spirits & disagreeable [-] I may say dreadful [-] Ideas it introduced
were such as till then I had no conception of.'[79]

Also struggling with low spirits, the patient Mr Elliot explained how his
mental symptoms were the most troubling part of his disorder. He confided in
Cullen that 'About two years ago I was sore troubled with causeless doubts &
fears; strange fancies ... and almost the whole train of disorders that accompany
nervous complaints'. Although he had since followed the doctor's instructions
to take 'pukes and powders', he stated that his symptoms had returned and his
mind was once more 'fester'd with nonsense': 'all these doubts & wanderings of
the mind seem to rage as much as ever'. In the conclusion of his letter, Mr Elliot
explained the origin of his renewed nervousness:

> Most of these complaints I know were raised by grief for the loss of my wife who died
> in the beginning of August; If you can do me any service it will be the greatest char-
> ity, for I am now so pestered with this disorder, yet not often sick; that it is certainly
> worse than death, thus to live in this way; and if I find no relief from what you shall
> please order, [I] must refer my case to God almighty, being satisfied that if you can do
> me no good, no mortal on earth can.[80]

Thus, whereas many non-sufferers frequently dismissed the reality of nervous
complaints, believing that they were only a figment of 'sufferers'' imaginations,

patients were surprisingly willing to acknowledge the mental dimension of their malady. Far from compromising the legitimacy of their complaint, the mental and oftentimes 'fanciful' component of nervous disease appeared to them as a significant symptom of their complicated disorder.

Given the presumed strength of the connection between the mind and body in the eighteenth century, it was only natural for doctors treating nervous disorders to acknowledge the pathological significance of both mental and emotional complaints. More interesting is the way in which these doctors also acknowledged the physical consequences of imaginary symptoms. For example, the physician Patrick Scott remarked in a case note that one of his patients was

> observed to have great lowness of spirits, & thoughtfulness, broken sleep, deep sighing & moaning, peevishness so that every thing offended, doing & saying things that before was quite opposite his inclination, his appetite at this time very irregular, sometimes voracious, his digestion at same time very bad with great flatulency and sour Belchings; avoiding company, had numberless imaginary complaints, and when forced into company seemed to increase the taciturnity into an habitual silence so that a word could not be got from him.

These symptoms culminated in a fit wherein the patient was 'strongly convulsed', his face became a 'purple colour, and he temporarily lost all power of 'speech, memory [and] judgment'.[81] The mere fact that the doctor mentioned his patient's imaginary symptoms as a precursor to this fit indicates that he did not doubt the authenticity of his patient's sufferings, or the significance of his illusory complaints.

Some nervous patients were greatly alarmed by the severity of their mental symptoms. One patient, after consulting Cullen about his nervous condition in 1781, wrote again eight years later to describe the escalation of his disorder. The majority of his concerns regarded his mental symptoms:

> My complaints just now are these – Upon taking up a bundle of miscellaneous papers to arrange them properly in two minutes my Head is confused – Upon writing a page of an account the same – I can sum one page but not two at a time – The most necessary business of setting down money received & paid away is that thing I abhor the most ... Instead of thinking what is proper to be done first every thing rushes into my mind & nothing is done properly.

He then complained of his increasingly volatile temper claiming, '[I] will laugh one moment & like to weep the next'. Most worrisome, he confided to Cullen, was that sometimes 'without any cause I will when standing suddenly leap up turn round in the air & strike myself on the cheek & Breast – Then I think I am going mad which is the principal reason for wishing a consultation'. The fears expressed by this nervous patient cannot be minimized. The depth and heart-breaking sincerity of his anxieties are fully revealed in the final paragraph of his letter:

> I wish to know how I am either to get perfectly well or better – and if I was dying as
> I should like my Physician to tell me[,] so in this case I should like to be told whether
> or not I shall ever enjoy perfect health – The idea of Drowning has occurred to me
> but 1ˢᵗ I had no Right & 2d it would be Cowardly.[82]

Cullen's patient, Thomas Bushby, also feared that death would be his only relief
from his 'lowness of spirits and ever attendant nervous symptom[s]'. As he wrote
to the doctor, 'my anguish under this depression of spirits is so great I can[not]
avoid exclaiming must I indeed parish? or what more can be done for such an
unfortunate wretch?'[83] Nervous patients contemplating death or suicide as a
result of their depressed spirits were extreme cases. Yet regardless of whether
nervous patients acknowledged their mental symptoms in a calm or distressed
manner, none of them believed that their complaints were 'all in their heads'.
Rather, mental symptoms were regarded by nervous sufferers and treating physicians as psychological symptoms of physically disordered nerves.

Many of Cullen's patient letters reveal a profound sense of guilt over nervous suffering. Far from exhibiting prideful boastings or any sense of superiority
for suffering from a nervous disease, many patients believed that their illness
was punishment for irresponsible or immoral behaviour. The patient John
Warrandice acknowledged his own fault in bringing about his nervous hypochondriac symptoms; after feeling better for a while during a long journey away
from home he wrote to Cullen,

> I forgot my former complaints and used too much freedom with my constitution. I
> was anxious about getting home and allow'd myself too little sleep ... For a good part
> of the Journey my only dinner was a bit of bread and a draught of Porter: and twice
> at night I drank too much wine. The consequence of all this was – that a short time
> after I returned home my old terrors came upon me in the night and continued with
> me in a great measure thro the day – the merest triffles filled me with fear ... And by
> this means my life was rendered very uncomfortable.[84]

Here it is clear that Warrandice believes he is at fault for the recurrence of his
nervous symptoms. Far from being proud or smug about his ailment, Warrandice
was instead secretive and slightly embarrassed: 'my natural bashfulness kept me
from communicating my case to any body – but I had the address so to manage
matters that few or none suspected me of being ill'.[85] Warrandice's shame over his
hypochondriac disorder is further explained in his letter when he acknowledges
his additional culpability for his disordered nerves:

> When I arrived at the age of fourteen, thro the bad example of my companions I got
> into a custom that greatly strengthened the disorder.⁺ [Here he footnotes 'self-abuse']
> It now appeared by a weakness at the heart – pains in the small of my back – a dif-
> ficulty of breathing & a constant fear of death.[86]

Such embarrassing information would be difficult to divulge. The mere fact that Warrandice included this information in his letter proves the seriousness with which he took his hypochondriac disorder: the hope of a cure was worth the short-term embarrassment.[87]

Warrandice was not the only one to reveal such sensitive information in his case history. Mr Pinkerton's personal physician, writing to Cullen for advice noted of his patient that

> from the age of twelve he has been troubled with very frequent nocturnal pollutions which have weakened his nerves and constitution in a very great degree – Giddiness in the head especially when walking, flushings in the face, cold tremors, slight aliena-tions of mind, vain terrors and anxieties, weariness, and faintness with sometimes a sense of suffocation in the brain, form a list of his chief complaints. [88]

In a similar vein the patient J. Nicholson wrote to Cullen in 1785 regarding pains in his legs, back and head along with the 'general relaxation of [his] nerv-ous system'. He explained, 'my complaint is from excess of venery in my youth and a continuation of it'.[89]

The sense of guilt voiced by so many nervous sufferers in their letters to Cul-len was not always tempered with embarrassing information. Some sufferers felt surprisingly ashamed over fairly innocent past behaviour, which they believed contributed to their poor health. For instance, the twenty-five year old Rever-end Charles Charleton complained to Cullen in 1785 that 'the least exertion, hurry or surprise affect my nerves in the most sensible manner, accompanied with tremors in my hands &c'. The likely cause of these ailments, he confessed to Cullen early on in the letter, was that 'I have lived rather a sedentary life, particu-larly when at College during the vacations'.[90] Here the Reverend's confession is honest and heartfelt; he is not taking pride in his ability to afford a sedentary or lazy lifestyle, but is instead telling on himself, and exhibiting a sense of guilt over his slothful student years.

Another minister writing to Cullen from Orkney Island displayed similar embarrassment over his nervous disorder, although he acknowledged that it was not the result of any sort of intemperance. He begged the doctor 'that immedi-ately on perusal you will tear the subscription & date from this letter. For many reasons I wish no one in the world but yourself to be acquainted with my disor-der'.[91] Describing his condition, the twenty-three year old wrote,

> Ever since I remember my nerves have been weak. There was always a visible tremor in my hand, which, when my spirits were any way agitated, or my body heated by exercise, became excessive. About nine years ago ... I was insensibly seized with an uncommon sort of weakness in my head. I cannot describe it to you, any other way, than by telling you that I was apt to imagine myself in a dream, rather than in real life.

He continued, informing Cullen, 'The association of my ideas is always irregular, & sometimes I think, partakes of folly'. Plagued by poor sleep and vivid nightmares he related how at night

> the most unaccountable ideas arise in my mind, my heart is chilled with horror, the bed seems to sink under me, & every thing alludes my grasp . . . My temper is fretful [and] inconstant. Study distress[es] me, & passion almost throws me into convulsions.

In addition to these mental and emotional symptoms the minister listed the physical effects of his malady: 'I have every morning had a most disagreeable taste in my mouth, & always, when I waken, spit up a great deal of yellow, glutinous stuff'. He also suffered from pain in his left shoulder, indigestion and 'frequent gripes in the belly'. Concluding his letter, the distraught minister wrote, 'My nerves are evidently weaker now than ever ... What I wish to know of you, sir, is, what you think will be the event of my disorder, whether you think it possible to cure, or even to alleviate'. The depth of his distress was evident from his final claim that 'if I die, I should leave behind me a wife, & two fatherless children'.[92]

For some patients embarrassed by their nervous conditions, the idea of constitutional or inherited nervousness could help to absolve them of any guilt or perceived responsibility. Interestingly, the number of cases in which nervous disease was supposedly caused by an inherited family constitution rose at the same time that the reputation of nervous disease as a fashionable malady was losing ground; for, as will be discussed in the final chapter of this study, romanticized notions of superior sufferings were replaced in the final quarter of the century by the far less-glamorous implications of self-indulgence and laziness. One patient writing to Cullen in 1789 regarding a nervous complaint acknowledged that he had 'used much freedom with my Constitution' – a freedom it seems that may have been sexual in nature given his discussion of frequent mercurial treatments. Yet personal vice was not to blame for his condition. Instead, he explained, 'I imagine my Nervous system has not originally been strong – My parents were not strong – I had always a great flow of spirits without any corresponding low ones'.[93] That same year the Reverend Mr Surteer from University College, Oxford wrote to Cullen about a nervous complaint, complaining that he was 'much subject to nervous infirmity' and had a 'general irritability' of habit. Assigning no particular cause to his disorder, Mr Surteer professed that he had 'always had a constitutional Instability which never failed to shew itself on the slightest Occasion'.[94] Far from bragging about the high living or extreme thinking which may have instigated their nervous ailments, it seems many nervous patients towards the end of the century sought refuge in the blamelessness of a hereditary condition.

Doctors also increasingly discussed the hereditary nature of nervous disease. For instance, interviewing the mother of a nervous patient, Mr Anstruther, Doctor Alexander Douglass wrote to Cullen,

I find by Mrs Anstruthers account that his fathers family were subject to nervous
complaints & considerable inequality of spirits, some of them to a remarkable degree,
& by what I can gather from her I have little doubt of the hereditary disposition ...[95]

Likewise, in one consultation by correspondence, Cullen asked a colleague about
one of their mutual nervous patients who was suffering from ongoing headaches,
'Is the Delicacy of nerves that appears in this Lady in any measure a family constitution?'[96] Such questions appear ever more often in case notes from the final
quarter of the century.

Whether hereditary or personally acquired, nervous disease was frequently
a lifelong affliction. Several adult patients writing to Cullen claimed to have suffered from nervous complaints since childhood. Warrandice believed that his
troublesome hypochondria originated in his infancy. As he claimed,

from the earliest period of my life I can remember I have at times been afflicted with
a disorder of the nervous or hypochondriac kind. When I was a child it appeared
chiefly in the night by filling me with fearful and gloomy ideas which awaked me with
great terror. My parents have told me that this was occasioned by a fright some young
fellows in the neighbourhood gave me when an infant.[97]

Due to the chronic nature of nervous disease, it was common for patients to
suffer for decades without a successful cure. The physician of one middle-aged
nervous patient suffering from 'headaches, watchfulness, anxieties, dimness
of sight, loss of memory and a confused, indistinct, wavering apprehension of
things' acknowledged his patient's frustration, claiming that 'he has been in the
above situation twenty years, has consulted numberless Physicians, & vainly
tried all their different prescriptions'.[98] Likewise, after composing a lengthy list of
symptoms including 'wind in my stomach and bowels', 'flying pains in my head',
'wandering thoughts and wild imaginations', a tendency to become startled at
the 'least noise' so that 'my heart will beat for sometime', 'an aversion to company
and love of solitude', 'frequent startings in my legs, arms and thighs' and 'deep
melancholy thoughts', the despondent nervous patient Mr Finny wrote, 'I am
about 50 years of age, and have been in this melancholy situation for ... these
twenty or thirty years by past'.[99] Another patient, Mr Shields, informed his Bristol physician that he had suffered for so long while in search of a remedy that he
was close to giving up hope of ever finding a cure:

I am resolved to take no medicines having already in the West Indies tried almost all
nervous medicines, tonics, bitters, & the cold Bath &c. to no manner of purpose. If
this climate with the waters of Bristol, Bath or Spaw &c. & with a proper regimen
won't relieve me, I shall go no farther.[100]

Still, most nervous patients exhibited admirable fortitude in their ongoing quest
for health. Nervous patients writing to Cullen consistently emphasized the great

lengths to which they had gone in order to recover. One such patient wrote to Cullen in the summer of 1785 that he had been following the doctor's recommendation of exercise on horseback to the letter: 'I have been strictly attentive to it, never letting one day slip without riding at least once, if not twice, or perhaps oftener'.[101] Similarly, in his attempt to convey the severity and deep-rootedness of his 'disordered state of the nerves', Thomas Christie provided Cullen with a long list of treatments that had failed to procure relief:

> The cold bath did me no service ... No bracing, strengthening, stimulating medicine ever did me any effectual service – sometimes I have found them of bad consequence. I have avoided Indolence so carefully – I have exercised myself, to such a degree, by frequent long journeys upon horse back to the extent of a Thousand Miles – by walking liberally &c&c, as might have strengthened and hardened any one – but this never carried off the sensibility.[102]

Consulting Cullen in 1789, one Mr Smith wrote of his horseback-riding regimen, 'I find myself much better for it, my head & stomach are easier, but I do not find myself relieved with regard to my thoughts. I have been prevented from riding by a very absurd apprehension ie. [that] I should during that exercise be carried off [in] some sudden attack'. Nevertheless, Smith announced his brave resolve to continue the regimen: 'I am very confident that this exercise will be of the greatest benefit to me, & I am determined to continue it as much as I can'.[103] Patients also showed a willingness to travel great distances for medical consultations. After providing a meticulous list of symptoms one nervous patient writing from Boreland, eighty miles south of Edinburgh, wrote, 'If you think you could be of more service to me by my coming into Town & informing you personally of many of my Complaints I certainly will. I would be glad to do any thing to be relieved of such uncommon Complaints'.[104] Other patients were willing to cross oceans in search of a cure. In 1785 one physician wrote to Cullen regarding the case of a girl from Louisiana suffering from 'an uncommon Sensibility of the whole Nervous System' whom he had met on a boat to Bordeaux. After unsuccessfully travelling to France with her father in search of an 'eminent' physician who might be able to relieve her nervous symptoms, she was about to return home. The physician writing to Cullen informed him that he had recommended that the girl and her father travel instead to Britain to consult him as their final resort. He wrote,

> The poor man [the girl's father] has certainly made too great a sacrifice in the Circumstances of Life that he is in, as being a Person Advanced in Years, and having left his wife and a large Family behind for the sake of this one Daughter to return after so long a voyage without reaping some advantage from consulting the Physicians in Europe.[105]

The girl did, in fact, continue in her search for a cure, consulting Cullen within the month.

The vast majority of case notes and patient letters to physicians display this type of sincere concern, fortitude and eagerness to get well. Nevertheless, popular stereotypes of nervous patients in the second half of the century persistently portrayed them as selfish sufferers, happily obsessed with their poor health. Philip Thickness's *Valetudinarians Bath Guide* (1780) even half jokingly referred to physic as a 'fashion', claiming that 'it is the amusement of idle people, who not knowing what to do with their time, bestow it upon their preservation'.[106] Though very much in the minority, some eager sufferers did exist. In such cases, nervous patients often became consumed by thoughts of their poor health. Self-help guides were particularly dangerous in the hands of these sufferers, as dwelling on nervous ailments was commonly acknowledged by physicians to make them worse. One letter to Cullen from a nervous patient's personal physician clearly exemplified the danger of indulging in too much medical reading. In the introduction to his letter the physician wrote that his patient

> has in general been healthy, but supposed to have a moveable state of nerves, for some time past uncommonly anxious about his health, inquisitive about nervous complaints & reading books upon that subject, which seem to have made some impression upon his mind.[107]

In this case, the patient's personal indulgence by dwelling on and constantly investigating his nervous feelings resulted in a far more severe case than if he had tried to resist them.

Occasionally troublesome nervous patients would disregard or irresponsibly attempt to modify their physicians' instructions. For instance, after repeatedly seeking Cullen's detailed medical advice, one of Cullen's regular nervous correspondents proceeded to write to the doctor complaining of his most recent recommendations:

> Tea you say will be rather hurtful – For some years past I have seldom drunk above two ordinary cups in the morning and the same in the afternoon. – To the former I generally eat an egg & plenty of bread and butter – and in the afternoon I cou'd be brought to give it up – but unless there was a real necessity for it I wou'd not be fond of giving up my two cups at either time because I find them comfortable and I know of nothing I cou'd get so good. If you say however that this point must be given up – Pray point out something else in place of them.[108]

Writing at the beginning of the nineteenth century, the physician Thomas Beddoes expressed strong irritation with such patients who were unwilling to make dietary sacrifices in order to improve their health. In the first volume of *Hygeia*, Beddoes grumbled that 'a child is ridiculed for thinking that he can *eat his cake and have it.* Are not grown people equally ridiculous, if they complain of ailments at the same time they are doing everything in their power to bring them on?'[109]

Equally troublesome to nerve doctors were patients who indulged in the minutiae of their complaints. For instance, one nervous patient writing to Cullen in 1776 and complaining of 'some slight Pains in my head, with now and then a little noise and giddiness; and at times a sinking, with wind in the stomach and bowels' went on for an entire paragraph explaining all aspects of his dietary regimen. After explaining the types of vegetables he liked to eat, the quantity of meat and number of glasses of wine he usually took with dinner, and the seasonings he used with every meal, he finally got to the point of his letter: 'May I now and then eat moderately of fish, and might I not substitute Honey in the place of Butter at Breakfast?'[110]

While self-indulgent, uncooperative and bothersome patients are uncommon among surviving case records, it is interesting to note how frequently they appear in books intended for the public. Forbes Winslow's 1839 collection of medical biographies, *Physic and Physicians*, related anecdotal stories about several physicians' irritation while treating nervous patients who revelled in the attention that their disorders conveyed. For instance, Winslow wrote of the physician extraordinary to George III, Doctor Matthew Baillie's frustration with one supposedly nervous patient:

> After listening, with torture, to a pressing account from a lady, who ailed so little that she was going to the opera that evening, he had happily escaped from the room, when he was urgently requested to step up stairs again; it was to ask him whether, on her return from the opera, she might eat some oysters. 'Yes, ma'am,' said Baillie, 'shells and all'.[111]

The Glasgow physician John Moore, known for his satirical writings regarding fashionable manners in late eighteenth-century London, also made light of nervous sufferers and complained of such irritating patients as the 'old lady [who] cannot dine with comfort till [the physician] has felt her pulse, looked at her tongue, and told her whether her chicken should be roasted or boiled'.[112] These stereotypes also appeared in fiction of the late eighteenth and early nineteenth century. Readers of Jane Austen's *Emma* were undoubtedly familiar with the supposed petty dietary concerns of hypochondriacs like Mr Woodhouse, who was unable even to enjoy a slice of wedding cake without first consulting his apothecary about its digestibility.[113] Designed to entertain readers, these popular books intentionally portrayed nervous sufferers in a comical light. As will be discussed in the final chapter of this study, these derogatory portrayals increased over the course of the century as physicians, moralists and politicians alike began to equate nervousness with national degeneration.

Number, Sex, Age and Class of Nervous Sufferers

While historians have fruitfully investigated the cultural significance of nervous sufferers in the eighteenth century, surprisingly little is known about the basic demographics of real nervous patients in Britain, including their number, sex, age and class.[114] The remainder of this chapter explores answers to these questions, again highlighting the frequent divisions between the discourse and reality of nervous disease.

For most medical practitioners, it appears that the number of nervous patients in relation to patients suffering with other diseases was relatively small. The Royal College of Physicians in London houses ten casebooks belonging to Sir Henry Halford ranging from 1787 to 1791. Of the total 230 cases discussed in these books, only twelve (about 5 per cent) of the patients were listed as hypochondriac or hysteric.[115] Likewise, the London physician John Coakley Lettsom's records from the London General Dispensary show that of the 1,650 patients treated at the Dispensary from 1773 to 1774, thirty-six, or about 2 per cent, were hysteric.[116] According to the published disease reports of the Finsbury Dispensary for the month of July to August of 1805, approximately 7 per cent of all admitted cases were hypochondriac.[117] Robert Willan's *Reports on the Diseases in London, particularly during the Years 1796, 97, 98, 99 and 1800* included 'Lists of cases which occurred in my own practice'. In these lists, Willan provided the number of sufferers for each disorder on a month-by-month basis. Though seemingly straightforward, Willan's lists complicate matters by his inclusion of 'Asthenia', which he defines as 'the disorders, in general, denominated nervous', alongside traditional diagnoses of nervous disease including hysteria, hypochondria and melancholia which were defined most generally as chronic ailments caused by an 'uncommon delicacy or unnatural sensibility' of the nervous system.[118] He also listed dyspepsia, or chronic indigestion, as a separate disease, although many other physicians regarded it as simply an aggravating cause or symptom of nervous disease. As noted in Chapter 1, separating such diagnostic entities was a frustratingly vague process for all physicians; as one doctor and aspiring author on a treatise on nervous disease privately confessed to his mentor, he was not sure what cases to include in his book, especially since conditions like dyspepsia and Hypochondriasis were 'always mistaken' for the other.[119] Operating within this context of general professional confusion, Willan's ambitious attempt to strictly delineate diagnoses and to create hard statistics provides rare and valuable insight into the prevalence of nervous disease in a private practice. Willan divided the diseases encountered in his practice every month into acute, periodical, chronic and childhood diseases. Over the five years covered by the report, he treated a total of 8,116 chronic patients, including 820 nervous cases. Thus, nervous diseases composed approximately 10 per cent of the total

chronic diseases that he encountered during the period. While these numbers
are hardly overwhelming, the fact that cases of nervous disease were consistently
catalogued alongside such other diseases as smallpox, fevers and consumption
attests to the seriousness with which it was taken by the medical faculty, despite
its diagnostic ambiguity.

Doctor Clarke's Medical Report from Nottingham General Hospital, published in *The Edinburgh Medical and Surgical Journal* in 1808, is one of the
most systematic and telling sources regarding the sex and age of nervous sufferers. In his report, Clarke listed a total of ninety-two diseases encountered at
the hospital from 1807 to 1808, among which were hysteria and hypochondria.
Clarke's data reveal that over the course of the year the hospital treated a total
of thirty-four hysterics and seventeen hypochondriacs. Clarke also reveals the
precise number of male versus female sufferers, listing thirty-two female and two
male hysterics, and four female and thirteen male hypochondriacs.[120] Physicians
commonly acknowledged that the number of female sufferers far outnumbered
the males, due to women's supposedly stronger sensibility and tender frames. In
addition to confirming a higher rate of female nervousness, these statistics also
support the nerve expert Robert Whytt's claim that specific nervous diagnoses
of hysteria and hypochondria were most often intended as a simple reference
denoting the sex of the sufferer. Other than this sexual difference, Whytt argued,
the symptoms of hysteria and hypochondria were nearly identical:

> It is true that in women, hysteria symptoms occur more frequently and are often
> much more sudden and violent, than the hypochondriac in men; but this circum-
> stance, which is only a consequence of the more delicate frame, sedentary life, and
> particular condition of the womb in women, by no means shews the two diseases to
> be, strictly speaking, different.[121]

While Clarke's numbers confirm general notions about hypochondria as a male
disease, and hysteria as a female disease, the few patients crossing these boundaries are an interesting anomaly, and prove the way in which definitions of such
disorders remained porous and indeterminate well through the eighteenth century. The statistics from Nottingham General Hospital are also unusual due to
their inclusion of the ages of sufferers. Again, Clarke's data support contemporary medical conclusions regarding the age of hysteric and hypochondriac
sufferers; the largest number of hysterics were in their twenties and early thirties,
whereas the majority of hypochondriacs were in their forties. Among the 2,404
patients admitted to Nottingham General Hospital over the course of the year,
the fifty-one nervous cases make up only 2 per cent of the total.[122]

The statistics from Clarke's one-year report are consistent with the numbers
ascertained by Guenter Risse in his study of the register of the Edinburgh Royal
Infirmary from 1770 to 1800. Risse's review of the Infirmary records determined

that approximately 1 per cent of patients admitted were diagnosed with hysteria, and one half of a per cent were diagnosed with hypochondria. His study of the sex of sufferers also supports notions of hypochondria as a male diagnosis and hysteria as a female diagnosis, though again, it reveals some curious overlap; 98 per cent of the total 157 diagnosed hysterics were women, and 75 per cent of the diagnosed hypochondriacs were men. The ages of sufferers at the Royal Infirmary were also consistent with other data, revealing that most hysterics were in their early twenties, while the limited sample of hypochondriac sufferers ranged from twenty to forty years of age.[123]

These statistics are useful for several reasons. First, while according to these numbers nervous sufferers generally made up only a small proportion of the overall number of patients (generally one to 5 per cent), the consistency with which they were diagnosed cannot be overlooked. Just as the medical textbooks used at medical schools like the University of Edinburgh regularly discussed nervous disease, so too did nervous disease routinely appear in public and private practices. This consistency lends much credibility to the status of nervous disease as a medically grounded disorder rather than a social construction or fleetingly fashionable diagnosis. Perhaps even more importantly, these numbers destroy the notion of nervous disease as a purely upper-class malady, as it was portrayed in popular discourse of the eighteenth century and has continued so in much of the historiography. Because hospitals in the eighteenth century catered exclusively to poor charity patients, the constant presence of nervous disease in hospital registers reveals that this diagnosis was not reserved exclusively for the rich. Moreover, the regularity with which hospital physicians and medical students conducting clinical rounds discussed nervous, hysteric and hypochondriac cases of charity patients in their notes, lectures and dissertations, proves that they were well accustomed to the presence of lower class nervous patients. As will be discussed in the final chapter of this study, publishing medical practitioners commonly blamed the existence of these poor nervous sufferers on their supposed immoral tendency to live beyond their means in the style of their social superiors. Interestingly, however, case reports for poor nervous patients in hospitals never accuse them of having acquired their disorders by mimicking the lifestyles of their superiors. Rather, the nervous, hypochondriac, hysteric and melancholic cases discussed in such records reveal causes and symptoms identical to those discussed in wealthier patients' private consultations. Anxiety, fear and other passions are generally the attributed instigators of nervous conditions among hospital patients, while costiveness, wind, weakness, tremors and irrational fears are also among the symptoms that they displayed. For instance, in 1772 'E. Johnston', a member of Edinburgh's Royal Medical Society, read to his fellow members the case of a hypochondriac coal-miner treated in the Royal Infirmary. Johnston began by detailing the patient's symptoms:

> I.C. aged 24 is affected with a sensation of uneasiness beginning in the lower part of his Belly & from thence creeping upward to the Epegastric region, flatulence, acidity of the stomach ... vertigo, faintishness & lowness of spirits; sometimes also he feels a sensation of creeping over his whole Body followed by such an unusual agitation of Mind as often to occasion Weeping.

Johnston then related the patient's own history of the origin of his disorder, before opening the floor to a discussion of treatment therapies:

> He says that about 4 months ago when at work at a COAL-PIT he was on his candle's going out seizd with faintishness & such a degree of insensibility that he with the greatest difficulty got out of the pit, & that since that time he has been liable to the above complaints.[124]

Another case example discussed in the Royal Medical Society in 1784, related the story of the hypochondriac 'I.H. (of a melancholic temperament)' who suffered from chest pains, anxiety, weakness, heart palpitations, difficulty breathing, back pains, frightful dreams and tremors 'about eight months since, in consequence of great distress of mind'.[125] Similarly, another female case of hypochondria explained that the patient 'ascribes her complaints originally to a fright'.[126] Just as with wealthier private patients, general mental anxiety was frequently presented as the instigator of poor patients' nervous symptoms.

Many publishing physicians, particularly social critics, insisted that the spread of nervous disease to the lower classes was a recent phenomenon, resultant from the contagion of luxury infecting the lower classes in the second half of the century. Despite these claims, it is clear from even such records as the only surviving register book from the Bath General Hospital covering the years 1742 to 1752 that this is not the case. Twenty-eight out of the 1,596 patients listed in the register, or 1.75 per cent, were listed as nervous.[127] This percentage is fairly consistent with hospital statistics later in the century, and proves that the presence of poor sufferers in the late eighteenth century was nothing new. The appearance of nervous sufferers in hospital registers also attests to the seriousness with which doctors took nervous disease. Hospital admission procedures were rigorous, and only the most worthy patients – and diseases – were accepted. Because patients were objects of charity and the number of beds in infirmaries was limited, physicians were forced to select the patients they would accept from the many that applied for admission. Acceptable patients needed to be 'deserving' of charity by demonstrating that they were employed or at least morally upright when well. Patients also needed to suffer from disorders that would benefit from hospital treatment. 'Incurables', or patients destined to die or remain permanently afflicted by their malady such as blind or cancerous patients, were not admitted, as physicians would be unable to save them, and because deaths in the hospital would reflect poorly on the institution's reputation.[128] All patients seeking admittance to charity hospitals were required to obtain a recommendation from one of the financial donors to the hospital testifying to their deserving natures. They were then forced to undergo an interview with hospital staff so that the latter could further determine the suitability and desirability of their particular case. If admitted, patients were compelled to obey hospital rules which enforced strict diets, particular sleeping hours, regular prayer, and obliged them to submit to any and all treatments prescribed by their treating physician. In addition to being curable, patients admitted to teaching hospitals like the Edinburgh Royal Infirmary also had to be useful for instructional purposes, as they were the subjects of the physicians' clinical lectures. Consequently, the patients admitted needed to suffer from disorders which medical students were likely to encounter in their future careers. In light of these rigorous admissions procedures, the presence of poor nervous patients achieves added significance. The fact that nervous sufferers were considered serious enough cases for hospitalization confirms the perceived gravity of nervous disease; the choice of nervous patients as objects of clinical study attests to the ongoing presence of nervous sufferers outside of the infirmary walls, and the willingness of nervous sufferers to subject themselves to such rigorous and competitive admissions procedures demonstrates the strength and sincerity of their desire for treatment.

The fact that nervous disease was not exclusive to the upper class is also evident from the surviving records of Cullen's practice. Of course, there is no doubt that many of the patients writing to Cullen belonged to the upper echelons of society. As Risse has noted of Cullen's patients by post, '[his] list of correspondents reads like a Who's Who in Scotland'.[129] Yet as Risse additionally acknowledges, Cullen's correspondence also contains a large number of letters pertaining to nervous sufferers beyond the aristocratic sphere. For instance, in 1778 Cullen treated the nervous manufacturer James Mill for the second time, after he was again 'attacked with ... a violent fit of my nervous disorder', involving a quickened pulse, trembling and 'violent pulsations in different parts of the body'.[130]

In another case, Doctor Thomas Mack consulted Cullen regarding the case of a farmer, Mr Acrum. According to the doctor, Mr Acrum's disorder originated a year earlier after he was 'attack'd by some Footpads who robb'd him of his money and bruised him most cruelly'. This traumatizing experience, together with his already 'weak irritable nervous System' was suspected by the doctor to have increased 'the general Relaxation' of his nerves. The obstinacy of Mr Acrum's relaxed state was of particular concern to the doctor, who insisted that his patient had always lived a temperate life, and, given his occupation, was 'accustomed to regular exercise'.[131] As with the instances of poor hospital patients, patients of the 'middling sort' were treated as sufferers in their own right, and never discussed in the context of their emulation of the leisured class.[132]

The popularly held notion that nervous disease belonged exclusively to the sedentary upper class came under increasing attack by the late eighteenth century. The self-proclaimed nervous sufferer, James Boswell, set out to destroy this misconception, informing readers of his column, 'The Hypochondriack', that 'Melancholy, or Hypochondria, like the fever or gout, or any other disease, is incident to all sorts of men, from the wisest to the most foolish'. He then attested that had encountered 'as dull and as course mortals ... as ever appeared upon earth, who had all the symptoms of it'.[133] Many medical professionals voiced a similar opinion. In 1782 the physician William Heberden further undermined the notion of nervous disease as a purely upper-class malady. Arguing that everyone experienced some degree of hypochondria or hysteria, he claimed, 'Few persons, if any, have been blessed with such a constant cheerfulness, as not to have sometimes felt a languor and dispiritedness, without any manifest cause'.[134]

Thomas Trotter's *View of the Nervous Temperament* (1807) spoke candidly about what he perceived was a growing number of nervous sufferers in the middle classes. He described how 'Men of Business' increased their chances of suffering from nervous disorders by spending their days inside of offices and hunched over desks at the expense of fresh air and exercise. Trotter disdainfully explained how shopkeepers were particularly delicate and prone to these ailments:

> Not a few of them behind the counter, approach in external form towards the female constitution; and they seem to borrow from their lah customers an effeminacy of manners, and a smallness of voice, that sometimes makes their sex doubtful. Such degeneracies in corporeal structure, cannot fail of engendering a predisposition to diseases of the nervous kind.[135]

Cullen's correspondence includes cases of nervous members of the mercantile profession, such as the hypochondriac William Hampton, who, 'engaged in Trade at Birmingham' 'prejudice[d] his health' by pursuing his business 'with unvaried attention.'[136] Interestingly, none of these letters make any mention of the sufferers' unmanly weakness or effeminacy. Although this suggests (not surprisingly) that Trotter exaggerated his depiction of nervous 'men of business', his use of this caricature implies that his public audience was already aware that nervous disorders were not exclusive to the upper class. Trotter's derogatory depiction also evinces his growing discomfort with nervous males. Although this concern was more pronounced in the *View*, his awareness of the large number of male sufferers was not new. His earlier *Medicina Nautica* (1803) openly addressed the proliferation of nervous disorders amongst sailors:

> That a body of men, by education and habit accustomed to adventure, braving danger in every hideous form, and surpassing hardship, famine, and fatigue in every shape ... should be subject to complaints more nearly allied to the tender female than the

robust masculine constitution, would appear a paradox, did not daily experience confirm the fact.[137]

According to Trotter, the reasons behind the high rate of nervous disease among seamen were many; too much drinking aboard ship could easily lead to indigestion and liver complaints 'to which quickly succeed the horrid train of hypochondriacal and nervous disorders'; living abroad, particularly in the East or West Indies could induce nervous disease due to 'living on high-seasoned food, so common in both Indies' as well as a 'gradual disposition induced from the excessive heat of the climate'; mercurial treatments for syphilis, 'however judiciously managed' supposedly disposed sailors 'to nervous weakness'; 'violent hysteria' was oftentimes caused by 'long cruises in bad weather, joined to severe and irksome duty in the foggy and variable climate of the channel'; the nostalgia and homesickness experienced by navy men forced into service through impressment was diagnosed by Trotter as 'only a variety of hypochondriasis'; and passions like lovesickness, jealousy and disappointed ambition also ran rampant among navy men, making them dangerously susceptible to such complaints.[138]

Cullen's correspondence confirms the presence of nervous naval and military men, offering an equally varied assortment of disease aetiologies. For instance, in 1780 one physician submitted a sixteen-page letter to Cullen, describing his nervous patient, Captain Guise, and his unfortunate decline into madness. According to this letter, Guise's nervous symptoms began while he was stationed in Gibraltar in 1752. Rendered 'unfit for duty' he gradually returned to work only to be attacked with 'different nervous symptoms' ten years later, including general weakness, cold extremities, faintishness and 'disturbed thoughts'. Attributing these symptoms to the climate, the garrison physicians and surgeons granted him leave to return to the colder climate of England. Unfortunately Guise's symptoms only worsened upon his return. By the late 1770s his emotional despair, giddiness in his head, inability to sleep and 'disturbed imagination' reached such a point that the doctor determined that his hypochondriac symptoms had been replaced by symptoms of pure insanity.[139]

Slightly less extreme was the case of Colonel Burden, who was diagnosed with a combination of dyspepsia and hypochondriasis resultant from some 'excess in drinking' and exacerbated by anxiety over his forthcoming marriage. Among his symptoms were a distended belly, wind, cold sweats, general nervous agitation and a 'remarkable dejection of spirits'. These symptoms were temporarily palliated by the use of laxatives, limewater, Bark and exercise, but were soon revived by 'some little excess in venery, or some other constitutional circumstance'.[140] Suffering from similar excess, one Captain Wilson was seized with 'a great oppression on the spirits with indigestion and frequent difficulty of breathing' after being 'two or three times infected with the venereal disease'.[141]

Writing to Cullen on his own behalf, Captain Furguson complained in February 1775 of 'flying pains' in all parts of his body and limbs, general listlessness, inflamed eyes, rhumatick pains in his jaws, neck, teeth and ears, a loss of appetite, giddiness in his head and clammy sweats, which he attributed to 'very unsettled nerves'. Illuminating the origin of his disorder he stated, 'I am inclined to impute this Disorder to a weaken'd circulation & to a relaxed obstructed bilious habit partly occasioned by the west Indies & partly by having thrown myself three months ago into a cold bath with the remains of a rash upon me ... '[142]

Whatever the reasons behind male nervousness – effeminacy, hard living, climate, or excess - it is surprising to note how many nervous men there actually were, both in and out of the military setting. While popular discourse commonly spoke of 'nervous females', and even the medical discourse discussed the much higher rate of female over male sufferers, the number of male sufferers evident from surviving postal correspondence and hospital registers is significant. Furthermore, although it is impossible to glean precise numbers of male versus female sufferers from Cullen's correspondence due to imprecise and frequently entirely unstated diagnoses, the number of men complaining of nervous symptoms appears greater than the number of nervous women.

Despite their apparent clinical banality, the occasional male patient expressed embarrassment over suffering from a disease popularly believed to belong to the female sex. For instance, one Mr James Dallas writing in Cullen in 1789 described his nervous complaints and extremely irritable temper with great self-disdain: 'I am as with Vapour: weak as any delicate female'[143] Yet unless they were hysteric, which very few were, most nervous males did not reference the feminine aspect of their disease. In practice, popular discourse allying nervous disease so closely with feminine weakness and delicacy did little to undermine the notion of male sufferers as individual sufferers in their own right.

Conclusion

Popular discourse on nervous disease in the eighteenth century consistently joked about patients flaunting or even faking fashionably disordered nerves. Yet case notes from private practices and charity hospitals together with nervous patients' personal writings and letters to their physicians reveals the shallow nature of these stereotypes. Despite such glaring differences between the discourse and 'reality' of nervous disease, the two cannot be fully separated. For it is also clear that cultural beliefs and stereotypes about nervous disease tangibly shaped the patients' experience. Popular discourse accusing nervous patients of faking their complaints forced many to speak defensively about their symptoms and to feel the pressure of proving their reality. Likewise, moral discourse decrying the vices which led to nervous disease caused many patients to feel extreme shame over their condition, even prompting some to suffer in private. In this manner, popular discourse about nervous disease shaped the ways in which sufferers understood, experienced and even treated their illness.[144] It is for this reason that obtaining a medical diagnosis was often so important to patients. Writing to Cullen in 1778, the patient Nicholas Ryzack expressed the significance of a precise diagnosis to the success of his recovery:

> My ignorance of the Cause of my Disease I am afraid is a very great Impediment to my Cure. You assur'd me in the strongest Terms that you did not think it Venereal but you did not tell me what you did think it. Do Good Sir oblige me in complicit Terms with your Opinion hereon. It may answer a good purpose – It cannot answer a bad one. If you think it gouty, Rheumatic, Scorbutic, Nervous, or whatever other Disorder my Regimen shall be made comfortable to your directions for any of these cases ...[145]

As Lisa Smith has explained, 'the experience of pain was intricately connected to its meaning'.[146] Patients first had to know what they suffered from in order to know how to think about their ailments, and how to act upon them.

The treatment of nervous disease was also heavily shaped by cultural discourse. Popular understanding of how the body worked affected the treatments that patients received as well as the patient's perceptions of successful treatment. Patients who subscribed to highly visual theories of overly taut or relaxed nerves were likely to find relief in treatments which bowed to this perception; exercises which supposedly stretched tight nerves could bring relief to some, whereas drinking tinctures of steel could relieve patients who believed that their fibres were weak and overly-relaxed. For patients whose understanding of the body was based upon a mixture of nervous sensibility and the humours, treatments such as bleedings, vomits, oozing issues and blisters were most likely to harbour relief.[147] Likewise, patients who believed that their disorders were the result of the overstimulation of certain nerves had great faith in the relief that travel and a new set of sensory impressions could bring.

To consider the pathological reality of nervous disease apart from the culture that diagnosed it would be a disservice to medical history. Yet the opposite extreme – describing nervous disease as a mere cultural construction – is equally dangerous; as Clark Lawlor stated so perfectly in his discussion of consumption and literature, 'complete relativism is a throwing out of the biomedical baby with the cultural bathwater'.[148] The actual patient experience of nervous disease in the eighteenth century straddled the realms of objective symptomology and subjective discourse about the body and the meaning of nervousness. For sufferers, the reality of their disorders was a complicated mixture of perception, affection and physical sensation.

This chapter has provided a clearer picture of the 'reality' of nervous disease for eighteenth-century sufferers. Although no two patients were exactly alike, the surviving medical records reveal several surprising inconsistencies between the discourse of nervous disease and its lived experience. While patients composing public accounts of their ailments were likely to portray them as a flattering statement about their character or intellect, the vast majority of private medical records reveal a serious pathological concern over disordered nerves, void of social commentary. Far from nervous disease being a purely upper-class malady, poor nervous patients maintained a consistent presence in charity hospitals; far from sharing the glamorous symptoms exhibited by fictional sufferers and nervous authors flaunting their sensibility, nervous sufferers writing to Cullen complained openly of exceptionally unflattering symptoms like burping, profuse sweating and painful flatulence; and far from basking in the supposed superiority conveyed by their nervous sufferings, most patients exhibited a profound sense of guilt over their ailments and a strong desire to recover. The methods by which patients tried to recover is the subject of the following chapter.

4 THE PURSUIT OF HEALTH: THE TREATMENT OF NERVOUS DISEASE

In his popular self-help guide *Domestic Medicine*, the physician William Buchan opened his discussion of nervous disease with the claim that, 'of all diseases incident to mankind, those of the nervous kind are the most complicated and difficult to cure'.[1] There is little doubt that most physicians treating nervous disease agreed with Buchan's statement. While some mercenary 'third-tier' medical practitioners like the surgeon Adam Neale brazenly heralded their ability to 'effectuate a perfect cure' of nervous disease, most well-trained and well-educated physicians never made such empty promises. Edinburgh's famed nerve expert and Professor of Physic, Robert Whytt, warned readers of his *Observations on the Nature, Causes, and Cure of those Disorders which have been Commonly Called Nervous, Hypochondriac, or Hysteric* (1764) that nervous disorders 'scarce ever admit of a thorough cure'.[2] William Cullen similarly noted to one of his nervous patients that it was 'not possible to give a new set of Nerves', but that 'a proper management and a few remedies will do a great deal either to prevent ailments or to render them much less troublesome'.[3]

This chapter explores the various means by which the cure of nervous disease was treated and rendered less troublesome in the late eighteenth century. It begins with the manipulation of the 'non-naturals', or, the external factors capable of influencing the body's internal health: regulation of diet, exercise, sleep, emotions, air, evacuations and emotions. It then investigates the less esteemed yet still highly employed method of treatment by medication. As in Chapter 2, this section highlights significant tensions between first- and second-tier practitioners who insisted on the superiority of the non-naturals over medications, and the third-tier practitioners who more often proclaimed the unequivocal benefits of a quick pharmaceutical fix. While this chapter investigates treatments from late in the century, it also considers self-help guides and treatment advice from practitioners earlier in the century whose works remained in print throughout the period.

Just as the status of a medical practitioner could affect his chosen method of treatment, so too could the status of patients affect the treatment that they received. The final treatments discussed in this chapter consist of aggressive therapies readily administered to poor nervous patients in the hospital setting including heavy bleeding, blistering and electric shock therapy. Because hospital patients were objects of charity, they had little choice but to submit to such treatments or be dismissed. Consequently, eighteenth-century infirmaries offered physicians the opportunity to experiment with more hands-on and arguably more unpleasant remedies than they would readily employ on wealthier private patients upon whose patronage they depended, and who were able to afford long-term natural therapies involving repeated consultations.[4]

Of course, the therapies endured by even the wealthiest of nervous patients were often unpleasant. Many affluent patients were prescribed, and even requested, aggressive and painful treatments. This was especially the case when their ailments failed to respond to more mild forms of cure. Likewise, as this chapter will show, the medications consumed by nervous patients of every class were generally repellent; many acted as purgatives and emetics, and nearly all laid claim to offensive tastes and smells. Even the most mild treatments such as diet, exercise and travel could be time-consuming, expensive, inconvenient and difficult to maintain. The continued willingness of nervous patients to undergo these treatments demonstrates the sincerity of their concern for their health and the strength of their faith in the period's medical science.

As this chapter will show, all nervous therapies, including prescriptions for cheerful company and seemingly flippant trips to the spa during 'the season', were firmly rooted in eighteenth-century medical theory. Of course, fashion and the demands of wealthy patients oftentimes did force first- and second-tier physicians to alter their prescriptions from such treatments as trips to spa towns mid-century to more fashionable seaside resorts at the end of the century, and from a strict emphasis on regimen mid-century to an increasing, though guarded, use of strengthening and palliative remedies towards the end of the century. Nevertheless, it will reveal how most doctors held fast to their medical beliefs, willing to negotiate with – but not to sacrifice their medical theory to – fashion.

Because nervous disease was most broadly understood in the eighteenth century as an uncommon delicacy or unnatural sensibility of the nervous system, treatments naturally consisted of efforts to strengthen this debility, and to lessen 'the too great sensibility' of both the patient's body and mind.[5] Like the symptoms of nervous disease, treatments were specific to every patient. The precise diet followed, mode of exercise taken and medications swallowed by nervous patients were dependent upon their individual constitutions. No single remedy could promise a consistent or fool proof cure of all nervous symptoms. This was due, not only to the varying constitutions of nervous patients, but also to the diverse origins of their nervous debility, such as gastronomic overload, excessive passion, particular frights or sudden impressions made on the nervous system, sedentary lifestyles, or hereditary constitutional disorders, to name but a few. Consequently, even Whytt's instructive *Observations* alerted readers that

> In treating... of the cure of those diseases, I shall not attempt to lay down any general method to answer in all cases or circumstances, even for the same symptoms; but shall endeavour to point out that particular treatment, which seems best suited to the case, according to the various causes from which it may arise.[6]

A patient's treatment was constantly modified and fine-tuned in an ever-evolving and oftentimes never-ending search for a cure. The road to recovery was not easy or certain. As Whytt advised his colleagues, it was best to warn patients that 'it is frequently beyond the power of art to eradicate the disorders we now treat of'. It was 'further necessary', he continued, 'to acquaint every patient, that without a long perseverance in a course of medicines, diet, and exercise, no great or lasting benefit can be expected'.[7] Perseverance was crucial to the success of any treatment. As Cullen reminded the physician for one nervous patient suffering from low spiritedness, faintishness and a 'sensation as if his Brain was tumbling out': 'we must acknowledge that much attention will be requisite on [his] part, & time must be allowed for the effectual operation of the Regimen we mean to propose, and of the Remedies we prescribe'.[8] The most popular regimens and remedies prescribed for nervous patients are discussed in turn below.

Eat Less and be Merry: Manipulating the Non-Naturals

Armed with few successful methods of treatment, doctors since the age of antiquity stressed the importance of preventative medicine.[9] Regulation of the 'non-naturals', including diet, exercise, hours of wakefulness and sleep, retentions and evacuations, emotions and the quality of the air one breathed were the primary medical recommendations for maintaining a healthy lifestyle. In addition to preserving health, the non-naturals also appealed to the Galenic tradition of treating disease by restoring harmony to imbalanced constitutions. Hence gouty over-eaters were advised to alter their diets, consumptive patients were encouraged to try a change of air, and feverish patients were instructed to sweat out their sickness with exercise; as William Buchan warned, 'nothing tends to prolong an intermitting fever, [more] than indulging a lazy indolent disposition'.[10] Despite their name, the non-naturals were valued in the eighteenth century for their natural approach in disease treatment and prevention. In a fast-paced consumer culture plagued by quackery and incessant tincture gulping, an emphasis on the non-naturals seemed, to traditionally minded physicians, refreshingly grounded. Much of the appeal of the non-naturals came from their basis in ancient medicine. As ancient medicine provided the framework for formal medical educations well into the eighteenth century, the use of these timeless methods were the mark of a medical gentleman.

The non-naturals were particularly well suited to the treatment of nervous disease. Supposedly caused by such vices as over-eating, sedentary living and excessive feeling, basic methods including the regulation of diet, exercise and emotions were an obvious choice for affecting a successful, safe and long-term cure. Consequently, educated first- and second-tier medical practitioners most commonly advised a careful attention to the non-naturals for the restoration of balance to nervous patients' debilitated systems.

The willingness of nervous sufferers to keep regular hours was crucial to restoring this balance. In his *Essay of Health and Long Life* (1724), George Cheyne decried the practice of staying up late and sleeping during the day as 'pernicious' to one's health and 'plainly contrary to the Indications of Nature'. 'Nothing', he claimed, 'is more prejudicial to tender Constitutions, than lying long a Bed, indulging in lethargical and drowsy Sleep, or lolling or loitering awake'.[11] John Wesley, the founder of the Methodist church and ardent admirer of Cheyne's medical advice, recommended in his own medical guide *Primitive Physick* (1747) that tender persons 'ought constantly to go to bed about nine, and rise at four or five'.[12] Cullen similarly advised his nervous patient Miss Naven that 'any bodily fatigue is very improper and therefore much dancing... late at night or lying long in the morning are both bad for nervous complaints'.[13] Cullen's correspondence reveals that nervous patients were regularly reminded of this advice. In another letter to a nervous Mrs Cochran, Cullen stated that 'sitting up late at night, & lying long abed is common to most people of weak nerves & is very bad for them'.[14] Another physician, Dr John Heysham, writing to Cullen regarding his hysteric patient Miss Percy, noted disapprovingly that she was in the habit of sitting 'up late reading... & of course indulges in bed in the morning'.[15] People who overslept or napped lazily during the day were as guilty of detrimental indulgence as gluttonous overeaters. Edward Baynard drew this connection explicitly in his poem, *Health* (1716), which was in its twentieth edition by 1789:

> When sleep does first desert you, rise;
> Next, wash the Gum from off your *Eyes:*
> Cold *Water* pure will clear the Sight,
> Comfort the Eyes and keep them bright.
> Indulge not Drowsiness, unless
> It does proceed from Weariness.
> 'Thout some Fatigue, there's no sound Sleep,
> 'Tis eating without Appetite.[16]

Throughout the eighteenth and into the nineteenth century, eating without appetite and heavy drinking were indiscretions believed to invite nervous disease. As a particularly sensitive organ, an overburdened stomach was destined to disrupt the rest of the body.[17] Warning the public of this fact, the temperance enthusiast Thomas Trotter wrote in 1807 that 'he that laughs and drinks with every one, grows sad in time; and early decreptitude, and nervous debility, are his certain portion'.[18] Physicians treating nervous disease generally recommended the consumption of simple and plainly dressed foods that were easy on the stomach. As Cullen advised one nervous patient in 1775, 'Everything known to prove heavy on the stomach must be avoided'.[19] Given their proclivity to digestive complaints, physicians encouraged nervous patients to consume easily digestible meat like chicken in place of heavier meats like venison, beef and pork.[20] Most doctors recommended that meat be served boiled and plain; anything salted 'or dressed with gravie ' was known to be 'of most pernicious consequence' for sensitive stomachs.[21] Fish was also recommended for nervous sufferers. White fish was preferred above all other types. As the physician Benjamin Bell counselled one nervous patient in 1788, 'Fresh white fish of every kind may be taken with safety, particularly Turbot – Haddock – and Flounder – But Salmon & Lobsters – and all kinds of salted fish should be avoided'.[22]

In addition to limiting the type of meat consumed, nerve doctors also encouraged sufferers to limit the frequency with which they ate meat. While the Bath physician William Falconer acknowledged that eating meat could provide 'a greater quantity of nourishment' than vegetable food, he later tempered this claim, warning readers that 'high-seasoned meats, and animal diet, both of them contribute to keep the nerves constantly agitated and in a state of stimulation'.[23] Occasionally physicians recommended entirely vegetarian diets for nervous patients. Early in the century, Cheyne, who struggled with his own weight and diet (at one point reaching thirty-two stone, or 448 pounds), recommended in his *Essay* that patients eat only light meats, while hailing vegetarianism as the ideal healthy diet. Cheyne also became a vegetarian, touting his milk and vegetable diet as a recipe for health. His claims did not go uncontested. Dr Kinneir, a physician publishing soon after Cheyne, spoke of 'the inconveniences that may attend the prescribing of a vegetable and milk diet indiscriminately to all persons and in all cases alike'.[24] Likewise, one Dr Wynter wrote a personal letter to Cheyne, condemning his unorthodox methods:

> Tell me from whom, fat-headed Scot,
> Thou didst thy system learn;
> From Hippocrates thou hast it not,
> Nor Celsus, nor Pitcairne.
> Suppose we own that *milk* is good,
> And say the same of *grass*;
> The one for *babes* is only food,
> The other for an *ass*.

> Doctor! One new prescription try,
> (A friend's advice forgive;)
> Eat *grass*, reduce thyself, and *die*;
> Thy *patients*, then, may *live*.[25]

Despite such bitter criticism, Cheyne's *Essay* was a huge success, running through four editions in its first year alone, and remaining in print a century later.[26] Cheyne's milk and vegetable diet became so well known by the middle of the century that Whytt was obliged to address the regimen in his *Observations*, where he diplomatically noted that this diet could 'be of great service' to some nervous patients, although it was not appropriate in every case. The reason for this, he explained, was that he had encountered some nervous patients who, 'when wholly confined to milk and vegetables, were not only troubled with faintness and lowness of spirits, but with great flatulence'.[27] Reiterating the importance of structuring dietary recommendations to individual patient constitutions, Whytt wrote,

> Every valetudinary person ought... to keep by those kinds of meat and drink, which he finds by experience to be lightest and most agreeable to his stomach. But whatever aliments may be used, moderation should be constantly observed, as people are generally less hurt by the quality, than by the quantity of what they eat and drink.[28]

The nerve doctors also heavily regulated alcohol. The elite physicians discouraged strong liquors like rum and brandy, advising patients to replace these beverages with water whenever possible. Although diluted wine was occasionally recommended by physicians to stimulate a patient's spirits, excessive amounts of wine were believed to debilitate the nervous system.[29]

Despite the dangers of alcohol, most publishing nerve doctors agreed that tea and coffee were the beverages most likely to induce a nervous disorder. Medical publications decrying the consumption of tea and coffee crescendoed in the 1760s and 1770s as these luxuries, once restricted to the rich, trickled their way into the cups of the poor. John Coakley Lettsom jumped on the prescriptive bandwagon with his dissertation, *The Natural History of the Tea-Tree with Observations on the Medical Qualities of Tea, and on the Effects of Tea-Drinking* (1772), noting that the dangerous consequences of the beverage were already commonly known: 'It stands charged by many able writers, by public opinion, partly derived from experience, with being the cause of many disorders; all that train of distempers included under the name of NERVOUS are said to be, if not the offspring, at least highly aggravated by the use of Tea'.[30] The London physician William Heberden argued that even the smell of tea was enough to encourage nervous sufferings, citing as evidence 'three persons employed in examining and smelling tea, [who] have suspected that it occasioned tremors and other hypochondriac ills'.[31]

Ultimately, moderation was the primary rule of thumb for nervous patients seeking dietary advice. Buchan put it quite succinctly in his *Domestic Medicine*, declaring that 'all excess should be carefully avoided'.[32] This prescriptive note was carefully followed in practice. As Cullen advised one nervous lady in 1768, 'she must consider that what is not half enough to another; may be an overburden to her & she must always keep within the bounds of her appetite whatever it is'.[33]

Moving and Shaking: Exercise for Healthy Nerves

First- and second-tier physicians also recommended exercise as an important way to prevent, manage and cure nervous complaints. As with diet, the use of exercise to combat nervous disease was firmly rooted in medical tradition. Cheyne's *English Malady* (1733) noted that 'there is not any one Thing more approv'd and recommended by all *Physicians* and the Experience of all those who have suffer'd under *Nervous* distempers... than *Exercise* of one Kind or another'.[34] Although explanations of human physiology evolved during the century, understanding of the physical benefits of exercise remained relatively constant. Alexander Sutherland provided a particularly visual account of the way in which exercise could strengthen, tone and improve a patient's ailing innards:

> The body of man is made up of tubes and glands fitted to one another in so wonderful a manner, that there must be frequent motions, concussions, and agitations to mix, digest, and separate the juices, to cleanse the infinitude of pipes and strainers, and to give the solids a firm and lasting tone. Exercise ferments the humours, forces them into their proper channels, throws off redundancies, and helps nature in those distributions which are necessary for life.[35]

A steady stream of spirits flowing through the body strengthened and toned relaxed nerves and weakened constitutions. Sutherland confirmed the value of exercise once and for all with his claim that 'Julius Caesar was of a weak delicate constitution by nature, which he hardened by exercise'.[36]

Exercise was especially important for nervous patients suffering as a result of inactive lifestyles. Whether patients were victims of sloth or of sedentary employment, exercise could help to repair the inevitable damage caused by years of inactivity. Explaining the importance of exercise to the nervous Lord Moray Cullen wrote, 'at sometime our Machine must go far wrong if it is allowed to stand still'. In case his patient missed the hint, Cullen added, 'I wish my Lord Moray would stir a little more than he does'.[37] In another instance, a London physician was forced to inform his patient that 'walking within doors on a smooth floor is not a sufficient exercise'.[38] Energizing patients to follow an exercise routine was not always an easy task – particularly in the case of such patients as Mr Bradley Smith who described one of the primary symptoms of his nervous complaint as an exceptional 'aversion to exercise'.[39] Yet for as long as doctors

had recommended exercise for nervous complaints, they had encountered stubbornly inactive patients. Francis Fuller's *Medicina Gymnastica*, first published
in 1705 and in its ninth edition by 1777, marvelled at the extraordinary lack of
willpower exhibited by some nervous patients, claiming,

> It is a matter of wonder that the Spasms, the Tremors, the Shiverings, the Watchings,
> and all the very numerous Plagues of an Hysterick Person should not be able to rouze
> People into a Quest of Health, upon Measures suitable to the Causes of things; that
> such Painful experience should not animate 'em, into a Resolution to exchange the
> Pains of a sedentary, for the... pleasures of an Active Life.[40]

For sufferers truly unable to make time for regular exercise, such as businessmen
or the exceptionally studious 'who in reading and writing sit so much with their
body bent forward', physicians were willing to compromise their prescriptions;
Whytt recommended that they 'read or write mostly standing' so as to allow for
an unobstructed flow of healthy bodily fluids.[41]

The forms which useful exercise could take were many. Buchan advised
patients that since everyone responded differently to various types of exercise,
each person 'ought to use that which he finds most beneficial'.[42] Like many of his
Edinburgh colleagues, Whytt recommended the use of the flesh brush, claiming,
'friction of the legs, arms, trunk of the body, and *abdomen*, with a flesh brush,
with flannel or a coarse linen cloth, is a kind of exercise that strengthens, pro-
motes the circulation, and is particularly beneficial when the bowels are weak'.[43]
Further advocating the flesh brush, Whytt informed his fellow physicians that it
was particularly useful for patients suffering with flatulence. The professor and
physician John Rutherford also strongly endorsed the flesh brush for this reason,
elaborating upon its effects in one of his clinical lectures:

> I have never found any remedy so well as rubbing the abdomen for half an hour in any
> of these nervous Disorders for the fibres of the guts contract very unequally and this
> inequality in their contraction is the principal cause of the Hypochondriac symptoms
> in the abdomen and I have observed that when the patient was very much distressed
> with these symptoms, if rubbing was applied he soon felt the wind shifting from place
> to place which at last was expelled either upwards or downwards & then the patient
> was immediately relieved.[44]

Cullen similarly prescribed the use of the flesh brush in nervous cases. Mrs
Oswald, a patient suffering from a 'too great mobility of her nerves', was told by
Cullen that rubbing her arms and legs with a flesh brush every morning would
'answer for some exercise and be other ways usefull'.[45]

For the equally unathletic, Cheyne recommended riding in a chaise or char-
iot, as this activity would ensure that the *Hypochondres* were properly 'shaken
and exercised'.[46] A similarly soft exercise regimen was recommended by Dr Bell
to a nervous patient in 1788 for use in poor weather: 'In bad weather some kind

of chamber-exercise becomes necessary – For this purpose A Swing is perhaps better than any other'.[47] While indoor exercise was not valued as highly by physicians as other more vigorous outdoor activities, it appears that swings were a welcome prescription for many sufferers. After recommending a swing for a patient suffering from a cough and mysterious pains in her side, one Dr Wood wrote to his colleague, 'She not only bears the swinging well, but delights in it'.[48]

Despite the occasional use of swings or carriage rides, the majority of exercise regimens were rigorous. Ebenezer Gilchrist's *The Use of Sea Voyages in Medicine* (1756) offered a particularly trying exercise regimen. Praised by Whytt, and in its third edition by 1771, Gilchrist's book recommended sailing as a remedy for 'vapours in all degrees of it, from a low-spirited illness to the highest nervous distemper'.[49] Suggesting that nervous patients sail for several weeks to several months at a time, he wrote, 'It will prove more effectual, I think, than to send them to drink spaws, or milk... at least, when all these have availed little, and after tedious courses of medicine, I have tried it with success'.[50] According to Gilchrist, the exercise afforded by a sea voyage could provide substantial physical benefits for travellers. The tossing motion of the ship forced passengers into relentless exercise as 'one set or other of muscles is constantly kept in action alternately, through the whole body, in order to preserve equilibrium'.[51] This was not the only benefit of sailing. As Gilchrist maintained, 'Sailing... is a compound exercise, of gestation, and that of a particular kind; a preternatural spasmodic motion in vomiting'. Singing the praises of a good vomit at sea, he wrote,

> Vomiting, by driving a greater supply of blood and spirits into the parts, warms and strengthens them; and the long continued nausea, giving a lasting contractility, restores the tone of the stomach, and its appendages; which from natural weakness, or other vice, are unable to do their office...[52]

Above all, sea sickness could be used with more frequency and safety than an emetic: 'The sea sickness can be sustained with safety hours, days, weeks, a longer time by far than we dare attempt to promote vomiting, or a nausea, by any medicine thrown into the stomach, and affecting it immediately'.[53] Sailing was not a remedy for the lackadaisical; as Gilchrist stressed in the introduction to his book,

> It is a remedy for those only who really stand in need of a remedy... and to comply with it to the utmost that sometimes may be necessary, will require a degree of reason and fortitude, beyond what the small feelings of slighter ills, or a mere modish affectation of being ill, can ever inspire.[54]

One dogged patient described the benefits of sailing where prior courses of cold bathing and nervous medicines had failed. Although sailing along the coast of India did little to relieve his symptoms, his fortitude paid off once he encountered a hailstorm near the Cape of Good Hope. He explained, the increased weight of the atmosphere, together with a perpetual and accelerated motion (for there we had tempestuous weather and high seas) contributed greatly to my relief: and before we had stretched twenty degrees to the eastward of the Cape, I thought the disease almost eradicated.[55]

As a more mainstream and slightly less intimidating exercise option for treating nervous complaints, Gilchrist also recommended horseback riding, claiming that it was 'thought to be of most use to restore health, and where it agrees, is a manly cheering exercise, and therefore is more especially adapted to the low spirited and hypochondriacal'.[56] Most doctors of the century, including Cheyne, recommended horseback riding as the best method of physical exertion. For patients too weak to endure an excursion out of doors, or in case of bad weather, Cheyne recommended the use of a chamber horse, which he declared he had 'tried by Experience' and which was 'well known in London'.[57] Composed of several layers of boards, each separated with a series of springs, the chamber horse allowed seated patients to bounce up and down, thus mimicking the movement of riding on horseback. The continuing popularity of the chamber horse by the end of the century is evident from their advertisement in even such mainstream sources as the *Cabinet-Makers London Book of Prices* (1788). This catalogue listed a basic chamber horse with four heights of springs as just over ten shillings, with additional heights available for purchase at one shilling apiece.[58]

While the chamber-horse was useful in bad weather, real horseback riding was much preferred. Dr Richard Mead's *Medical Precepts and Cautions* (1751) insisted that 'all sorts of bodily exercise are necessary; and in particular it will be of great service to play at bowls or tennis, to toss the arms briskly to and fro with lead weights in the hands; but nothing is better than riding daily on horseback'.[59] The beneficial effect of horseback riding was further explained by Sutherland in 1764: 'by riding the pendulous viscera are shaken, and gently rubbed against the surfaces of each other; meanwhile the external air rushes forcibly into the lungs'.[60] That same year Whytt noted in his *Observations* that of all kinds of exercise available to such patients,

> Riding on horseback has been justly esteemed the best: It has been particularly extolled by *Sydenham* in hypochondriac and hysteric disorders. It greatly promotes digestion, sanguification, the distribution and secretion of all the fluids; and strengthens the whole body, as well as the stomach and bowels. Riding is preferable to walking, as it shakes the body more and fatigues it less.[61]

As late as 1807 Trotter's *View of the Nervous Temperament* noted that 'the value of *exercise on horseback*, is so well known, that it may seem superfluous to mention it here'. 'But', he claimed, 'in the prevention and treatment of nervous and bilious diseases, it is supereminent'.[62]

Diversion, Distraction and Delight: Exercising the Mind

In a medical dissertation of 1784, one student explained how nervous patients were 'particularly fond to talk of their own health, to the state of which they are remarkably attentive, and from which [they] can rarely divert their thoughts, whether to business or amusement'.[63] It was widely accepted among practitioners that the tendency of nervous patients to dwell on their poor health often exacerbated their mental and physical symptoms. Consequently, diverting the attention of nervous sufferers from their complaints was a key aspect of their cure. In addition to its physical benefits, horseback riding was highly valued an effective method of mental distraction. Falconer claimed that riding was of particular value to self-obsessed hypochondriac patients 'on account of its relaxing the mind, by abstracting the attention from being fixed on the disorder, a circumstance that constitutes the principal and distinguishing mark of this complaint'.[64] Gilchrist's *Sea Voyages* likewise acknowledged the importance of diverting the attentions of nervous patients, touting the way in which the 'terror' arising from a patients' 'apprehension of danger' in stormy seas was 'many times a principal means of cure'.[65]

Doctors recommended a wide range of activities for diverting the attention of nervous patients. In addition to horseback riding and fear of a watery death, the enjoyment of music, sociable conversation and cheerful company were frequently prescribed. For instance, the Scottish natural philosopher John Anderson noted in his *Institutes of Physics* (1777) how musical tones could 'excite vibrations in certain parts of the body', and, in turn, 'excite corresponding sentiments, and passions in the hearer'.[66] Armed with this knowledge, composers and musicians could capably use 'their skill in musical expression' to 'command' the passions and nerves of their listeners, and manipulate them to a healthier state.[67]

Like music, light-hearted conversation and banter could also distract patients. Gregory even acknowledged the importance of chatting with patients during scheduled medical consultations in order to prevent them from engaging in unrestrained rants over their ailing nerves. He recommended that during consultations medical men

> divert the [patient's] mind, without seeming to intend it, from its present sufferings, and from its melancholy prospects of the future, by insensibly introducing subjects that are amusing or interesting; and sometimes he [the physician] may successfully employ a delicate and good-natured pleasantry.[68]

It was in an effort to divert his own thoughts from an untoward focus on his bodily complaints that James Boswell informed readers of his column, 'The Hypochondriack' that he fostered a love of reading. Boswell insisted that biographies were particularly helpful in their ability to withdraw 'my attention from myself to others', stating, 'I look upon the *Biographia Britannica* with that kind of grateful regard with which one who has been recovered from painful indisposition by their medical springs beholds Bath, Bristol, or Tunbridge'.[69] Boswell's friend and fellow sufferer, Samuel Johnson, also recommended diversion for nervous melancholy. In a letter to a nervous friend in 1764 Johnson offered his best medical advice:

> make use of all diversions, sports of the field abroad, improvements of your estate or little schemes of building, and pleasing books at home or if you cannot compose yourself to read, a continual succession of easy company. Be sure never to be unemployed... and give up no hours to musing and retrospect. Be always busy.[70]

Sociability was an integral part of the cure. As Johnson wrote in yet another letter to a suffering friend, 'solitude excludes pleasure'. Hence, he vividly advised, some amount of social interaction was 'necessary to give vent to the imagination, and [to] discharge the mind of its own flatulencies'.[71]

Not all patients were willing participants in this therapeutic sociability. One frustrated hypochondriac wrote to Cullen complaining of his ongoing 'weakness of both body & mind' and his doctor's insistence that he go 'to town, where it was hoped the company of my companions & amusement might be of service to me'. After three months in town, the patient decided that his health would receive greater benefit from the open air of the countryside. His doctor disagreed: 'that Gentleman still said I was Hypochondraical & that solitude was bad for me & in consequence I was detained in town till near the end of May'. The disgruntled patient proceeded to write an eight-page rant about this ineffectual treatment, his physician's failure to comprehend his complaints, and his despair over the fact that all of his 'hopes of recovery' had been 'unfortunately disappointed'.[72]

The importance of diversion and amusement in the treatment of nervous disorders was strongly conveyed in a series of letters between one Dr Joseph Saunders and Cullen regarding the patients, Mr and Mrs Gordon. Frustrated in his attempts to relieve the couple of their nervous and stomach complaints, Saunders recommended that they consult Cullen. In advance of their personal consultation, Saunders offered Cullen a letter detailing the background of their cases, focusing primarily upon the complaints of Mr Gordon. Saunders informed Cullen that in recent months Mr Gordon had

> Increased a habit, which he has a great tendency to in bad health, that of keeping his bed & a dislike to company & exercise; in this time he generally slept in the day time, sweat profusely, & tossed & tumbled about in his bed restless all night. He lost his appetite so that he could taste no food, without bringing on violent reachings to vomit, by which he was quite sunk.

Mrs Gordon suffered similar problems. At the conclusion of his letter, Saunders informed Cullen, 'All these complaints were greatly increased by the loss of a favourite child this Winter'.[73]

Days later, Saunders wrote to Cullen again 'at the joint desire of his [Mr Gordon's] friends. Concerned that the Gordons wanted to spend the winter with their two daughters in Edinburgh, Mr Gordon's friends insisted that he would be better off in their own company. As one of his friends wrote,

> He has been in use to live here in Winter, where his near relations of Mrs Gordons are very numerous his friends here are all of opinion that this circumstance conduces not a little to his health.

After forwarding this message to Cullen, Saunders noted that Mr Gordon's companions excelled at 'persuading him to get out of bed & forming partys for his amusement & luring him out to get exercise'. After expressing his willingness to 'submit the whole' to Cullen's judgment, Saunders reiterated, 'you will perceive that publick places of amusement would afford him no entertainment, he finds that only in private partys of his Friends and intimate acquaintances'. He likewise informed Cullen that neither of the Gordons 'know of my having wrote you on this subject'.[74] The obvious concern which the Gordons' friends and physicians had for their social welfare reveals the seriousness with which diversion and social interaction were believed to influence health.

Because of the importance of diverting nervous patients, hospitals were typically regarded by physicians as improper places to effect a cure. Although infirmaries offered the benefits of structured hours of sleep and meticulously regulated diets, their lack of variety and amusement could easily outweigh such advantages. Trotter noted in his *Medicina Nautica* (1803) that naval hospitals were

> very little to be preferred... in the treatment of this disease. They afford no amusement to seamen... All energy of mind is lost within these walls, and must be, till some means are devised by officers of address and intelligence to shake off that languor and indolence which we observe so general in the wards.[75]

Andrew Duncan, a physician at the Edinburgh Royal Infirmary similarly insisted that

> An hospital is a bad place for hypochondriacs. They have too much time to brood over their complaints and... they suppose themselves affected with all the complaints they hear of. The best remedy is certainly... [the] exertion of mind and body.[76]

Some hospitals, including the Edinburgh Royal Infirmary, attempted to divert nervous patients with chamber horses, walks in the hospital yard and mandatory participation in hospital chores like cleaning the wards and making beds.[77] Nevertheless, it was widely acknowledged that the monotony of hospital living was ill suited to the treatment of nervous patients. Of course, as objects of charity, nervous hospital patients had few other options.

For wealthier patients outside of the hospital setting, travel was an ideal diversion. In his *First Lines* Cullen noted how 'a journey, both by its having the effect of interrupting all train of thought, and by presenting objects engaging attention, may often be useful' for nervous patients.[78] Travel had a long history as a useful means of diversion and cure for nervous sufferers. Even Robert Burton's *Anatomy of Melancholy* (1621) insisted that there was 'no better physick for a melancholy man than change of aire and variety of places, to travel abroad and see fashions'.[79] Buchan extolled similar benefits of travel for nervous sufferers, claiming that a 'change of place, and the sight of new objects, by diverting the mind, have a great tendency to remove these complaints'. Thus, 'for those who can afford to take them', Buchan advised a long journey or voyage by sea.[80]

Spa towns were a popular destination for nervous sufferers travelling in search of a cure. Places like Bath, Harrogate and Leamington offered patients a diverting change of scenery, social opportunities and supposedly curative waters. The number of travellers flocking to leisure and spa towns increased dramatically over the course of the eighteenth century. As Anne Borsay has revealed, the number of visitors to Bath increased from 8,000 early in the century to 10,000 in 1766 and 25,000 by 1791.[81] In 1790 Horace Walpole went so far as to claim that 'one would think the English were ducks; they are for ever waddling to the waters'.[82] Satirical literature and prints depicting nervous sufferers in the eighteenth century consistently poked fun at patients who suspiciously insisted on their need for a therapeutic trip to the spa during the 'season'. The joke in such cases was that patients were at the spa under the pretence of needing to 'take the waters' when in reality they only wanted to partake in the lively culture of the resort town. It is easy to understand why nervous sufferers fell victim to such mockery. Because prescriptions for diversion, cheerful company and amusement were so commonly prescribed in nervous cases, feigning these maladies appeared to many non-sufferers as a convenient excuse for a vacation. Certainly some 'nervous sufferers' were hardly sufferers at all. For instance, one highly irritated John Byng grumbled that all he found in a seaside resort were young ladies 'expecting to drown their nervous fears, and hysteric wanderings, in the sea, assisted by the use of gentle dancing with soft speeches from beaus, and the indulgence of polite conversation'.[83] The hypochondriac philosopher Adam Smith also acknowledged the possibility of feigned ailments. In a letter to his friend, the lawyer and politician Alexander Wedderburn, Smith wrote,

> It gives me great concern to learn by Mr Cunningham that Mrs Wedderburne's state of Health obliges you to pass some months at Spaw. I would hope, however, that necessity is only the pretence, and that amusement is the real purpose of your jour-

ney, which will at any rate remove you from a scene of Business and anxiety to one of Pleasure and dissipation.[84]

Yet to deny the sufferings of all nervous patients who were eager to participate in the shopping, balls and assemblies offered by spa towns is to misinterpret the purpose in these medically prescribed vacations. The diversion and delight that a trip to the spas could afford nervous sufferers was worth just as much, if not more, than the medicinal effects of the waters.

Engaging in leisure activities was not only a means of distracting nervous patients from harassing thoughts of their malady; it was also a pro-active measure. In a paper delivered to the Royal Medical Society, the speaker, Patrick Miller, elaborated upon the physical effects of joy. Joy, he claimed, 'Increases the action of the heart and arteries' which in turn meant that a 'larger quantity of blood' travelled to the muscles, thereby giving 'the feeling of increased vigour and activity'.[85] He continued,

> How much this state of mind, or affections allied to it, contribute to good health, must have appeared to every attentive observer – To this head, must be referred the good effects which Music, pleasant society, travelling, and the like, have had on different diseases – particularly Melancholy, Hypochondriasis... and other diseases in which languor and debility of body and dejection of mind form a principal part.[86]

It was in hopes of these good effects that doctors throughout the century encouraged and prescribed the indulgence of nervous sufferers in the 'pleasures of society'.[87]

The diversion of travel could also remove patients from the stresses of daily life, which were often the supposed cause of their disorders. Indeed, nerve specialists consistently warned against uninterrupted study or attention to business. For instance, Heberden's posthumously published *Commentaries on the History and Cure of Diseases* (1802) explained,

> It will indeed sometimes happen, that some degree of these miserable [nervous] sensations will be produced by a too great weight of business; the vexations of which in some evil hour may entangle a man so much, as to disable him from extricating himself by his own struggles, unless for a while he eases himself of the load by retiring to some such place as Bath, where the manner of living will effect the cure, though the reputation of it may be put to the account of the waters.[88]

Likewise, Cullen's prescription for the nervous Mr Miller advised that

> much application to Business and especially at one time long continued hurts the stomach & spirits, both by the employment of the mind and the sedentary state of the body. Such application therefore should be moderated and rendered easier by the frequent interposition of amusement and exercise.

In particular, Mr Miller was urged to take a journey 'once or twice a year directed so as to give the greatest variety and amusement'. [89] Balance between work and play was crucial to healthy nerves.

Climatic Cures: Getting a Change of Air

Recommended for patients in need of escape from stressful city living, travel also offered city-dwelling patients an escape from harmful city air. London air was notoriously insalubrious. Heberden described how in London 'there are amazing quantities of soot, ashes, powdered flints (in the form of dust) and horse dung perpetually floating in the atmosphere. Such substances applied to the surface of the lungs have a weakening effect upon the body'. [90] Lettsom likewise described how the crowded city's atmosphere was 'loaded with human effluvia'. [91] Cheyne's *Essay* addressed the particular effects of London air on nervous sufferers. Especially in the winter, he claimed, 'London is cover'd over with one universal nitrous and sulphurous Smoak, from the Multitude of Coal Fires'. During this season, he recommended, 'weak and tender people, and those that are subject to nervous or plumonick Distempers, ought... to go into the Country, or to be home soon after sun-set, and to dispel the Damps with clear, warm Fires, and chearful Conversation'. [92] Well through the century, travel to the countryside, and by the end of the century, travel to the seaside, were recommended to all sufferers in need of fresh air.

Seaside resorts became more commonly prescribed destinations just as spa towns began to lose their appeal among elite sufferers offended by the city's inter-class sociability; wealthy patients were no longer willing to bathe in the supposed scum of their social inferiors. [93] At first glance it appears that doctors who began to recommend trips to the seaside instead of the spas were merely catering to the whims of their fashionable clientele. Given the voluminous number of medical publications affirming the virtues of chalybeate spa waters for nervous complaints, it is difficult to understand the doctors' willingness to alter their advice so suddenly. There is little question that at least to some extent, patronage-dependent doctors were forced to cater to the demands of their wealthy patients. [94]

Yet again, pleasing patients did not necessarily come at the expense of professional integrity. For despite the increasing popularity of seaside resorts, the benefits of chalybeate waters were not forgotten. Bottled spa waters grew in popularity over the course of the century, allowing patients to reap their benefits from afar. Furthermore, knowledge of the supposed medical benefits of seawater far preceded the seaside's late-eighteenth and early-nineteenth-century status as a fashionable destination. [95] Seawater was not the only curative feature of coastal destinations. John Anderson, the appointed physician to the Margate Sea Bathing Infirmary, praised the particular virtues of the 'purifying and nutritive quality of the air' at Margate.[96] Gilchrist also emphasised the benefit of ocean air and a strong sea breeze for nervous sufferers, claiming that, 'From an unequal pressure of the air, in a percussive way, it is that many low spirited and hypochondriacal people, feel greater constancy, and elevation, in windy blustering weather'.[97]

In addition to the healthy effects of breathing clean air, a change of climate could also restore health. In his *Remarks on the Influence of Climate* (1781), Falconer acknowledged the physical and psychological effects of climate on the human body. He further insisted upon the climate-induced tendency of Englishmen to become melancholic and depressed, declaring, 'the English, and indeed some other nations in nearly the same latitude, often put an end to their lives in the bosom of happiness. This seems to resemble a disorder of the climate, and to be interwoven into the constitution of the people'.[98] Nervous complaints were supposedly at their worst during the cold, dark and damp winter months. As Trotter explained, 'the human nerves in such patients are like barometers: it is thus the fall of the year, in November and December, [that] is proverbial for lowness of spirits and melancholy'.[99] Records from the Edinburgh Royal Infirmary confirm that it was precisely during this time that admissions for hysteric and hypochondriac patients peaked.[100]

Nervous patients commonly associated their complaints with the climate. The nervous Robert Ligertwood complained to Cullen in 1781 that 'I have been much distressed with my Nerves & Stomack, & during the continuance of Frosty weather I was greatly borne down...'[101] Likewise, the Reverend Mr Surteer wrote to Cullen that 'in moist weather my nervous indisposition is greatest', and one Dr Raymond asked Cullen for advice on the treatment of a patient for whom 'the Winter seasons always increase his complaints and bring on tremors in the Nerves'.[102] Consequently, in addition to escaping the polluted and debilitating air of the metropolis, nervous patients with the means to do so commonly travelled to warmer climates during the colder seasons. Cullen's correspondence records many British patients travelling to France, and even as far as Bermuda. One particularly zealous nervous patient in 1776 wrote to Cullen that he had travelled from London to New York to Bermuda to South Carolina and back to London in search of a climatic cure, though it appears from his letter that his travels were unsuccessful.[103]

Whether travelling in search of healthy air or an escape from the stresses of daily life, dieting, or following a consistent exercise regimen, most nervous sufferers engaged in the manipulation of one or more of the non-naturals over the course of their treatment. The severity of a patient's regimen necessarily varied according to the severity of their disorder. There is little doubt that a long distance journey on horseback was more taxing than an afternoon spent bouncing on a chamber horse, or that a rough sea journey required more fortitude on the part of a nervous sufferer than a trip to the spa. Yet regardless of their severity, all of these treatments were firmly backed by medical theory; medical tracts contained as much evidence in support of the healthy effects of entertainment and travel as it did for strict diets or exercise. Far from simply catering to modern fashions or patient whims, doctors prescribing anything from a vegetarian diet to a trip to the South of France did so in the confident belief that they were appealing to the traditional therapeutic methods.

It is impossible to comment conclusively on the effectiveness of these remedies. There is little doubt that patients suffering primarily from digestive complaints would have found relief in a change of diet. It is also likely that some grief-stricken and melancholic patients would have successfully tempered their misery with sociable conversation or a change of scenery. Not all patients were so fortunate. As one long-term sufferer complained to Cullen,

> I have avoided Indolence so carefully – I have exercised myself, to such a degree, by frequent long journeys upon horse back to the extent of a Thousand Miles – by walking liberally &c&c, as might have strengthened and hardened any one – but this never carried off the sensibility.[104]

The enormous range of supposed symptoms and causes of nervous disorders meant that every patient's case was unique. Consequently, the recommended treatments and regimens for nervous sufferers were highly varied. The outcomes of these prescriptions were equally diverse. Yet for patients unable or unwilling to effect relief through a change of regimen, pharmaceutical remedies presented an alternative pathway to health.

Tinctures, Pills and Decoctions: Consumable Cures

As discussed in Chapter 2, most first- and second-tier physicians well versed in the medical theory of the ancients stressed the inferior nature of medicinal remedies compared to regulation of the non-naturals. Buchan defended his scanty list of nervous medications in *Domestic Medicine* on precisely these grounds:

> It would be an easy matter to enumerate many medicines which have been extolled for relieving nervous disorders; but whoever wishes for a thorough cure must expect it from regimen alone; we shall therefore omit mentioning more medicines, and again recommend the strictest attention to DIET, AIR, EXERCISE, and AMUSEMENTS.[105]

Doctors consistently stressed the impossibility of obtaining a thorough or long-term cure through medication alone, and expressed irritation with patients who lazily relied on consumable remedies instead of willpower and a change of lifestyle. As Trotter lamented,

> It has been unfortunate for the medical profession, as well as patients themselves, that persons labouring under nervous disorders, have too much expected from the pre-

scription of the physician, and the shop of the apothecary, what is only to be obtained from their own caution and circumspection.[106]

Occasionally patients bemoaned their own lack of fortitude in this matter. In 1789 the nervous Bradley Smith wrote to his physician that while he believed he had found some relief from his medication, 'probably I should have derived still greater advantage from it had I … used proper exercise'.[107]

Yet if properly paired with diet, exercise and diversion, physicians exhibited at least a tempered faith in the strengthening and palliative powers of certain medicines. Interestingly, whereas most elite physicians publishing on nervous disease expressed disapproval over the use of drugs in nervous cases, in practice, their use of prescription remedies was common. The surviving case notes of the famed physician Sir Henry Halford reveal that on average he prescribed three drugs for each of his hysteric and hypochondriac patients.[108] The reasons behind this apparent inconsistency are threefold. First, patients often demanded drugs. As Buchan complained,

> Patients who labour under nervous diseases, are generally very fond of medicine; and when they are not swallowing drugs, they think themselves neglected. For this reason the doctor must either give medicine, or lay his account with being dismissed.[109]

One physician writing to Cullen on behalf of a patient suffering from 'feelings of distress' revealed the pressure that he was under to deliver an appropriate prescription. Upon anxiously asking Cullen to prescribe his patient some sort of medication he wrote, 'I beg you would order something, that she may not think she is… neglected. [I]f it is something that will relieve her it will be so much the better'.[110] The pressure to prescribe only grew over the course of the century, as newspaper advertisements for proprietary medicines increased, enticing patients with the promise of alluringly exotic and fast-acting fixes. When treating wealthy patients upon whose continued patronage their livelihood depended, physicians were often forced to compromise, prescribing drugs and negotiating treatments which were acceptable both to themselves and to their patients.

Yet as with doctors who recommended trips to fashionable seaside resorts, doctors who succumbed to their patients' demands for drugs were not necessarily neglecting their professional principles. While physicians firmly believed that medicines could not effect a perfect cure on their own, they did have faith in the ability of some to at least partially strengthen weak and debilitated systems. Thus, the second reason that physicians prescribed pharmaceutical remedies was due to their sincere belief that these medications could, when used in conjunction with the manipulation of the non-naturals, effectively compose a minor part of a patient's treatment. The third reason that physicians prescribed medications was to provide immediate relief for their suffering patients. Although palliative remedies offered only temporary reprieve, it was considered the duty of a good physician to relieve patients from discomfort wherever possible. As the physician William Rowley explained, 'A number of diseases, not perfectly curable, can be mitigated; the art extends no farther; but to deny relief because we cannot effect a radical cure is inhuman'.[111] The willingness of doctors to prescribe these palliative remedies attests to the seriousness with which they regarded their nervous patients' pain.

The most commonly prescribed strengthening medications were Peruvian bark, steel, vitriol and rhubarb. The most commonly prescribed palliative medications included opium, camphor, musk and asafoetida. While useful for treating nervous disease, these medications were also commonly prescribed for other disorders. Peruvian bark was used for treating fevers and 'most periodical disorders', rhubarb was employed in cases of colics and diarrhoeas, and camphor was known to treat inflammations and rheumatic pains.[112] Despite being imported from as far away as China and South America, the majority of these exotic medications were regularly stocked in eighteenth-century physicians' medical chests, and were even recommended by Buchan for inclusion in private family medical stocks. While popular, the taste of these drugs was often objectionable, and side effects were frequent. The continued willingness of patients to endure and even request these remedies illustrates the strength of their desire to recover from what they clearly believed was as medically curable a disorder as rheumatism, diarrhoea, or fever.

Strengthening Medicines

As perhaps the most commonly prescribed medicine for nervous disorders, Peruvian bark was valued for its strengthening effect on the nerves. The chemist William Lewis noted in his *Experimental History of the Materia Medica* (1761) that 'by its bitterness, astringency, and mild aromatic warmth, it strengthens the whole system, and proves a medicine of great utility in... chronical diseases proceeding from a laxity and debility of the fibres'.[113] Bark was prescribed to relieve patients of general nervous weakness and specific nervous symptoms including flatulence, giddiness, faintness and indigestion.[114] Andrew Duncan commented on the immense national consumption of the remedy in his *Annals of Medicine for the Year 1796*, estimating that approximately half a million pounds of bark were used in England from 1788 to 1793 alone.[115] Part of the bark's authority lay in its long history as a strengthening remedy; Indians recognized its medicinal virtue as early as 1500, and it first appeared in Europe as a remedy in 1649.[116] As its name suggests, bark was, in fact, bark from a middling-sized tree grown in Peru. It was imported to England in pieces of a 'rusty iron colour'. Bark could be chewed directly, boiled and formed into pills by an apothecary, or, more commonly, prepared as a decoction or infusion. To make a decoction, the bark was first pulverized into a fine powder resembling cinnamon, then boiled in water until 'the whole of its virtue is pretty readily got out'. The concoction was strained, and the resultant liquid was swallowed. To make an infusion, powdered bark was mixed with water, wine, brandy or rum, and let to stand for twenty-four hours before being filtered. The recommended doses for these medications varied widely, ranging from Whytt's recommendation of a tablespoonful with four or five spoonfuls of water twice a day, to the medicinal warehouse Bath and Company's recommendation of filling an entire 'large tea cup twice, or three times in a day' - a quantity which would no doubt be good for business.[117] Regardless of the size of the dose, patients were expected to continue on a course of the bark for several months at a time.

The persistence required for such a lengthy prescriptive regimen is all the more remarkable in light of the apparent taste of the bark. Described as 'considerably bitter, astringent, [and] very durable in the mouth', Lewis' *History of the Materia Medica* recommended taking liquorice to mask its offensive taste, whereas Whytt recommended the spirit of lavender.[118] The potential side effects of bark included sickness, sharp bowel pains and a general looseness of the bowels, although these effects were said to lessen over time as the patient's body became accustomed to the medication.[119] Despite its supposedly remarkable strengthening powers, bark was most commonly prescribed in conjunction with other strengthening remedies and lifestyle changes. As Thomas Skeete advised his readers, 'it must be obvious... that a careful regulation of diet and exercise here, as at other times, is necessary to insure the efficacy of the Bark'.[120] The fact that patients were so consistently reminded of this fact suggests that they were frequently all too willing to trust their recovery to the power of medicine.

Touted for its ability to 'remarkably strengthen the stomach and bowels, and indeed the whole body', steel was also commonly prescribed for nervous sufferers.[121] In addition to strengthening the system, steel was also useful for 'quickening circulation, raising the pulse [and] rendering the blood more florid'. The preparation of steel medications varied widely; iron filings could be partially dissolved in a 'quarter of a pint or more of strong vinegar' and drunk. They could also be prepared by a confectioner and candied with sugar, a method that Lewis described as 'very commodious for taking'.[122] Easiest on the stomach, and the form most commonly prescribed for nervous patients was the tincture of steel. Mixed by apothecaries, this tincture was composed by soaking three ounces of iron filings in wine for one month. Aromatic spices like cinnamon and mace were added to the concoction to make it more palatable.

As with bark, the recommended doses of steel ranged considerably; Whytt related the case of one patient who took 230 grains of iron filings daily and another who could only bear six to eight grains in a day. For patients taking iron filings directly with vinegar or sugar, an average daily dose was about fifteen filings, taken two or three at a time every couple of hours.[123] Like bark, steel also caused bothersome side effects including 'great sickness and perturbation'. These effects could be lessened 'by beginning with very small doses', but generally disappeared as patients became accustomed to the treatment.[124]

A gentler method of employing steel in nervous cases was through the use of the iron-rich spa waters. While nervous patients often bathed in spa waters to relax their bodies and minds, spa water was also consumed. Whytt explained the virtues of the waters:

> The chalybeate waters, altho' they contain but a very small proportion of iron, are often observed to have remarkable effects in strengthening the body. Particularly, the waters of *Bath* in *Somersetshire* have been of great use to many, who, from a weak state of the stomach and bowels, were affected with low spirits and other nervous complaints.[125]

Specific spa waters were recommended for different complaints. Whereas Whytt recommended Somerset, Alexander Thompson noted in his article on Scottish baths, 'I have found the use of the Aberbrothock water of singular advantage, in lowness of spirits and other maladies, where the nerves are said to be affected; for which I have also seen the Kincardine water beneficial'.[126]

Physicians regulated the consumption of mineral waters as carefully as any other drug. Adam Smith declared in a 1776 letter to David Hume that 'A mineral water is as much a drug as any that comes out of the Apothecaries Shop. It produces the same violent effects upon the body'.[127] Doctors carefully prescribed the times that patients should drink the waters, as well as the amount they should consume. The *New Bath Guide* (1785) noted that most patients drank the waters in the morning, from six to ten o'clock, in the quantity of one to three pints in a day.[128] The Bath physician William Oliver's concurred with this advice, also suggesting that a course of drinking should last for five to six weeks.[129] Given the supposed strength of their medicinal powers, overindulging in the Bath waters could be dangerous. For this reason, physicians often reminded patients of the necessity of obtaining medical advice before drinking the waters. As the *New Prose Bath Guide* cryptically warned visitors in 1778, 'TAKE NOT THE BATH WATERS UNTIL YOU HAVE TAKEN GOOD ADVICE; for they are Waters not to be trifled with'.[130] In his *Directions for the use of the Harrowgate Waters* (1773), William Alexander acknowledged the temptation of many invalids to overdose on the waters, claiming that some people

> are apt to imagine they can never take too much of any thing that is good for their health; therefore they take as much of the water as their stomachs can possibly bear; and thus often bring diseases upon themselves as bad, and perhaps worse, than those they expected to be relieved from.[131]

In this way, Alexander explained, some patients nearly died in their attempt to expedite a cure.[132] Such reports are highly doubtful, and probably served as more of a ploy to scare patients into seeking formal medical advice than any candid observation.

While probably not deadly, consumption of spa water was unpleasant due to its high sulphur content. In his attempt to describe the offensive taste of the mineral waters near Moffatt, the Scottish surgeon George Milligen was rendered nearly speechless:

> I have no words fully expressive of the taste of these waters; most people who drink them resemble it to something sulphureous, as gun powder, the scourings of a foul gun . . . Some express it by the taste of a rotten egg; but none of these justly come up to the genuine taste of the mineral water.[133]

Still, patients 'took the waters' in increasing numbers over the course of the century. For patients unable to make the journey to Bath or any other spa town, spa waters were bottled and available for order. While the practice of selling bottled spa water originated in the late seventeenth century, it grew enormously in the eighteenth. By 1746 one London retailer offered water from Bath Spa three times a week.[134] Water warehouses and merchants who dealt exclusively with the trade of bottled water were only a small part of the overall trend; druggists, tavern-keepers and tea and coffee merchants also sold bottled spa water. Ledgers belonging to the famous Thomas Twining show that in addition to his tea and coffee, he also annually sold over 1,000 flasks of spa water from 1717 to 1722.[135]

The mineral water trade was not limited to the waters of Bath spa. By the middle of the eighteenth century, the waters of Buxton, Holt, Bristol, Malvern, Hampstead and Epsom, to name but a few, were also bottled and sold. Indeed, in 1774 one of Cullen's patients wrote to him to 'beg the favour of a line from you the first opportunity, informing me... of what you thought further necessary to my wish for health; and if you thought... sending for a small quantity of Buxton spaw water in Bottles might be of any service'.[136] Waters from foreign spas in France, Germany and Holland also became popular over the course of the century. This trend only decreased at the very end of the century as sea bathing and the consumption of seawater and artificially made soda and seltzer waters surpassed them in popularity. Providing one of his nervous patients with a recipe for this therapeutic seltzer water, Cullen suggested 'dissolving from ten to twenty grains of a pure salt of tartare in a pint of water & impregnating the same water by a proper apparatus with a quantity of fixed air taken from chalk'. Useful for preventing 'stagnation in the bowels', seltzer water was best 'taken from the quantity of an English pint to a quart every day'.[137]

Rhubarb could also appease stomach and bowel complaints. Valued as a mild laxative capable of ridding the body of impurities, it also appealed to nervous sufferers for its supposed ability to strengthen the stomach and bodily fibres. Only the root of the plant was used medicinally. Imported from Turkey, Russia and the East Indies, rhubarb was typically dried and available for purchase in small pieces at all apothecary shops. The smell of rhubarb was deceptively light and aromatic; the taste was bitter and acrid, allegedly adding a sharp smell to a patient's urine.[138] Like bark, rhubarb was often powdered and consumed in a tincture. Some patients chewed the root on its own, as in the case of the nervous John Warrandice who informed his physician that he typically chewed 'a little rubarb twice a week or so'. The effects of this remedy, according to Warrandice, were unconfirmed: 'whether then this may seem to weaken my sensibility or not I can't say'.[139]

The final most popular strengthening remedy prescribed by physicians was the acid elixir of vitriol, or, sulphuric acid.[140] Commonly recommended for patients 'afflicted with wind', elixir of vitriol was touted for its ability to strengthen the stomach and aid digestion.[141] John Quincy noted in his *Pharmacopia Officinalis* that this medication was of particular use for people recovering 'from debauches and over-feeding'.[142] Cinnamon, orange peel and rose petals were often included in the elixir to cover its otherwise acidic taste. Of this remedy, Buchan recommended fifteen to thirty drops mixed with water, taken two to three times per day.[143]

Palliative Medicines

Opium was an often-employed remedy for pain relief in the eighteenth century. Used even by Hellenistic physicians, it was credited with the ability to create

> assurance, Ovation of the Spirits, Courage, Contempt of Danger, and Magnanimity... [it] prevents and takes away Grief, Fear, Anxieties, Peevishness, Fretfulness... lulls, sooths, and (as it were) charms the Mind with Satisfaction.[144]

Extracted from white poppies, opium was a 'gummy resinous juice' of 'dark reddish brown' colour with a 'faint disagreeable smell, and a bitterish, somewhat hot, biting taste'.[145] As Lewis explained, it could render the solids 'less sensible of every kind of irritation' and provide temporary relief for 'debilities of the nervous system'.[146] Opium was also valued for its ability to combat the low spirits, grief and unease so common in nervous cases. Despite these medicinal virtues, the long-term use of opium could have dangerous effects, including a

> great relaxation and debility, sluggishness, heaviness, loss of appetite, dropsies, tremors, acrimony of the humours, frequent stimulus to urine, and propensity to venery.

Addiction was also a problem. Lewis warned readers that

on leaving it off, after habitual use, an extreme lowness of the spirits, languor, and anxiety, succeed; which are relieved by having again recourse to opium, and in some measure by spirituous or vinous liquors.[147]

Decrying the tendency of nervous patients to appeal to drugs and quick fixes, Trotter expressed his concern over the particular danger of opium addictions:

When opium happens to be soothing to weak nerved people, from their quick sensations, it is apt to be the more craved for, and converted into habit. The languor and dejection which follow its operation pave the way for repetition of the dose, till general debility succeeds.[148]

Trotter noted several cases of 'fashionable women in high life, of the nervous temperament, who had got into the baneful habit of using opium as a *cordial*. Some had become so addicted 'as to carry a vial of laudanum constantly with them'.[149] Despite these warnings, opium was commonly prescribed throughout the century for its unparalleled pain-relieving abilities. Because of the amorphous qualities of nervous diseases, discovering and treating the 'root cause' of patients' nervous ailments was no easy task. Consequently, the ability of opium to relieve patients of any and all mysterious symptoms made it an extremely valuable tool for otherwise helpless medical practitioners. In his receipt book the London chemist Ambrose Godfrey quoted one physician as saying 'if it was not for Opium he wou'd not Practice'.[150]

Opium could be consumed directly, usually one grain at a time, or as a tincture in water or wine. The Royal College of Physicians' Pharmacopoeias for London and Edinburgh advised the addition of cinnamon and cloves to any tinctures in order to mask the opium's unpleasant smell. Opium could also be taken as a pill. Recipes for opium pills varied; one 'elegant pill' was composed of 'thirty-two parts of almond soap, four of strained opium moistened with a little wine, and one of essence of lemons, beaten together'. Another recipe called for 'one part of opium, four of extract of liquorice, three of Spanish soap, and two of powdered Jamaica pepper'.[151]

Like opium, camphor was also a highly employed palliative remedy by eighteenth-century nervous sufferers. Extracted from the bark and root of a bay tree found in East India and Japan, this gummy substance had a 'fragrant smell, somewhat approaching to that of rosemary, but much stronger; and a bitterish, aromatic, pungent taste'. Camphor was known to produce 'very uneasy sensations about the stomach' when taken on its own, and most often prescribed with opium. Taken together, these remedies caused profuse sweating, which was believed to rid the body of any 'impurity of the humours'.[152] In nervous cases, a small amount of camphor was usually dissolved 'in watery liquors, and thus fitted for being commodiously taken, by grinding it with sugar, almonds... and adding water by degrees'.[153] The Gloucester chemist Daniel Cox recommended that the camphor be mixed with 'four times its quantity of refined sugar' before adding 'a large spoonful of spirit of wine or brandy'. His recommended dose was anywhere from one half to two ounces.[154]

As an even more exotic nervous remedy, musk gained quick popularity for its ability to relieve pain, raise the spirits, relieve spasms including hiccups and stomach cramps and to encourage refreshing sleep. According to the *Experimental History*, musk was 'found in a little bag, situated near the umbilical region of an oriental quadruped, which is said by some to bear the greatest resemblance to the goat'.[155] The best musk was imported from China, although inferior varieties were available from Russia and Bengal. Musk was described as having a 'bitterish subacrid taste; and a fragrant smell, agreeable at a distance, but so strong as to be disagreeable when smelt near to'.[156] This bad smell was supposedly one of the only negative effects of the drug, although it was acknowledged to particularly 'offend and disorder' nervous patients with 'constitutions of great sensibility'.[157] Musk was prepared as a tincture, steeped in wine. The generally accepted dosage was a sizeable twenty to thirty grains every four to six hours.

Extracted from the root of a Persian mountain plant, asafoetida was commonly prescribed with musk and opium, and was valued by nervous sufferers for its antispasmodic qualities, and its 'good effects in flatulent disorders'.[158] Originally milky and white, asafoetida became brownish in colour and achieved a thicker, resinous consistency once it was exposed to air. Given its 'strong fetid smell approaching to that of garlic' and 'nauseous bitterish biting taste', asafoetida was usually taken as a pill so as 'not to give any taste' as it passed.[159] Asafoetida could also be purchased from apothecaries' shops as a tincture, and was usually mixed with alcohol and water.

Proprietary Medicines

Store-bought medications multiplied in eighteenth-century Britain, with newspaper advertisements touting cures for everything from gout to dental problems, and venereal disease to all imaginable nervous symptoms.[160] P. S. Brown's study of the medical advertisements in eighteenth-century Bath newspapers revealed that over 7 per cent of the advertisements from 1744 to 1800 were intended to relieve mental symptoms and diseases of the nervous system.[161] This high rate of advertising is a clear testament to successful sales, a fact further confirmed by Trotter's claim that 'all nervous persons are uncommonly fond of drugs; and they are the chief consumers of advertised medicines, which they conceal from their medical friends'.[162] Newspapers like the *Bath Chronicle* repeatedly advertised medications like Dr Lowther's Nervous Powders and Mr Rymer's nervous tincture, intended for 'nervous affections and corporeal weakness, dizziness & buzzing noise in the head, faintness, low spirits, etc'.[163] The price of proprietary medicines varied considerably, although the majority sold for one to five shillings.[164] This price would have been significant yet manageable. In light of John Trusler's 1786 budget estimate for a family of six, the cost would have amounted to slightly more than the cost of the week's supply of bread.[165]

The composition of proprietary medicines was often nearly identical to the drugs prescribed by physicians. Such similarities are puzzling in light of physicians' generally professed opposition to store-bought remedies. Yet as many members of the medical faculty claimed, the value of medicines depended on their correct application more than their composition. As one anonymous physician in London wrote to a friend in Bath, 'Diseases are not cured by Medicines and Receipts, but by a learned and methodical Use of them, whereunto Empiricks cannot attain'.[166] Given the competitive medical marketplace of the eighteenth century, it is also likely that physicians were opposed to proprietary medicines because they competed with their own services. Still, in light of the medical faculty's reluctance to recommend drugs as a primary form of treatment, their scepticism over the efficacy of store-bought medications cannot be attributed solely to professional safeguarding.

Indeed, the tendency of proprietary medicines to promise perfect cures in every case was in direct contrast to the basic medical tenets of patience, perseverance, moderation and healthy living espoused by most learned practitioners. S. Solomon claimed extravagantly that his 'most excellent medicine the Cordial Balm of Gilead' could provide speedy relief and a remarkable cure in all cases of 'delicate, weakly, and relaxed constitutions, lowness of spirits, hypochondria, horrors, tremblings, [etc.]'.[167] Likewise, Joshua Webster recommended his celebrated English diet drink for an unlimited number of disorders including Hypochondriasis, promising that 'if the diet drink be *regularly* taken, and *persevered* in for some *considerable time*, a cure will infallibly be accomplished'.[168] As most well educated physicians treating nervous disease consistently acknowledged, no medicine could perform a perfect cure. These promises appeared particularly irresponsible to first- and second-tier physicians in light of the worrying tendency of patients merely to patch their poor health with palliative medicines rather than effect true and long-term cures with diet and exercise. Quackish claims that proprietary medicines would unilaterally 'strike at the root' of patients' disorders 'and not at the branches' were blasphemous to most traditionally educated medical practitioners who knew otherwise.[169]

In addition to the irresponsible tendency of proprietary medicines to encourage quick fixes, physicians also worried about their potential to cause addictions and alcoholism. The amount of alcohol in these medications was often substantial, and patients could easily overindulge without professional supervision. In his 'Hints Respecting the Effects of a Little Drop' Lettsom advised patients to set aside their medicines in favour of natural and non-alcoholic cures:

> Regard not the prevalence of a bad habit, or the fallacy of language, for a little drop
> of spirit, is a drop of poison. You have heard of cordials, stomach tinctures, bitters,
> nervous drops, hysteric water, and other alluring titles, but alas! the drop sparkles
> only to deceive.[170]

Despite such warnings, nervous medications continued to proliferate as nervous sufferers continued to buy. For patients desperate to feel better, the allure of proprietary medicines outweighed physicians' alarms.

Homemade Medicines

Patients frequently made their own medications. Several self-help medical guides offered simple remedies for nervous patients without the money to purchase proprietary medicines or the means to seek professional medical attention. For instance, William Chamberlaine's *The West-India Seaman's Medical Dictionary* (1785) provided simple instructions for 'a *very small number*' of 'really *useful*' medications for sea merchants without the time or money to consult a physician, or for men onboard ships without a surgeon.[171] Of this select group of remedies, Chamberlaine recommended a teaspoonful of the spirit of lavender on a lump of sugar for 'lowness of spirits, nervous head-aches, tremblings, and other nervous complaints' commonly encountered at sea.[172] Believed to calm the stomach and aid sleep, the spirit of lavender was also recommended in the *Family Medical Compendium* (1790) for 'all kinds of languors and weakness of the nerves'.[173]

Not all homemade remedies were so agreeable; the *Compendium* also provided instructions for tar water. Invented by the Irish Bishop George Berkeley in 1744 as a remedy for fevers, gout, scurvy and dropsy, this unpleasant medicine was also used as a 'slow yet effectual' remedy for hysteria and hypochondria.[174] The physician John Rutty praised tar water in a letter to another physician claiming that 'in some chronical hypochondriacal cases it has done great things, & particularly restored Appetite & Rest where other medicines failed'.[175] Designed to raise the pulse and to cause 'some considerable evacuation, generally by perspiration and urine, although sometimes by stool and vomiting', tar water worked in a Galenic manner to 'expel the morbific humours'.[176] The recipe for tar water was simple: 'Take of tar, two pounds; water, one gallon. Stir them well together with a wooden rod; and after standing to settle for two days, pour off the water for use'.[177] Nervous patients were instructed to take a total of one pint of tar water per day on an empty stomach.

Less offensive than tar water, Wesley's *Primitive Physic* recommended tincture of valerian to ease riled nerves. This tincture was prepared by cutting to pieces

> Six ounces of wild Valerian-Root, gathered in June, and fresh dried. Bruise it by a few
> strokes in a Mortar, that the Pieces may be split, but it should not be beat into Pow-

der: put this into a Quart of strong white Wine; cork the Bottle and let it stand three Weeks, shaking it every Day; then press it out and filter the Tincture through Paper.

Wesley assured his audience that the tincture would not carry an offensive odour. As he helpfully noted, 'The true, wild Valerian has no bad smell: if it has, Cats have urined upon it, which they will do, if they can come at it'.[178] Patients were instructed to take an ounce of the tincture every morning with hot water, cream and sugar.

The willingness of patients to make and take the tincture, or any other more objectionable nervous remedies, attests to the seriousness with which they took their disorders, and their belief that they were suffering from a medically treatable disease. More importantly, the fact that remedies for nervous disease appeared in so many self-help guides, including Wesley's *Primitive Physic*, which was designed for the 'common people' and the 'bulk of mankind', proves that nervous disease was not exclusively suffered by the rich.[179] Chamberlaine's inclusion of a remedy for nervous complaints within his brief medical dictionary for merchants at sea also proves the presence of nervous disease outside of the realms of fashionable society, and suggests that the eighteenth century witnessed a larger group of sufferers than was typically acknowledged in the period's popular discourse.

Efficacy of Medication

It is difficult to determine the efficacy of any eighteenth-century remedies from a modern perspective. One of the primary complications inherent in determining their effectiveness is the disparity between historical and contemporary definitions of success. In the eighteenth century, emetics and purgatives were believed to 'work' if they provoked the intended physical response. Patients' beliefs regarding the efficacy of their treatment were also dependent upon their understanding of human physiology. Those subscribing to a humoural vision of the body were likely to believe that productive emetics and purgatives were effectively voiding their bodies of harmful fluids. Patients who imagined that their nerves were weak and flaccid might also believe that these potentially violent remedies would have a bracing effect. Hence, a remedy like tar water could be 'successful' for its notable ability to cause vomiting, although in actuality these 'strengthening discharges' would have done little to toughen a patient's nerves.

While more palliative than curative, it is likely that some herbal remedies employed by eighteenth century physicians worked with good effect. Lavender is still valued by modern herbalists for its ability to relieve upset stomachs, insomnia and gas; valerian root is recognized as a sedative, and rhubarb is still considered an effective laxative.[180] There is also little doubt that opium and alcohol would have masked many patients' pains.

Some relieved nervous patients did attribute their improvement to medication. William Nevin, writing to Cullen regarding 'dreadfull' bladder pains, began his letter by thanking the doctor for his earlier 'prescription for a nervous complaint for which I own myself greatly obliged to you'. He stated that he was already 'a little better of that Nervous Disorder' when his new complaint began.[181] Other patients seeking medical advice indicated that their medicines that were initially useful, but had lost their effectiveness over time. As Mr Rae wrote to Cullen in 1777,

> You'll probably recollect that when I was in Edinburgh last December I took your opinion concerning an unhappy complaint I then labored under and which I think you call'd Nervous, after using your prescription for about ten days which was purgative I got somewhat better and continued so for about two months but afterwards relapsed and have since endured much perplexity in my mind where the disorder seem altogether to seat itself.

He then asked Cullen to recommend a different remedy 'which might be serviceable'.[182] Similarly, the physician to another nervous patient wrote to Cullen that although his patient had been treated with gentle emetics, the Bark and aromatics, nothing had afforded him 'any more than a Temporary Relieff'.[183] In these instances, although medicine was minimally effective, it did not provide lasting relief or a permanent cure.

In most cases, patient letters and medical case notes suggest that medications met with little curative success. Of course, the very nature of these sources, written by, or on behalf of, still-ailing patients, presents an obvious negative bias, if the medications had worked, the patients would not seek additional treatment. Still, negative feedback was plentiful. In the case of one nervous Mr Weetwood, Cullen wrote, 'I think [he] can hardly be relieved by any medicine & he must be satisfied with the easy means of relief which his experience has taught him'.[184] Another doctor indicated that his nervous patient had endured his condition for twenty years, consulted 'numberless Physicians, & vainly tried all their different prescriptions'.[185] Case records for a hypochondriac at the Edinburgh Royal Infirmary similarly noted that the patient had employed multiple medications 'without relief'.[186]

Often medicines had a different effect than intended. For example, one letter to Cullen from another physician described how a particular nervous patient had 'swallowed a great quantity of Bark and other medicines, without any good effect. Indeed the Bark never agreed with him, for instead of bracing it always proved laxative'.[187] Some medications actually caused harm. In a case from 1770, a nervous patient already suffering from 'a great depression of spirits' together with 'sighing, a nausea, and a total aversion to food' became additionally plagued by a headache, failing memory, cold sensations, and an accelerated pulse which his doctor attributed to 'the heating qualities of a nervous medicine he had pro-cured from an advertisement'.[188]

The failure of a drug to cure a patient's nervous disorder did not necessarily signal to physicians that it was ineffective. Because medications were most often prescribed in tandem with other treatment therapies, it was often presumed that the efficacy of treatments were co-dependent. For instance, melancholic nervous patients had to first gain control over their passions before medication could work. Socialization and amusement typically took precedence over pharma-ceutical remedies. For example, in his treatment of a melancholic patient the physician John Andrew prescribed bark, camphor and laxatives to 'no effect'. Unfortunately, the doctor noted, his patient was 'in that low way' where 'he wishes to see no body and his nearest friends are most disagreeable to him which makes it very difficult to administer any medicine that might be of use'.[189] In cases where other aspects of a patient's regimen were in order and a prescription still did not work, physicians usually assumed that the failed drug was wrong for the patient's particular constitution. In such cases, dosages were tweaked, and different medications were tried. Still, the secondary status held by pharmaceuti-cal remedies within the ranks of most physicians' prescriptive artillery suggests that they were not regularly successful.

Occasionally patients were unable to determine the effectiveness of their medications. One nervous patient wrote to his physician that he was in the habit of taking a 'compound spirit of Lavender of which I take a little upon sugar when I find myself growing low, & fancy it does me service, for on those occasions I am apt to attribute more virtue to it, than it really possesses'.[190] Doctors did not dis-miss this power of patient faith in drugs. Rather, they often exhibited more faith in the potential placebo effect of remedies than in the effect of the actual drugs prescribed. In his *Treatise on Female, Nervous, Hysterical, Hypochondriacal, Bil-ious, Convulsive Diseases, &c*, Rowley acknowledged the importance of patient belief, noting that 'where there is no faith, there is no cure'.[191] Alternatively, John Gregory attacked what he viewed as a misplaced faith in drugs in his *Lectures on the Duties and Qualifications of a Physician* (1772). Railing against many mod-ern medicines and expressing his irritation with patients who staked their faith in the mysterious complexity of prescribed drugs over simple common-sense remedies, Gregory wrote,

> A firm belief in the effects of medicine depends more on the imagination, than on a rational conviction impressed on the understanding; and the imagination is never armed by any object which is distinctly perceived, nor by any truth obvious to com-mon sense. Few people can be persuaded that a poultice of bread and milk is in many cases as efficacious as one compounded of half a dozen ingredients, to whose names they are strangers.[192]

John Haygarth's *Of the Imagination as Cure and as a Cure of Disorders of the Body* (1800) discussed the placebo effect even more explicitly. As a respected physician to the Chester Infirmary and member of the Royal Society for London and Edinburgh, Haygarth insisted upon the power of patient faith to produce legitimate medical effects. To test his hypothesis, Haygarth treated five hospital patients suffering from chronic rheumatism with fake magnetic therapy. Four of the five patients reported that they were 'much benefited' by this fake treatment, with one patient being able to walk much better, and another reporting an ongoing tingling sensation for two hours. The significance of this experiment, Haygarth explained, was unwavering proof that 'a patient ought to be always inspired with confidence in any remedy which is administered'. The trials also justified the occasional efficacy of quack medicines: 'magnificent and unqualified promises inspire weak minds with implicit confidence'.[193] In addition to the power of patient faith in drugs, Haygarth also explained the power of their faith in medical practitioners:

> we may discern the great advantage of medical reputation. This explains what has been frequently observed, that the same remedy will produce more beneficial effects when prescribed by a famous physician, than by a person of inferior character.[194]

Cullen's fame undoubtedly had this effect for many nervous sufferers. One patient even wrote to Cullen expressing the way in which she had such faith in his abilities that even the receipt of his letter worked like a remedy: 'I reckoned myself effectualy cured when I received it'.[195] Likewise, another patient wrote to Cullen in 1775, 'I believe it is just observation that to have confidence in the physician is of great benefit to the patient'.[196]

Although Haygarth's experiment dealt exclusively with patients suffering from chronic rheumatism, he did not overlook the significance of his experiment to nervous patients. Referring readers to Falconer's award-winning *Dissertation on the Influence of the Passions Upon Disorders of the Body* (1788), Haygarth noted that Falconer's work 'confirms the doctrine I wish to establish, by proving how much they [hysterical and other nervous disorders] lie under the influence of the Imagination'.[197] Convinced of the physical reality of nervous disease, Haygarth was equally convinced of the power of the mind to cause and cure its physical symptoms. Thus, while frowned upon by first- and second-tier physicians for their failure to treat physical symptoms directly, medicines could be esteemed for their ability to treat the body via the mind.

Beneficial Pain: Aggressive Physical Treatments

With regard to eighteenth-century medications, it seems that the more offensive the remedy, the greater the faith in its efficacy. Cramping, vomiting and uncomfortably sweating patients could at least suffer in confidence, knowing that their medications were working aggressively. The same was true for the unpleasant non-pharmaceutical therapies endured by nervous patients such as blistering, bleeding, enemas and electrical treatments. In addition to the potential placebo effects of these painful remedies, physicians believed that they could also powerfully affect the body by diverting the patient's mind. Whytt explained the particular value of violent remedies in nervous cases: 'nervous disorders occasioned by strong impressions on the mind, are often prevented, lessened or cured by exciting other sensations or passions of a superior force'. According to Whytt, a wide range of diseases and symptoms were responsive to aggressive therapies:

> Epileptic fits have been cured by whipping. - Convulsions from the toothach are removed by blisters; - vomiting has been stopt by putting the hands suddenly in cold water; and a common hiccup is instantly cured by whatever excites surprize, or strongly engages the attention.[198]

Thus, in addition to the direct therapeutic benefits supposedly derived from aggressive treatments, the unpleasant and often painful nature of these methods contributed to their curative clout by distracting patients from their original complaints. This therapeutic reasoning was the same as that for more enjoyable diversions. The medical student William Gibbons included both varieties of distraction in his list of useful activities for hypochondriacs, recommending 'cheerful company; exercise; traveling... sailing in a balloon; flagellation, &c'.[199]

Guenter Risse has revealed the willingness of Cullen and other elite physicians to attempt more aggressive treatments on poor hospital patients than on wealthier private clients, who were more often prescribed palliatives and changes in regimen. Risse explains this disparity by arguing that within hospitals, a diagnosis was of primary importance, whereas in Cullen's private practice, paying patients were the most important factor.[200] In order to maintain his private clientele, Cullen was under pressure to keep his patients happy. Furthermore, wealthy private patients were able to afford more gentle and long-term remedies. With money to spend on repeated consultations, these patients could afford to tweak the non-naturals gradually, and to resort to more aggressive and potentially painful treatments only if these methods failed.

Alternatively, hospital patients necessitated quicker, and hence, more aggressive treatments. Furthermore, hospital doctors were under no obligation to please their patients. As objects of charity, poor nervous patients could either endure their given treatment or be dismissed. Although such an ultimatum seems surprisingly cruel for a physician like Cullen so highly regarded for his sensibility, it was justified on several grounds. First, hospital physicians were continually wary of patients feigning disease in order to gain admission. The nutritious food provided by the hospital was often better than what patients could personally afford. Likewise, the relative comfort and warmth of a hospital was also frequently superior to that of their own homes. This prompted additional concern among physicians about patients faking ailments during the cold winter months. Harsh remedies would ensure that only the truly ill would seek admission and remain in the hospital. For instance, when one physician suspected a fourteen year-old boy of feigning his ailments after he sought admission to the hospital twice for fainting fits in 1780, he ultimately threatened to place a hot iron on the boy's body. According to this physician, the mere threat of the iron meant that the 'impostor' immediately felt better.[201]

Secondly, and again as Risse has argued, Cullen assumed that the hospital's working-class charity patients were 'inherently more hardy' than the delicate and often sedentary patients that he encountered in his private practice.[202] Strengthened by labour and untainted by the corporeal curse of luxury, their systems were less delicate than those of the upper class, and could cope with more aggressive treatments. Thirdly, the fact that infirmary patients were largely intended as illustrative teaching material for budding young medical students on hospital rounds meant that doctors were eager to exhibit the full gamut of nervous remedies. From diet and exercise to bleedings and electrical treatments, the infirmary was the proper place for students to learn all that could be done for nervous patients.

While aggressive therapies were readily employed in the hospital setting, they were not exclusively used on the poor. Although they were not typically the first course of action, physicians and private patients were entirely willing to employ these methods in cases of obstinate nervous disorders. Blisters, issues, setons and bleedings commonly appeared in public hospital and private practice records alike. Bleeding was perhaps the most common aggressive therapy employed in treating nervous disease. It was particularly popular for treating hysteric patients with a supposed excess of blood in their systems. As Risse related in his research of the Edinburgh's Royal Infirmary, Gregory let twenty-eight ounces of blood from one hysteric patient over the course of five weeks, while in another instance Francis Home bled eight ounces from an hysteric immediately upon her entering the hospital. Cullen's private practice also reveals a significant number of nervous patients receiving, and requesting, bloodletting treatments. Indeed, one hypochondriac patient wrote to Cullen asking for nervous medications and directions for medicinal bathing, before hinting that a bleeding might also contribute to his relief: 'For some time past I have thought that the taking a little blood might be of service and this I am the more confirmed in that within these few days my eyes seem a little blood-run'.[203]

Patients were often bled for nervous headaches, which were attributed to an excess of blood. For instance, the nervous Miss Ellison was bled repeatedly by her physician when she experienced 'fullness and tightness in her head'.[204] Six months later, her physician proudly recorded that his treatment was effective: 'with occasional Bleedings the sense of fullness in the vessels of the head has not been so frequent'.[205] Hospital records also reveal nervous patients having leeches applied to their temples for headache relief.[206] Leeches were not only used on the head; in his 'Remarks on the Hypochondriacal disease and on the use of leeches in it' published in a 1781 edition of *The London Medical Journal,* the physician John Henry Shoenheider explained how one of his patients suffering from costiveness, flatulence, vertigo, haemorrhoids and low-spiritedness was treated with six leeches applied around his anus. As Shoenheider concluded, the leeches 'produced a copious flow of blood, which continued for several days, after which the costiveness and other symptoms were effectually removed'.[207]

Like bleeding, blistering was also used to relieve nervous patients of corrupted or excess humours. While this ancient practice again reveals interesting overlap between traditional humoural theory and nerve theory, the motives behind its use had changed. Instead of blistering patients purely in an effort to remove harmful humours as in ancient times, eighteenth-century nerve doctors administered blisters as counter-irritants, in an effort to draw the patient's attention away from their primary complaint. While readily applied to nervous hospital patients, blisters were also used in private practice. The medical student Robert King highly recommended them to all medical practitioners in his *Inaugural Essay on Blisters,* claiming that the 'action they produce, abstracts the excitement from the blood-vessels, and by diverting the attention from the melancholy subjects, the train of gloomy associations is broken off'.[208] In accordance with such advice the physician Alexander Douglas announced that as a result of 'the melancholy temperament' of his private nervous patient, Mr Anstruther, 'I have ordered his head to be shaved again & a blister to be applyd'.[209]

Blisters were formed by placing irritating substances on a patient's body. Recipes for these substances varied. At the Edinburgh Royal Infirmary, physicians placed dressings soaked in mustard flour and sulphuric acid on the patients' skin, keeping them in place with bandages for twelve to twenty-four hours until blisters formed. Another recipe for a blister-inducing plaister recommended by the London Pharmacopia directed physicians to 'take Spanish flies, one pound; plaister of wax, two pounds; prepared hogs' lard, half a pound... Having melted the plaister and lard, a little before they coagulate, sprinkle in the flies, reduced to a very fine powder'.[210] Potentially fatal if ingested, Spanish flies contained a poisonous chemical, which made them a natural irritant and the most important ingredient in this recipe. After forming, blisters were drained periodically. Dry cupping was yet another means of creating blisters; with this method, heated cups were placed on the skin, and the resultant suction caused blisters to rise.

Blisters were believed to do the most good if placed on sensitive areas of the body such as the neck, between the shoulder blades, or on the crown of the head.[211] Cullen's correspondence includes several cases where patients were instructed to shave their heads and apply blisters, in an effort to relieve headaches.[212] Cullen also occasionally recommended this remedy for patients suffering from severe mental agitation. For instance, in his treatment of a patient who was suffering from weak nerves and 'giddiness' as a result of 'some shock', Cullen recommended a blister as his first course of action:

> I think it very proper that in the first place you should have your hair cut and your head shaven, and that hereafter you should continue to keep it close shaven. A day after your head is first shaven put a blistering plaister of about three inches diameter be applied to the crown of your head. Let the plaister be without any loose flies and let it lye on constantly for several days only lifting it once a day to dry up or wipe off any moisture that may be discharged.

The patient was instructed to keep this blister for 'eight or ten days'.[213]

Aggressive treatments like blistering and bleeding were frequently conducted together. For instance, the physician Alexander Browne explained how he had treated one hysteric 'young Lady' suffering from 'faintishness and Languor and severe headaches', low spirits, 'a pain in her side and flatulencies after eating' with a combination of bleeding, blistering, diet and exercise:

> She has had two leeches and a blister applied upon the spine between her shoulders, with some cooling laxative medicines. Her diet has been light and easy of digestion consisting principally of white meats and cooling vegetables [and] when she could be prevailed upon to go out of the house she has rode on horseback and in a carriage as the weather would permit.[214]

Beyond addressing her physical symptoms, it is likely that this extensive treatment was meant to consume her attention and direct her thoughts away from her symptoms.

Setons, or running sores, were another counter-irritant, highly regarded for their ability to balance the system and divert nervous patients' attentions. Setons were made by threading an irritating piece of thread or horsehair through the skin. These threads were pulled back and forth throughout the day in order to prevent the sore from healing, and to promote drainage from the wound. In more serious cases, doctors used issues; like setons, issues were formed by threading bulky twine or an irritating object like a small bead through the skin. This created a greater amount of discharge than produced by a single thread.[215] Cullen prescribed issues for many of his private nervous patients. One such patient suffering from debilitating headaches was advised to undergo 'the shaving of the head and the application of a perpetual issue to the crown of it'. Yet, as Cullen suggested, 'if this should either fail in procuring a sufficient discharge, or give too much pain and uneasiness – a[n]... issue on the neck or one or both sides of the spine' could be used instead.[216] Some patients specifically requested issues. In a letter to Cullen in 1776, the nervous Thomas Christie wrote, 'I humbly propose to you, whether a perpetual issue or blister might not be very beneficial in my case – as it wd give free scope... to some portion of that humour which I take to be the cause of the Nervous symptoms'. Although he requested this treatment, Christie acknowledged its severity, asking Cullen 'If the continuance of an Issue... would weaken the Constitution – have a paralytic affects on the parts principally affected – or on the Nervous System in general'.[217] The willingness of so many nervous patients to undergo this daunting treatment attests to their belief in the severity of their nervous ailments.

As a newer form of treatment, electrotherapy was also used in nervous cases. It became particular popularity after 1745, when London's Royal Society encouraged members to investigate its virtues. Subsequently, during the second half of the century, the Royal Society's *Philosophical Transactions* published up to six articles a year on medical electricity.[218] By 1750 the Edinburgh Royal Infirmary was equipped with its own electrical machine.[219] Although electrotherapy was a fairly experimental treatment mid century, it was full of promise. In his anonymously penned *Desideratum: or, Electricity Made Plain and Useful* (1760), the minister and medical practitioner John Wesley noted that if medical men

> would only be diligent in making Experiments... I doubt not, but more nervous Disorders would be cured in one Year, by this single Remedy, than the whole *English Materia Medica* will cure, by the End of the Century.[220]

While to modern eyes the use of medical electricity appears shockingly unnatural, to eighteenth-century physicians, it was the ultimate natural medical treatment, allowing practitioners to harness the powers of the environment to reset a patient's bodily equilibrium. Although belief in an ethereal life force flowing through the nerves was largely discredited by the late eighteenth century, belief in a stimulating electric fluid flowing through the body was highly supported. Repeated experiments electrifying the limbs of dead frogs and seeing them 'jump' supported theories of electricity as a life force.[221] Conditions like paralysis were attributed to a deficiency of this force, requiring the application of electric shocks to the affected limbs in order to regain motor capabilities. Alternatively, an excess of electric fluid caused convulsive disorders and nervous fits. These conditions necessitated the application of 'negative electricity' achieved by drawing electricity from the body through sparks or electric auras.[222]

A course of medical electricity could be long and painful. Nevertheless, doctors and patients continually attested to its success. Cadwallader Evans, a medical student at the University of Philadelphia, submitted a paper to London's *Medical Observations and Inquiries* in 1754, relating the successful treatment of an American hysteric patient who had sought medical advice and taken nervous medicines for ten years without effect. He included an excerpt from a letter by the patient, detailing her desperate willingness to try any remedy:

> At length my spirits were quite broke and subdued with so many years affliction, and indeed I was almost grown desperate, being left without hope of relief. About this time there was great talk of the wonderful power of electricity; and as a person reduc'd to the last extremity... I resolv'd to try, let the event be what it might; for death was more desirable than life, on the terms I enjoy'd it.

During her first two weeks of treatment, she received eight electric shocks per day:

> indeed they were very severe. On receiving the first shock, I felt the fit very strong, but the second effectually carry'd it off... the symptoms gradually decreased, 'till at length they intirely left me.[223]

Later physicians recommended negative electrical treatments above the application of electric shocks. One anonymous physician treating a woman suffering from 'an uncommon Sensibility of the whole Nervous System' wrote of his patient,

> I think Electricity shd. be used once a Day or twice a Day, if that can be conveniently done – The best method is by not giving the shock, but by drawing Electrical sparks from the loins, thighs and legs. This may be continued for a month.[224]

Most physicians treating nervous cases with electricity advocated even milder forms of treatment. The medical student John Howell warned in his dissertation that the 'state of irritability of the system' in nervous cases meant that the electricity should be applied 'in its gentlest form'. He explained,

> The application of it by sparks, has, in many instances, brought on convulsions; and, in most cases of their application, the patient could not endure it. We must, therefore, begin with the aura, taken with a sharp pointed instrument, around the head; & it will be proper to augment its force as the patient can bear it.[225]

This treatment was administered by drawing the 'electric matter' from the patient's body by a pointed conductor. As Howell explained, patients felt a titillating effect, by which 'the sensibility and irritability are evidently augmented'.[226]

The London instrument maker Edward Nairne encouraged nervous patients to employ only the 'mildest methods', claiming that nervous disorders were 'sometimes aggravated by the application of too great a force'. For the removal of nervous head-aches he recommended that that electric conductors be only 'applied at a distance opposite the temples, and successively round the head'.

Only a 'gentle electrisation' was to be used in these cases as 'the effects of too much irritation are so exceedingly disagreeable'.[227] Aside from the painful effect of receiving too strong a shock, patients receiving electric therapy commonly complained of a 'persistently itchy feeling' following their treatment. Doctors attributed this sensation to residual electric particles inside of the patient's body, stimulating their nervous fibres.[228] While uncomfortable, these symptoms assured patients that the treatment was having an effect.

As with most other aggressive treatments, medical electricity was prescribed for hospital patients and for private nervous patients who were willing to withstand temporary discomfort in hopes of a cure. Private patients could seek electrical treatments from trained medical practitioners at places like the London Electrical Dispensary, which opened in 1793. Even wealthier patients could invest in their own electrical machines, which were conveniently designed with jointed conductors for self-application.[229] The willingness of patients to endure, request and even self-inflict these remedies again testifies to the depth of their suffering and the strength of their desire to recover.

Mixing and matching

Nervous sufferers typically engaged in a wide range of treatments. Most doctors recommended attention to several of the non-naturals at once. For example, in his prescription for a patient suffering from 'tremors of the nerves', 'headaches, watchfulness, anxieties, dimness of sight, loss of memory, and a confused, indistinct, waver apprehension of things', one Dr Raymond recommended attention to all of the non-naturals. The patient was instructed to 'rise early', and to engage in an hour of exercise such as walking, riding, or shuttlecock. He was advised to 'avoid all application of mind, violent passions, study, [or] business' and to 'search for amusement, for cheerful company, [and] for a climate that is warm & dry'. The bulk of Dr Raymond's prescription regarded diet; the patient was to avoid all foods that were 'heavy and hard of digestion', as well as 'all aliments which are apt to ferment such as all sorts of milks, cheese, &c&c'.[230]

In a similar fashion, patients taking medication typically tried several different prescriptions. For instance, suffering from a long list of symptoms including 'exquisite pain in the Hypochondria... pains thro' the rest of her body... frequent belchings of wind, restlessness, anxiety... want of appetite, sometimes vomitings, [and] costiveness, the hysteric Miss Betty Lindsay was prescribed an equally long list of medications. Her doctor noted that she had taken tinctures and undergone 'a course of Aromaticks, gums, bark, steel, opiates... & some topical applications &c'., although 'she found but little benefit from all these'.[231]

Physicians most commonly prescribed a mixture of treatment therapies. Writing to Cullen on behalf of a patient suffering from complaints 'intirely of the nervous kind' including 'giddiness in her head, violent shakings and every sensation of fainting away', William Ingham described the extensive course of treatment that he had prescribed. In addition to regular bleedings of four to five ounces, his patent had taken 'a variety of medicines [such] as asafetida, camphor, valerian bark, [and] cinnabar'. Ingham further noted that she 'had a perpetual blister at the top of her head and has now an issue'.[232] Similarly, another physician wrote to Cullen regarding a patient, Mr Macarthur, who was suffering from 'a great delicacy in the nervous system'. In an effort to treat the patient's 'complaint of winds and spasmodick contractions of the stomach', the doctor prescribed an 'antiscorbutick juice from the Edinburgh pharmacopeia', exercise on horseback, a diet void of 'flatulent food', and a trip to the chalybeate waters.

Some patients employed multiple modes of treatment merely for the sake of variety. The physician for one Mr Hogarth wrote to Cullen that his patient was taking a 'nervous mixture' in addition to the issue on his head, a restricted diet and a steady course of exercise on horseback. Despite this treatment, Mr Hogarth's low spirits were 'much the same', the wind in his stomach and bad appetite had 'encreased', and his pulse continued to 'flutter' upon any agitation. Writing to Cullen in 1781, the physician requested a recommended alteration of this regimen, which would bring more relief and offer some variety: 'your varying the mode [of treatment] would be agreeable, as people of his Disposition tire so soon of one form of Medicines'.[233]

Yet multiple therapies were most often employed due to the sheer obstinacy of nervous conditions. The nervous Miss Bell Shaw, described by her physician as having a 'weak [and] puny constitution' endured a particularly lengthy list of treatments for her ongoing 'nausea, frequent pains on the stomach', 'want of appetite' and costiveness, which had worsened since the death of her father. Advising Cullen of his unsuccessful efforts, Miss Shaw's physician informed him that she had been prescribed 'a light and nourishing diet', free of anything 'heavy or flatulent', 'gentle exercise' out of doors,

> various medicines of the nervous and antispasmodic kind, an asafetida, caster, valerian, ether rubbed on the temples, Blisters applied to the back, &c. but what seem'd of most service, was a dose of Laudanum every night at bedtime.[234]

In another obstinate case, the physician for a nervous Mr Davidson wrote to Cullen in 1779 indicating that his patient suffered from stomach complaints, 'violent' head aches causing 'giddiness & stupidity in the brain', 'noise in the Ears' and 'clouded' eyes. The doctor noted that Mr Davidson frequently 'force[d] himself to vomit for temporary ease', and that he was also 'very much relieved by a discharge of wind'. In addition to these do-it-yourself methods, the doctor indicated that Mr Davidson employed several medically prescribed treatments:

The patients regimen has been to drink valerian in infusion, he uses gum pills, has been blistered on the back legs & cupping with white mustard & a course of the Barks, which last has only been taked in small quantity, he has also bathed his feat in warm water once a day. But the disorder is unremoved ...[235]

Regardless of the treatment prescribed, the road to recovery for nervous patients was long and uncertain.

Conclusion

Whether gulping spa water or tar water, mixing tinctures or rushing to the apothecary shop, engaging in exercise or administering electrical treatments, eating lightly or dosing heavily, nervous patients endured a wealth of disruptive, time-consuming and often painful remedies. The spectrum of discomfort caused by nervous remedies was large, ranging from the strong physical pain of cupping and regular vomiting to the mere potential inconvenience of travel for a 'change of air'. Yet as this chapter has shown, all nervous treatments, including seemingly enjoyable activities and trips to the spa, were firmly rooted in medical theory. While all nervous treatments demanded patience and fortitude on the part of sufferers, the particular willingness of patients to undergo aggressive physical treatments attests most strongly to the seriousness with which they regarded their conditions. Although pauper patients in hospital settings were most readily subjected to aggressive treatment, wealthy patients capable of affording gentler and longer-term therapies also frequently opted for more aggressive, and hence, they hoped, more successful cures. In this way, although class was relevant to the type of treatment received by nervous patients, belief in the reality of nervous ailments and faith in the curative capabilities of medical science defied all socio-economic boundaries. Similarly, the presence of poor nervous patients in hospitals and the persistent discussion of nervous disease in health manuals intended for the middling classes challenges long-held notions of nervous ailments as the exclusive preserve of society's elite. While this examination of the medical treatment of nervous disease further undermines the accuracy of popular perceptions of nervous disease as a 'fashionable disorder', the following chapter argues that by the end of the century, nervous sufferings were decidedly démodé.

5 A DISEASE OF THE BODY AND OF THE TIMES

The second half of the eighteenth century witnessed a quiet revolution in public discourse about the nerves. In the 1750s and early 60s the public was still rapt in the romantic portrayal of nervous conditions presented by George Cheyne in 1733, revelling in the delicate swoons of Richardson's Pamela and Clarissa, with well-to-do ladies and gentlemen congratulating themselves on the superior quality of their nervous sensibilities. Melancholics were creative geniuses, and hypochondriacs were morally superior. By the turn of the century this story had significantly changed. Nervous disease no longer simply implied the progress of civilization; it implied over-civilization, luxury, vanity, sloth, national decline and artificial manners. Nervous sufferers who were once objects of praise, admiration and pity became instead objects of ridicule and scorn. This chapter explores both the medical and social debates that contributed to this radically changed climate of opinion.

Popular discussions of the nerves written and read by the middle- and upper-class laity abounded throughout the century, infiltrating moral, prescriptive, religious and political publications alike. Already in the first half of the century, the reading public was comfortable relating the nerves to wider social phenomena; the *Gentleman's Magazine* and *Scots Magazine* persistently associated nervous sensibility with refined modern manners; magazines and prescriptive literature for young ladies tirelessly referred to their appropriately delicate and feminine nerves; religious tracts emphasized the Christian fortitude of sufferers combating nervous disease, and political writings drew hyperbolic and flattering conclusions about Britain's superior civilization in relation to the nervously insensible colonials of its empire.

When looking at the trajectory of public discourse about nervous disease during the first half of the century, one would expect it to continue along the same fashionable course throughout the second half of the century. Yet the reality of the phenomenon was not so straightforward. From the 1760s onward there appeared a number of medical texts designed to separate the medical theory from the social implications of nervous disease. As discussed in Chapter One, the first of many such texts, Robert Whytt's all-encompassing treatise *On Nerv-*

ous, Hypochondriac, or Hysteric Diseases (1764), discussed nervous disease in an entirely dispassionate manner without reference to the class, wealth, or superior sensibilities of sufferers. After Whytt, other first-tier physicians followed suit, writing their own strictly academic texts on the nerves.

While first-tier physicians avoided social and flattering discussions of the nerves, many second-tier physicians actively denied the fashionable implications of nervous disorders. By the mid-1770s a growing body of medical evidence suggested that nervous disorders were on the rise among the poorer classes. Robbed of its exclusive social cachet, an increasing number of doctors (particularly social critics) began to portray nervous disease as less a disease of a luxurious few than of a degenerate nation at large. These physicians were part of a larger late eighteenth-century trend of melding professional medical expertise with moral advice intended to promote public health and to prevent further national decline. Given the fact that social critics generally wrote for a non-medical audience, it is not surprising to find that the second half of the century also witnessed a rise in the number of disparaging portrayals of nervous sufferers in non-medical texts.

Fashionable notions of the nerves did not suddenly cease in the second half of the century. Nervous and fainting heroines held popular appeal long after the publication of Whytt's treatise, with Henry Mackenzie's *Man of Feeling* (1771) and Fanny Burney's *Evelina* (1778) yet to be written. I it ......, ...larly among the publications of social .... and quack practitioners eager to attract a wealthy clientele, vestiges of older medical theories insisting upon the ...... nature of nervous sufferings continued through the century. Thus, nervous disease persisted from the 1760s to the 1790s as the object of occasional praise but growing censure. Yet by the turn of the century, the overwhelming majority of medical and social publications discussing nervous disease did so in a negative light – a view best characterized by Thomas Trotter's *View of the Nervous Temperament* (1807).[1]

Its investigation of the reasons behind the downward trend of the status of nervous disorders from Whytt's *Observations* in 1764 to Trotter's *View* of 1807, this chapter will focus on four themes both recurrent in the period's medical and social discussions of the nerves, and illustrative of its general developments: civilization, class, gender and politics. With regard to civilization it will show how, whereas in the first half of the century doctors and the general public interpreted the presence of nervous disease as a positive indication of Britain's increasing refinement, improved manners, and growing commercial strength, by the end of the century the heightened presence of nervous sufferers indicated the decline of civilization and a loss of virtue. Likewise, it will reveal how a supposedly increasing number of sufferers, particularly those of the lower class, buttressed pre-existing popular fears of over-civilization, proving that even the most plain-living members of society had become too exposed to luxurious habits.

This chapter will also demonstrate how women, once praised for their innately delicate nervous systems, were chastised later in the century for increasing the delicacy of their already vulnerable nerves through immoderate and luxurious living – a sin which, in light of a growing emphasis on hereditary nervousness, destined the next generation for even greater rates of nervous disease. Male sufferers were also victims of this changing view of nervousness. Whereas men were commonly praised mid-century for possessing weak nerves and humane sensibilities, the heightened threat of military invasion by the French towards the end of the century prompted popular fears of 'soft soldiers', and a consequent portrayal of nervous males as effeminate weaklings. The political implications of nervous sufferings also affected England's national self-image. During the middle of the century, Englishmen considered themselves perfectly balanced between the overwhelming effeminacy of the French and the embarrassingly rude health of non-nervous and unfeeling Scots.[2] Yet by the end of the century, Scottish heartiness was discussed in terms of approbation, as authors, medical and otherwise, lamented that the English had sunk even deeper into the pit of effeminacy than the French.

In addition to demonstrating the fading lustre of nervous disease over the course of the second half of the century, these themes also exhibit the period's complex interplay between medicine and society. The historiography of nervous disease in the eighteenth century has ably proven the strong role that societal factors played in shaping eighteenth-century medicine. Christopher Lawrence largely attributes the nerve theory taught by the eminent Edinburgh professors to the intellectual climate of the Scottish Enlightenment and to the philosophical teachings of men like Adam Smith and David Hume.[3] Likewise, Nicholas Jewson's discussion of the power of patronage to shape medical theory, along with Roy Porter and G.S. Rousseau's work on the fashionable implications of nervous disease, have convincingly expressed the effects of the commercial on the medical world. Porter and Rousseau's particular attention to nerve doctors like George Cheyne, James Makittrick Adair and the French physician Samuel Tissot has lent much credibility to their arguments in support of a culturally influenced medicine; the latter two physicians even explicitly referred to nervous disease as a 'fashionable disorder'.[4]

While nervous disease was often regarded as a 'distinguished disorder', its fashionable implications should not be allowed to overshadow its serious significance to the eighteenth-century medical world, or the reciprocal impression that medicine made on society. Thus, while this chapter acknowledges the ways in which physicians necessarily responded to and engaged with society in the construction of medical theories, it primarily seeks to demonstrate how nerve theory infiltrated and influenced society, providing the public with a medical lens through which to view, or magnify, social problems.

Linking Society, Sensation and the Soul: The Nerves in the Eighteenth Century

When Whytt assumed the post of professor of the practice of medicine at the University of Edinburgh in 1747, he brought with him a more formal and well-defined understanding of nerve theory than ever before. Published as a text for medical students, the medical theory set forth in Whytt's treatise quickly gained favour among learned physicians, dominating university-taught medicine for decades. Following his treatise, nervous disease gained added credibility as a serious physiological disorder rather than simply a social disease symptomatic of status and fashionable sensibilities.

Whytt's colleague and professional successor, William Cullen, also placed enormous emphasis on the role of the nervous system in modern medicine. While Cullen's private correspondence occasionally acknowledged underlying beliefs regarding the social implications of disordered nerves, his formal publications, as discussed in Chapter Two, contained only the strictly scientific aspects of the nervous system. The serious nature of these publications, in concert with the later serious writings that they inspired, provided little fodder for flattering social discussions of the nerves. Thus, together with Whytt, Cullen further strengthened the status of nervous disease as a genuine and pathologically significant medical disorder. The implications of this fortified reputation of nervous disease were visible even outside of the professional sphere. With his hugely successful private practice, Cullen's reputation was widely regarded among the British public. So too was his academic medical theory. The *Edinburgh Mercury* commonly informed its readership of the latest happenings at the medical school, and, as is clear from Cullen's correspondence, news of his system spread internationally through both word of mouth and a vast trail of references to his work in the footnotes of other physicians publishing for the public.[5] As the nervous system reached new heights in the Edinburgh medical school curriculum, nervous disease became an increasingly important and serious topic of discussion within both the medical and social realms of British society.

Part of the seriousness with which nervous disease was regarded stemmed from the sense that it was a growing problem. Of course, anxiety over the growing presence of nervous disorders was not entirely new to the period. In 1681 Sir William Temple noted that hypochondriacal disorders 'employ our Physicians, perhaps more than other Diseases'. That same year, Sydenham surmised that 'Hysterick Diseases, at least those that go under that Name, are half... the Chronical diseases'.[6] By 1733 Cheyne asserted that 'The Frequency of Nervous Disorders' was 'beyond what they have been in former times', composing 'almost one third of the Complaints of People of Condition in England'.[7] The sense that the number of nervous sufferers was growing continued throughout the century, with the perceived number of patients greatly outweighing the actual number of cases recorded. The *London Medical Journal* from 1781 took it for granted that all of its readers were aware of Britain's unprecedented number of nervous sufferers, claiming that, 'it is well known that nervous diseases are much more frequent now than they were formerly'.[8] By the nineteenth century the perceived number of sufferers had escalated to previously unimaginable proportions. Despite the fact that private case notes and hospital records reveal that during this time nervous patients generally composed only 1–5 per cent of the practices of treating physicians, doctors well-versed in notions of England's supposed moral decay were collectively under the impression that the numbers were much higher. In one of the most exaggerated estimates of nervous sufferers, Trotter claimed that

> In the present day, this class of diseases forms by far the largest proportion of the whole, which come under the treatment of the physician. Sydenham at the conclusion of the seventeenth century, computed fevers to constitute two thirds of the diseases of mankind. But, at the beginning of the nineteenth century, we do not hesitate to affirm, that *nervous disorders* have now taken the place of fevers, and may be justly reckoned two thirds of the whole, with which civilized society is afflicted.[9]

As a strong social reformer, there is little doubt that Trotter's generous estimate could buttress his calls for change. Yet these high estimates were not entirely self-motivated. As will be discussed, even medical students at the University of Edinburgh who had not yet opened their own practices assumed that the number of nervous sufferers was on the rise in the second half of the century.

Eager to explain the reasons behind this supposedly growing group, nerve doctors commonly looked to societal causes. Although discussing the congratulatory social implications of nervous disease was frowned upon by the medical elite after Whytt and Cullen, investigating the social causes of nervous disease was simply good practice. As discussed in Chapter One, the link between nervous disease and society was as old as the medical understanding of the nerves themselves. Late in the seventeenth century, the physician Thomas Willis identified the nerves as the conduits of sensation, responsible for relaying external impressions to the brain and soul. Consequently, man's environment, society and feelings were directly related to his physical health through his nerves, encompassing what Rousseau has termed an 'integrated physiology of man'.[10] 'Disordered nerves' became the assigned explanation for ailments presumably instigated by residence in unhealthy climates, indulgence in unhealthy lifestyles and unregulated passions. Consequently, nervous disease was commonly discussed in relation to refinement and modern consumer society with all of the unwholesome city living and nerve-weakening luxury that these entailed.

A Disease of Civilization

Cheyne proudly drew the connection between refinement, consumer society and disordered nerves in the *English Malady*, claiming that the rate of nervous disease had increased in England 'since our Wealth has increas'd, and our Navigation has been extended'.[11] Pride over the level of civilization implied by nervous disease was much discussed outside of the medical sphere. Twenty-four years after Cheyne's *English Malady*, an anonymous political author praised England's newly polite national character, claiming of sensation and the human frame that 'The more delicate it is, the more perfect; and the more perfect, the more we shew the dignity of our nature'. Citing the superior manners, philosophy and science of modern Englishmen, the author insisted that 'we owe the arts to this delicate texture of our nerves and fibres'.[12] While such positive connections were frequently forged between delicate nerves and civilization, they were most often posited in the first half or the middle of the century, when there was a sense that Britain had not yet reached its full potential at the pinnacle of civilization.

Yet as James Raven has explained, the 1770s to 1790s witnessed a popular backlash against modern civilization and luxury as the 'harbinger of indolence, effeminacy, insubordination, and social and political debility'.[13] At the same time, negative notions regarding the connection between civilization and nervous disease intensified in sincerity and urgency. There was a growing sense in both the medical and social sphere that England's level of refinement had finally peaked. By 1779 James Boswell reminded readers of his column in the *London Magazine*, 'The Hypochondriack' that

> Politicians and historians have told us from book to book, and from age to age, that all communities or states gradually rise from imperfect and coarse beginnings, till they attain to a certain degree of excellence and refinement; that then their progress is stopped, and instead of advancing farther, they, like Sysiphus's stone, roll back again into their original situation.[14]

As countless physicians warned the public, society had reached a point where healthy nerves were no longer compatible with modern manners. As early as 1765, the famed Edinburgh physician John Gregory worried that 'the softness and effeminacy of modern manners' had 'deprived' modern Britons of their 'natural defence' against 'debility and morbid sensibility of the nervous system'.[15] Non-medical writers discussing social ills also became increasingly anxious about the dangers that over-indulgence posed to the physical and moral health of the nation in the latter half of the century.

Modern manners and luxurious habits which had once implied refinement seemed increasingly irresponsible as the nation teetered on the precipice of civilization towards an immoral, degenerate and persistently nervous state. Like Boswell, the recovered nervous sufferer and historian Edward Gibbon hinted at the dangerous parallels between Britain's modern degenerate society and the fall of the Roman empire, noting how Rome's opulence ultimately resulted in the 'corruption of manners and principles' and how prosperity had ruinously 'relaxed the nerves of discipline'.[16] The *Female Spectator* also warned readers of the precarious state of civilization: 'LONDON has been call'd a second *Rome*, and we have flatter'd ourselves that the comparison has been just; but pray Heaven we may never be too like it in its decline'.[17] Anticipating the pernicious and unhealthy consequences of modern 'civilized' company, the *Female Spectator* decried countless modern amusements. The penchant for card playing in fashionable society was of particular concern to the editors of the magazine:

> Does it [gaming] invigorate the body, add to the elasticity of the nerves, or render the blood more pure and florid? – On the contrary... is not the body, by continuing so many hours in one posture, coop'd up, as it were, at a table, and without any significant motion, benumbed, and almost debilitated?[18]

Modern novel reading also came under persistent attack well through the turn of the nineteenth century by medical writers who warned against the overly inflamed passions which fiction could provoke. Gregory warned in 1774 that modern novels was likely to 'inflame the passions and to corrupt the heart', while in 1802 Thomas Beddoes insisted that the 'perusal of light books' tended to 'injure the perceptive and associating faculties, and by consequence to spread havoc through the nervous system'.[19] Similarly, in 1807 Trotter warned that

> The passion of *novel reading*... is one of the great causes of nervous disorders. The mind that can amuse itself with the love-sick trash of most modern compositions of this kind, seeks enjoyment beneath the level of a rational being... To the female mind in particular, as being endued with finer feeling, this species of literary poison has been often fatal; and some of the most unfortunate of the sex have imputed their ruin chiefly to reading of novels.[20]

Such medical and social writings in the final quarter of the eighteenth century reveal a surprisingly coherent collective belief that Britain had passed her prime in terms of civilization and nervous health. Though having moved beyond the primitive state of their ancestors, Britons had entered a state of artificial living. Given medical belief in the nerves as conduits between the external world and the body, doctors commonly blamed nervous ailments on these luxurious and intemperate lifestyles. According to most physicians at the end of the century, the cure for both the immorality of modernity and the nervous diseases that it had caused was moderation. Hence, second-tier nerve doctors late in the eighteenth and early nineteenth centuries like Beddoes and Trotter composed tracts on the nerves that were as moral as they were medical, imploring the public to return to a more simple way of living.[21] As Beddoes advised his countrymen,

> The English are more remarkable than any other people on the globe for the accumu-
> lation of *comforts*, and, indeed, unhappily we pique ourselves upon the distinction. I
> am not going to advise any one to discard his or her comforts all at once. I would only
> open a course of reflection, by which they may satisfy themselves that the reliance
> they place on externals is vain, and that those who have most comforts about them,
> are commonly the most comfortless of all mortals.[22]

Second-tier social critics were not the only medical practitioners to recognize the important link between moderation, virtue and health. First-tier nerve doctors like Gregory, Andrew Wilson and John Coakley Lettsom also took seriously their role as moral guardians, although their prescriptive messages for society did not infiltrate their academic publications on the nerves.[23] Wilson's *Rational Advice to the Military* (1780) warned of the ill health that would result from the 'incautiousness and indiscretion of individuals in the mismanagement of themselves'.[24] Equally instructive was Lettsom's *Hints Designed to Promote Beneficence, Temperance, and Medical Science* (1797), which described such matters as proper female behaviour and the dangers of drinking to excess, together with his *Hints Addressed to Card Parties* (1798), which insisted on the immorality of gambling. Likewise, Gregory's *Comparative View* (1774) remarked on such topics as the improper, unnatural and unhealthy tendency of modern mothers not to nurse their own children, and the danger that 'pursuits of commerce' posed to the health and virtue of the human species.[25]

Recognition of the connection between luxury, immorality and poor health was not exclusive to the medical profession. The Scottish judge and writer Henry Home argued that there was a general connection between 'down beds, soft pillows... easy seats', rich foods and rising mortality, claiming that 'It has not escaped observation, that between the years 1740 and 1770 no fewer than six mayors of London died in office, a greater number than in the preceding 500 years: such havock doth luxury in eating make'.[26] The diarist Catherine Powys similarly acknowledged the dangers of city living, writing privately in her journal that while in London she spent 'every evening [going] from Card Party to Card party, where the heat of each room is hardly bearable, which with the terrible late hours of the present Times, makes one not the least wonder, that most people, are complaining of ill health'.[27]

This 'ill health' was not limited to nervous disease. Conditions like gout and obesity were also frequently discussed with reference to modern luxury. Yet unlike other ailments, nervous disease was of particular danger to modern Britons for its psychological effect on sufferers; for in addition to physical symptoms such as heart palpitations, digestive problems and overall bodily weakness, nervous disease also wreaked havoc on sufferers mentally, leading to a nation of overly-sensitive, timid and weak-willed citizens, void of nationalistic spirit and traditional virtue. Thus, medical accounts of a growing number of nervous patients added further fuel to popular anxieties regarding the morality of modern consumer society and the physical and moral health of the nation.

A Disease of the Masses

The perceived rise of lower class sufferers was of particular concern to physicians and moralists. In the beginning of the century, doctors like Cheyne insisted that nervous disorders only plagued 'people of condition'.[28] Even as late as 1769 Gregory echoed this message, lecturing upon the way in which 'delicate' people suffering from strong impressions and consequent nervous disorders were generally of the 'better sort': 'this temperament commonly attends the rich, indolent and luxuriant. The labouring people are never attacked with nervous disease'.[29] Yet as the century progressed, doctors feared that the distemper was spreading to all ranks of society. In 1774, Cullen's student, the American physician Benjamin Rush, wrote that 'the hysteric and hypochondriac disorders, once peculiar to the chambers of the great are now to be found in our kitchens and workshops'.[30] The London physician Sayer Walker warned in *Treatise on Nervous Diseases* (1796) that 'these diseases are not the exclusive evil of the rich: they visit the cottage as well as the mansion'.[31] Likewise, in 1807 Trotter warned his reading public that 'nervous ailments are no longer confined to the better ranks in life, but rapidly extending to the poorer classes'.[32] Despite such bold claims, none of these physicians provided quantifiable evidence of this supposed surge in nervous cases. Yet however groundless these claims actually were, the fear and paranoia that they provoked were real.

This paranoia was not limited to the medical world. The proliferation of medical treatises composed for a lay audience in the eighteenth century meant that discussions about lower class sufferers quickly appeared in sources intended for the general public. Boswell's column 'On Hypochondria' in the February 1778 edition of the *London Magazine* denied the notion of the 'fashionable sufferer' in his remark that 'from having closely studied numbers affected with that disease; I must... beg leave to doubt the proposition, that it is peculiarly to be found in men of remarkable excellence'. Instead, he claimed, 'Melancholy, or Hypochondria, like the fever or gout, or any other disease, is incident to all sorts of men, from the wisest to the most foolish'.[33]

Medical explanations for a growing group of nervous sufferers were many. In his *Hints Designed to Promote Beneficence, Temperance, and Medical Science* (1797), Lettsom surmised that some poor patients suffered as a result of their contact with the rich. As he explained, domestic servants

> have been accustomed to the plenty of their master's table; and frequently receive indulgences to which the abject Poor have not been used: by this, and a continual intercourse with people of decent manners, they acquire a degree of delicacy of body, as well as sensibility of mind, that makes them less able to undergo difficulties, or exposure to the wide world.[34]

The supposed tendency of lower-class citizens to imitate the manners of their superiors, so frequently discussed from the 1760s onwards, only worsened matters. For instance, the drinking of tea and coffee, which doctors like Heberden warned would 'weaken the nervous system and the Brain' was, according to many physicians, increasingly adopted by the lower classes as a means of mimicking upper-class fashions. As Heberden lamented in his private notebook, while the 'present age has introduced many things our forefathers were ignorant of, Tobacco, Tea, coffee, sugar, silk, & many aromatics & a hundred other things', coffee drinking was a particularly pernicious modern habit. For, he argued, 'the Great among us, as they have the means, distinguish themselves from the Vulgar [by drinking coffee]; & these, to lessen the senses of inferiority, imitate them, & thus new manners are easily introduced'.[35] Similarly, in 1764 the physician Alexander Sutherland noted that 'from the prince to the peasant, Tea and Coffee are now in constant use. Never were nervous diseases so frequent as at this day. The question of Tea and Coffee cannot therefore be indifferent'.[36]

Lettsom's *Natural History of the Tea-Tree* (1772), discussing the detrimental effect of tea on the nerves, noted that it was primarily the upper class, or people with the 'most tender and delicate constitutions' who were 'most affected by the free use of Tea'.[37] Furthermore, Lettsom argued, 'The finer the Tea, the more obvious are these [nervous] effects. It is perhaps for this, amongst other reasons, that the lower classes of people, who can only procure the most common, are in general the least sufferers'. In an effort to explain the very presence of nervous disorders among the lower classes Lettsom wrote,

I am in general, but also very amongst them there are many who actually suffer much by it: they drink it as long as it yields any taste... and thus the quantity which they take, and the degree of heat in which it is drank, conspire to produce in them, what the finer kinds of Tea effect in their superiors.[38]

Nine years later, the physician Alexander Thompson noted in the introduction to his *Enquiry into the Nature, Causes, and Method of Cure of Nervous Disorders* (1781), that 'An opinion prevails that nervous disorders are more frequent in this country at present, than in any former period. This is commonly imputed to the drinking of tea, now so general among people of all ranks'.[39] Eager young medical students in the Royal Medical Society of Edinburgh also discussed the relationship between tea and a growing group of sufferers. After introducing the hypochondriac case of a day labourer, one medical student concluded his dissertation with the claim that Hypochondria 'is a disease which seems more prevalent in the present Age than in former ones... let it suffice to observe that the more universal use of warm debilitating Liquors such as Tea &c. in the present age may perhaps in some measure account for it'.[40]

Physicians clearly believed that the presence of nervous disease among the poorer classes was largely due to an amoral spread of luxury, with domestic servants invited to indulge in the comforts of their superiors, and the working classes greedily gulping large quantities of cheap tea. Tea was an easy way to measure the spread of luxury. As Lettsom calculated in the *History*, in the beginning of the eighteenth century, the East India Company imported less than 50,000 pounds of tea per year. By 1797 he claimed, these importations had increased to

> twenty millions of pounds; being an increase of four hundred fold in less than 100 years, and answers to the rate of more than a pound weight each in the course of the year, for the individuals of all ranks, sexes, and ages.[41]

Indeed, whereas England's population grew by 14 per cent in the final fifteen years of the eighteenth century, tea consumption increased by nearly 98 per cent.[42] By the turn of the century, it was clear that, like tea-drinking, nervous disease no longer held the exclusive status that it did one hundred years before. The reported rise in the number of poor sufferers lent systematic credibility to popular fears regarding the spread of luxury and declining morality; if a disease of luxury had infiltrated even the lowest and most 'simple' level of society, it was clear that fears of degeneration were fast becoming a reality.

In addition to fuelling fears of degeneration, the presence of poor nervous sufferers also inflamed existing anxieties among the nobility and upper-middling classes regarding the disintegration of traditional hierarchy and class difference. Already during the period, wealthy and retired businessmen were increasingly able to purchase expensive country estates that were once the exclusive preserve of the landed gentry, shopping on credit was becoming more common, and nabobs and the nouveaux riches were able to imitate the once-distinguishing manners of the nobility. The emulation of even middle-class habits by lower-class pretenders seemed to shake the foundations of an already teetering status quo. Beyond this, as Wayne Wild has explained, nerve theory 'facilitated social mobility by making "gentility" attainable to the middling class through the emulation of the new "sensibility"'.[43] The presence of paupers drinking tea and suffering from a disease that was once indicative of strictly upper-class sensibilities rubbed salt in the wound of an upper class that already feared the encroaching ruin of established hierarchy.

Medical preoccupation with the supposedly over-indulgent lower class sharply increased at the end of the eighteenth century, as doctors assumed increasing responsibility for the nation's moral health. While not new to the period, the link between moral and medical matters achieved renewed vigour as a result of the growing popularity of the mid-century's vitalist theories. Unlike mechanist physicians of the early eighteenth century who viewed the body as a collection of fluids, tubes and vessels which worked like a well-oiled machine in health, and whose malfunctions prompted disease, vitalist physicians in the latter half of the eighteenth century catered to a more holistic view, where external and environmental forces directly affected the internal body.

Cullen reflected this vitalist stance in his *Nosology* (1769), through his discussion of the proximal and remote causes of disease. Proximal causes of disease were malfunctions within the body like debility and spasms, which could be medically treated. Remote causes referred only to external origins of disease, including the non-naturals, cold, dirt, damp, miasma and contagion. These causes affected the body internally via the sensible nervous system.[44] Nerve doctors in the second half of the century subscribed to this holistic view of the body, emphasizing the role of sympathy between bodily organs, and the way in which nervous sensibility linked the physical health of the body with its social and atmospheric environment. The consequence of this holistic theory was a belief in the medical profession's ability to prevent disease through the manipulation of unhealthy environments and the remote causes of disease.[45]

The lower classes were suffering from disordered nerves as a result of inappropriate desire; lured by the temptation of luxury, they amorally adopted the manners of their social superiors at the expense of their health. Yet as more doctors noted by the end of the century, the poor were victim to a wealth of other dangerous diseases. The growth of cities in the eighteenth century resulted in close populations, slums and a proliferation of disease caused by filth and spread by either miasma or contagion.[46] Cullen's *First Lines* (1777) emphasised the way in which crowded places were susceptible to a 'human effluvia' that could lead to illness.[47] As supporters of this view surmised, moral attention to cleanliness, ventilation and order, together with the traditional regulation of diet and exercise, could help to prevent disease.

The military physician Sir John Pringle was at the forefront of the emphasis on the connection between morality, cleanliness and health. As early as 1752, Pringle's *Observations on the Diseases of the Army* listed uncleanliness alongside the poor regulation of the non-naturals, putrid air, heat, cold and moisture as the principal causes of disease 'most incident to an army'.[48] It was through proper personal and institutional discipline that environments would remain clean, and that people would conduct their lives in an orderly, judicious and healthy manner. After Pringle, and with Cullen's publications delineating the many causes of disease, interest in the regulation of cleanliness and virtue for the restoration and maintenance of health was applied to other heavily populated and medically problematic institutions including the navy, hospitals and jails.[49] As city populations grew to unprecedented heights at the turn of the nineteenth century, this reform was increasingly applied to the lives and urban dwellings of the poor.

Medical concern over the health of the poor reached a fevered pitch in the early Victorian period with Edwin Chadwick's *Report on the Sanitary Condition of the Labouring Population of Great Britain* (1842). Advocating public intervention to enforce proper drainage, ventilation and general sanitation in the slums, Chadwick believed that it was possible to break the supposed self-perpetuating and never-ending cycle of immorality, filth and disease among the lower classes. The poor, Chadwick argued, were 'improvident, reckless, and intemperate, and with habitual avidity for sensual gratification'.[50] Whereas in the eighteenth century, the lower classes were commonly associated with good health as a result of their simple diets and physical labour, in the nineteenth century, they were associated with poor health as a result of uncleanliness and moral laxity.[51] Unable to temper their desires, the poor were prone to over-indulgence, likely to quench their thirst with gin, indulge their laziness in unemployment, and wile away their days amidst the filth of their disease-ridden dwellings. Firm in their belief that health was the result of good morals and clean environments, nineteenth century physicians assumed the role of 'medical police', herding the poor into healthier styles of living. Although medical inspectors could enforce proper sanitation and behaviour, it was up to the middle and upper echelons of society to set a positive example for their social inferiors.

In this light, moderation, self-control and industrious behaviour were increasingly heralded as the mark of a civilized man in the late eighteenth and early nineteenth centuries: all qualities that were antithetical to nervous disease.[52] Furthermore, amidst this climate of institutional and moral reform, action and selfless activism were deeply admired, whereas antisocial or supposedly malingering valetudinarians were viewed as selfish drains on society's resources. As George Grinnell has explained, hypochondria in the Romantic era had become 'a symptom of excessive and misdirected sensitivity'.[53] Healthy citizens implied a strong and well-ordered civilization. Thus, in addition to closely regulating matters of health, doctors late in the century embraced a much wider role as society's moral guardians, reforming British institutions and morals in an effort to protect British civilization.

A Disease of the Weak-Willed

Whereas the sick role had long promised invalids comfort, sympathy and exemption from social responsibility, popular ideas were changing regarding the suitability of such behaviour in an enlightened age. Reclusive invalidism was in direct contrast with new Enlightenment ideals, which heralded social interaction as the basis of refinement and civilization. It was widely accepted among medical professionals and laymen that the cure of nervous ailments could only be achieved by a patient's active effort to get well. Patients who indulged their ailments by only half-heartedly following their doctors' prescribed regimen, or who spent their days worrying about their ill health, would only worsen their conditions and become a further burden on society. The *Female Spectator* warned its readership against dwelling on their poor health: 'so many people, by the fear of imaginary ills, create to themselves real ones; and others, by endeavouring to fly a danger which seems to threaten, run into far worse which they never thought on'.[54] Positive thoughts, 'an unshaken chearfulness' and a stoic, firm resistance to consuming notions of poor health were the only ways to prevent imaginary illnesses from becoming real.[55] The *Female Spectator* insisted that it was up to the patient to 'expel [such thoughts] as much as lies in our power' as 'sad thoughts will grow upon us if indulged'.[56] Similarly, the hypochondriac James Boswell advised a fellow sufferer that he should not allow 'hypochondria to gather strength, but should exert himself with all possible speed and activity to crush it in its beginning'.[57]

Medical practitioners often considered their patients culpable for advanced nervous disorders and responsible for their own recovery. Occasionally their case notes discuss patients who, they believed, were 'indulging', and therefore worsening, their nervous disorders. For instance, Thomas Thompson, the physician to the Prince of Wales, wrote of one hypochondriac patient, 'It appears... that since the death of his wife, which happened about five months ago, the clergyman, who has been long accustomed to a sedentary life, has too much abandoned himself to solitude and melancholy reflexions'.[58] The doctor recommended that his patient reconcile himself to the 'pleasures of society' claiming,

> If the gentleman can be diverted, by company and amusements, from ruminating on the cause of his affliction, and can be induced to ride much on horseback, no doubt need be entertained of his recovery, but without his compliance in these points, I am afraid all our endeavours will prove vain.[59]

As suffering from a nervous disease became increasingly associated with a lack of willpower or moral failure, recovering from one became a journey of moral redemption. The increasing prevalence of this opinion among medical professionals again highlights the growing role of doctors as moral guardians. As ever more medical practitioners warned at the end of the eighteenth century, nervous patients suffering as a result of luxurious living needed to renounce their opulent lifestyles, and patients indulging in self-pity needed to excite their fortitude in order to improve. Written at the end of the century, Robert Thornton's *Philosophy of Medicine* (1799) included an entire chapter on moral philosophy, in which he claimed,

> Trials arise, which demand vigorous exertions of all the moral powers; of patience, vigilance, and self-denial; of constancy and fortitude, to support us under danger and reproach; of temperance, to restrain us from being carried away by pleasure; of firm and determined principles, to support us under the different and trying circumstances of life.[60]

Heberden also firmly supported the increasingly popular belief that nervous patients could choose whether to 'indulge and give way' to their ailments, 'or to struggle against and resist them'.[61] Consequently, patients towards the end of the century were encouraged to overcome their disorder through a deliberate rejection of self-pity. Clearly aware of this tactic, the seemingly nervous patient John McKie wrote to Cullen in 1779 informing the doctor that in addition to his wind, tremours, 'giddiness & faintishness' he also suffered from 'low spirits which', he assured Cullen, 'I strive against as much as possible'.[62] A doctor's assistance was often necessary to achieve such resolve. In his award-winning essay of 1788, Falconer noted that for physicians treating hypochondriasis,

> The most judicious course seems to be, to endeavour to excite the fortitude of the sufferers by representing to them, that it is unworthy a brave and resolute character to be always complaining of misfortunes, which are in good measure the common lot of mankind, that it is more manly to struggle with ill fortune, than to sink without resistance beneath its pressure. Frequently a little raillery, if used with a great moderation and perfect good temper, will have an excellent effect.[63]

It was in this vein that the Bristol physician J. Woodforde wrote to the young medical student Anthony Fothergill, diagnosing him with hypochondria 'brought on by too intense application and the want of due exercise and amusement'. In an effort to treat this disorder, Woodforde recommended that Fothergill take a 'glass of julep & camphor' when his 'languor & depression' were 'very great', allow '2 hours for brisk exercise every day – whether in fencing, dancing, or riding a rough trotting horse' and 'Devote 2 or 3 evenings in a week to music or convivial meetings'. Yet most importantly, Fothergill advised Woodforde to strongly resist the disorder:

> These blue Devils must absolutely be brushed off or they will take possession of you and render you a moping useless being. But remember you are born to nobler ends – therefore banish spleen – banish melancholy - [64]

While more extreme than most treating physicians, Caleb Hillier Parry's treatment of nervous sufferers in the 1780s also exemplifies the medical profession's increasingly hard-hearted attitude towards these ailments. Recounting the case of two young hysterics who suffered repeated fits, Parry explained how he treated the young girls with a total lack of empathy:

> I told them, that this [hysteria] was a disease I was determined never to permit; and that on the next attack, I should be obliged to put in practice a remedy of so painful a nature, that the thought of it filled me with horror; but I trusted that there would be no return, and that the remedy would be therefore unnecessary. This conversation made a great impression on the minds of my young patients. No relapse occurred.[65]

Family members of nervous sufferers were also encouraged by Parry and other physicians not to over-indulge them with sympathy. For instance, Falconer noted how parents of hysterical children should punish them for hysterical fits instead of displaying worry or concern. As he argued, 'the displeasure of a parent, supposed to be likely to be incurred by the return of hysterical paroxysms, has contributed to prevent them'.[66] Parry repeatedly noted the importance of parental resolve in dealing with hysterical children. In a case of a fifteen or sixteen year-old hysteric who was 'uniformly indulged in every wish' by her father, Parry explained how

> having been long accustomed to observe what share moral causes had in producing or aggravating these complaints, I urged this man, as he valued the future happiness of his daughter, to change his method of proceeding, and, instead of this absurd indulgence, to give her a good shaking, or else to throw a bason of cold water in her face, immediately on the approach of the next fit.

Although the father was never able to bring himself to go to these lengths, he did, Parry reported, speak harshly to her during her next attack, only to find to his 'great astonishment' that she 'never had another fit!'[67]

According to Parry, friends of nervous patients should also be pro-active in discouraging their complaints, as offering unbridled sympathy would only encourage further suffering. Relating the story of one 'Miss W' who fell weak by reading aloud for nearly half an hour, Parry noted how she soon lost her voice, became too weak to exercise and could not be tempted by her friends to eat. The fault in this story, according to Parry, was with both the patient and her friends. By giving up exercise 'because it produced present inconvenience,' Parry argued, 'she forged one of the first links of that chain of infirmities by which she is now held in bondage.' Yet as for her friends, 'By encouraging the weakness of the patient, they confirm an indolent submission to maladies, which calm endurance and true fortitude would enable her ultimately to overcome'.[68]

Faith in the ability of patients to overcome their nervous ailments through the exertion of mental will did not imply that doctors thought their disorders were feigned. Rather, most doctors simply believed that the strength of a disorder could be tempered with positive thought. As Heberden explained,

> I would by no means... represent the sufferings of hypochondriac and hysteric patients as imaginary; for I doubt not their arising from as real a cause as any other distemper. However, their force will be very different, according to the patient's choosing to indulge and give way to them, or to struggle against and resist them, which is much more in his power than he is aware of, or can easily be brought to believe... For his striving to shake off this distemper is not contending about a frivolous concern, but whether he shall be happy or miserable; since it is of the essence of this malady to view every thing in the worst light; and human happiness, in many instances, depends not so much upon a man's situation and circumstances, as upon the point of view in which he contemplates them.[69]

Thus, patients could either dwell on their ailments, or mentally conquer them.

Ironically, the hypochondriac Samuel Johnson exhibited this uncompromising point of view in a letter to one of his sickly correspondents in 1771:

> do nothing that may hurt you and... reject nothing that may do you good. To preserve health is a moral and religious duty: for health is the basis of all social virtues; and we can be useful no longer than while we are well.[70]

Johnson's correspondence is full of comments regarding the self-absorbed nature of invalids. In a letter of 1783 he wrote, 'Disease produces much selfishness; a man in pain is looking after ease and lets most other things go'. In another letter five years later he complained, 'the first talk of the sick is commonly of themselves'.[71] As personal responsibility to maintain health became a pre-requisite for useful membership in society, nervous patients caught dwelling on or indulging in their poor health were increasingly subjects for ridicule, and less commonly regarded with sympathy. Corresponding with yet another friend suffering from 'a mind unsettled and discontented' Johnson wrote rather bluntly, 'I hope... that your complaints do not arise from the mere habit of complaining'. He then encouraged his friend to resist stewing in emotional malaise: 'there is no distemper... on which the mind has not some influence, and which is not better resisted by a cheerful than a gloomy temper'.[72] While in a much gentler manner, David Hume also encouraged his friend and fellow philosopher Adam Smith to overcome his hypochondriac complaints, and to reengage with society.[73] After Smith declined several invitations from friends on account of his ailments Hume wrote,

> I shall not take any Excuse from your own State of Health, which I suppose only a Subterfuge invented by Indolence and Love of Solitude. Indeed, my Dear Smith, if you continue to hearken to Complaints of this Nature, you will cut Yourself out entirely from human Society, to the great Loss of both Parties.[74]

Shirking social responsibility was increasingly seen as a personal failure as indulging in sickness was equated with unfashionable selfishness. Written at the end of the eighteenth century, Edward Gibbon's *Memoirs* exhibited this changing attitude through an exceptionally self-conscious discussion of his childhood nervous ailments. Before discussing the 'strange nervous affection' of his youth, Gibbon promised his readers that he would treat the subject with brevity:

> I will not follow the vain example of Cardinal Quirini who has filled half a volume of his memoirs with medical consultations on his particular case; nor shall I imitate the naked frankness of Montagne, who exposes all the symptoms of his malady, and the operation of each dose of physic on his nerves and bowels.[75]

Thus, after a few brief remarks regarding the incompatibility of his poor health with his scholarly pursuits, Gibbon informed his readers that his health improved with age: 'since that time few persons have been more exempt from real or imaginary ills: and till I am admonished by the Gout, the reader shall no more be troubled with the history of my bodily complaints'.[76]

Just as Gibbon eagerly disassociated himself from a self-indulgent description of his nervous disorder, many long-term nervous patients became ever more apologetic about their symptoms and apparent neglect of social responsibility. Mr Sandilands, a troubled hypochondriac who wrote several letters to Cullen from 1789 to 1790, was particularly eager to clear himself of any imputation of laziness, or indulgent infirmity. In one of his first letters to Cullen, Sandilands wrote,

> As I fear I may be blamed for indulging too much my disposition to solitude, I must beg leave to mention that my case seems singular in this that the smallest noise; the least motion disconcerts me. It is this extreme irritability of my Nervous system that makes me unhappy. It was this that made me quit my profession; & it is this that gives me up to an Inactivity which I should blush for if I knew how to remedy it.

After discussing his attempts and consequent inability to cure his low spirits and disordered nerves by exercise or social activity, Sandilands summarized his purpose in writing: 'My view was to endeavour to clear myself from the imputations of indolence & irresolution; & what I have written was under the strongest impressions of its Truth'.[77] In his effort to maintain Cullen's sympathy for his situation, Sandilands felt the need to describe his pro-active attempts to get better, and to insist on his unhappiness with his present poor health.

A Disease of the Softer Sex

Late eighteenth-century discussions of women and nervous disease also clearly exhibit a downward trend in the popularity of nervousness and over-delicacy. This discourse also highlights the strong interplay between medicine and society during the period. Whereas in the late seventeenth and early eighteenth centuries physicians developed nerve theories to explain observed cultural differences between the sexes in physiological terms, by the end of the century it appears that medical ideas regarding the spread of nervous disease and its hereditary nature pre-empted the public's increasingly antagonistic response towards feminine weakness.

As early as the seventeenth century it was acknowledged that women were more delicate and susceptible to the disorders which, in the eighteenth century were termed 'nervous', than men. For instance, the published case notes of Robert Peirce, a late seventeenth-century Bath physician and fellow of the Royal College of Physicians in London, reveal an overwhelming proportion of female patients suffering from the 'vapours' and hysterical disorders. Although they could be treated with drugs and bathing regimens, women suffering from nervous ailments were commonly believed to require the healthy, strong, stabilizing influence of a male companion to achieve a complete cure. Hence, for cases like that of the hysteric Miss Berisford, Peirce acknowledged his hope that 'her Mother, (by giving her to a good Husband) prevented a relapse'.[78] By the eighteenth century, the weakness of women compared with men was neatly framed in terms of the nerves. As Barker-Benfield has explained, Cheyne explicitly gendered the nerves, describing women's nerves as finer, weaker and more susceptible to strong impressions than men's.[79] In this way, nerve theory provided medical justification for existing cultural differences between the sexes. Men were made to reason, and women were made to feel; thus, men were best suited for business and work outside the home, whereas, according to most physicians throughout the century, women's nervous sensibility lent them a particular 'tenderness' and 'taste for moral excellence' well suited to raising children and 'forming the infant mind'.[80] In particular, women were physically designed to behave as compassionate and sensibility-ridden creatures, capable of softening the residually rough edges of their male companions.

As Robert Shoemaker has discussed, descriptions of appropriate gender roles in prescriptive literature of the eighteenth century were 'closely linked' to the physiological descriptions of gender differences set forth in medical texts.[81] James Fordyce's famous *Sermons to Young Women* (1765) embodied this view of female weakness and domesticity. Reminding his female readership that God made them from 'finer materials' and in a 'more delicate construction' than men, he insisted that 'war, commerce, politics, exercises of strength and dexterity, abstract philosophy, and the abtruser sciences' were the province of men, whereas the body and mind of women were more suited to everything 'which has the heart for its object'.[82] 'Feminine' delicacy of body and mind were prerequisites for attracting a husband. As Fordyce warned,

> Let it be likewise observed, that in your sex, manly exercises are never graceful; that in them, a tone and figure, as well as an air and deportment of the masculine kind, are always forbidding: and that men of sensibility desire in every woman, soft features, and a flowing voice, a form not robust, and a demeanour delicate and gentle.[83]

Gregory championed this romantic view of female delicacy in his *Father's Legacy to his Daughters* (1774). Composed after the death of his wife in 1761, the *Legacy* was intended to instruct his daughters on proper female conduct in religious, moral and romantic matters. Gregory's son later published the *Legacy*, one year after his father's death. It met with immediate success, selling 6000 copies in its first two years in print, with new editions still appearing late in the nineteenth century.[84] The conduct encouraged by Gregory in the *Legacy* encouraged a strict adherence to separate gender spheres; whereas men were designed more to think and reason, Gregory wrote to his daughters, 'The natural softness and sensibility of your [female] dispositions particularly fit you for the practice of those duties

where the heart is chiefly concerned'.[85] Women, Gregory insisted, were more
subject to sensibility, imagination, pride and vanity than men. Whereas Gregory
advised his daughters to resist most of these inflammatory female passions, he
did not issue the same warning with respect to sensibility. Instead he encouraged
this female tendency, claiming,

> When a girl ceases to blush, she has lost the most powerful charm of beauty. That
> extreme sensibility which it indicates, may be a weakness and incumbrance in our sex,
> as I have too often felt; but in yours it is particularly engaging.[86]

Beyond alerting his daughters to the power of attraction that sensibility and
emotional delicacy afforded, he also alerted them to the appeal of outward physical delicacy. To be sure, Gregory advised his daughters of the importance of
maintaining good inward health through a careful regimen of exercise and diet,
even warning them in particularly vivid terms that the 'luxury of eating... is a
despicable selfish vice in men but in your sex it is beyond expression indelicate
and disgusting'.[87] Yet despite the apparent importance that Gregory placed on
the health of his daughters, he encouraged them to keep their strong constitutions under wraps:

> Though good health be one of the greatest blessings of life, never make a boast of
> it, but enjoy it in grateful silence. We so naturally associate the idea of female soft-
> ness and delicacy with a correspondent delicacy of constitution, that when a woman
> speaks of her great strength, her extraordinary appetite, her ability to bear excessive
> fatigue, we recoil on this description in a way she is little aware of.[88]

Despite its popularity, the *Legacy* drew many critics, particularly late in the century in the context of a supposedly enlarged and growing number of nervous
sufferers. Mary Wollstonecraft was one such opponent. Her *Vindication of the
Rights of Woman* (1792) reviled Gregory's encouragement of feminine weakness and delicacy. Like most other reviewers, Wollstonecraft did not object to
Gregory's emphasis on women's innately heightened sensibilities. Rather, she
objected to Gregory's emphasis on exaggerating female characteristics to an artificial degree, encouraging women to, at least superficially, bend their feminine
natures to the will of fashion. Referencing Gregory in the *Vindication*, Wollstonecraft wrote, 'I respect his heart; but entirely disapprove of his celebrated
Legacy to his Daughters'.[89] For, she argued, Gregory's *Legacy* only 'contributed
to render women more artificial, weak characters, than they would otherwise
have been; and consequently [made them] more useless members of society'.[90]
Wollstonecraft took particular offence at Gregory's suggestion that women
downplay their physical health, claiming,

> Nature has given woman a weaker frame than man; but, to ensure her husband's
> affections, must a wife, who by the exercise of her mind and body... has allowed her

constitution to retain its natural strength, and her nerves a healthy tone, is she, I say, to condescend to use art and feign a sickly delicacy in order to secure her husband's affection?'[91]

At issue according to Wollstonecraft, was Gregory's 'system of dissimulation' whereby women were 'always to *seem* to be this and that', thereby becoming 'weak, artificial beings'.[92] According to Wollstonecraft, such 'unnatural' behaviour had larger consequences, undermining 'the very foundation of virtue, and spread[ing] corruption through the whole mass of society!'[93]

Published just one year before Gregory's *Legacy*, Hester Chapone's *Letters on the Improvement of the Mind* (1773) offered more subdued praise of female delicacy, carefully establishing the difference between natural and affected weakness, while emphasizing the need to regulate innate female sensibility with a healthy dose of reason. As Chapone argued, a 'vain' young woman growing up with the belief 'that tenderness and softness is the peculiar charm of the sex – [and] that even their weakness is lovely' would only foster this weakness, becoming artificial and socially offensive:

> Her fondness and affection becomes fulsome and ridiculous; her compassion grows [into] contemptible weakness... for, when once she quits the direction of Nature, she knows not where to stop, and continually exposes herself by the most absurd extremes. Nothing so effectually defeats its own ends as this kind of affectation: for though warm affections and tender feelings are beyond measure amiable and charming, when perfectly natural, and kept under the due controul of reason and principle, yet nothing is so truly disgusting as the affectation of them, or even the unbridled indulgence of such as are real.[94]

After quoting this entire passage from Chapone in his *Lectures on Female Education and Manners* (1793), the writer and moralist John Burton further expressed his annoyance that, 'to seem timid on the most trifling occasions – at the most ordinary accidents – and where there is no danger, is thought, by some Ladies, as not only graceful, but characteristical'. Burton urged his readers to consider 'whether this timidity be constitutional, or whether it proceed from affectation?'[95] The Evangelical philanthropist Hannah More's *Strictures on the Modern System of Female Education* (1799), which went through seven editions in its first year in print, complained that nervous sensibility was too frequently fostered and feigned by 'young women [who] were incessantly hearing unqualified sensibility extolled as the perfection of their nature'.[96]

Beddoes also decried the modern tendency to encourage false extremes of female delicacy. In his 1802 tract *Hygeia*, Beddoes disdainfully noted the way in which

> A mother, perhaps, here and there, (looking with more anxiety towards the means, by which a husband may be won, than those by which he is retained) will entertain fears

lest girls, brought up with a sovereign regard to health, should not be delicate enough for the present demand.[97]

In 1803, the London physician Sayer Walker still acknowledged the innate nervous weakness of women in his *Observations on the Constitution of Women and on some of the Diseases to Which they are More Especially Liable*, remarking that

> the lax fibre, the small and flaccid muscle, the delicate fabric of the nerves, the weak and yielding texture of the vessels, are some of the circumstances that unite in forming the constitution which is observed in the female.[98]

Nevertheless, unlike earlier writers, Walker was quick to qualify his statements regarding the appealing quality of feminine weakness, claiming that it was only attractive if 'indulged in a proper degree'. [99] Over-indulgence in sensibility and the passions, was, as most medical and moral writers of the period agreed, dangerous and irresponsible.

Early in the nineteenth century Trotter argued that natural feminine weakness was being exploited by artificial manners. While acknowledging the fact that 'nature has endued the female constitution with greater delicacy and sensibility than the male, as destined for a different occupation in life', he nevertheless insisted that it was fashion, not nature, that had encouraged weakness and sensibility to such an extent as to lead to the period's unprecedented proliferation of nervous disorders: [100]

> Fashionable manners have shamefully mistaken the purposes of nature; and the modern system of education, for the fair sex, has been to refine on this construction of frame, and to induce a debility of body, from the cradle upwards, so as to make feeble woman rather a subject for medical disquisition, than the healthful companion of our cares.[101]

According to Trotter, the fashionable manners exacerbating 'natural' female weakness were contributing to a loss of traditional virtue. Even seemingly minor issues like modern children's playful activities were indicative of the artificial and degenerate state of the female gender and the country:

> We indulge our boys to yoke their go-carts, and to ride on long rods, while little miss must have her more delicate limbs crampt by sitting the whole day dressing a doll. Ancient custom has been pleaded in favour of these amusements for boys, as we read in Horace: but it is no where recorded that the infancy of Portia, Arria, and Agrippina was spent in fitting clothes for a joint-baby.[102]

By encouraging weakness and delicacy even at this young age, women surpassed the natural boundaries of their feminine sensibilities. Artificial modes of living, in turn, exacerbated their innate physical weakness and nervous debility. Although it had long been acknowledged that women's delicate physiology qualified them for their role as compassionate mothers, moralists in the latter half of the eighteenth century began to fear that over-delicacy and artificial manners were diverting women from their maternal duties. Furthermore, as Linda Colley has explained, anxiety about keeping women 'contented within the domestic sphere... deepened as more and more of them appeared to be active outside of it'.[103] Consequently, the second half of the eighteenth century saw a flurry of publications decrying the tendency of modern women to neglect their maternal responsibilities through their participation in the unhealthy world outside of the home. In the anonymously penned collection of essays, *Dialogues of the Dead* (1760), 'Mrs Modish', a fictional caricature of modern woman, referred to diversion and amusement as the 'business of my life', complaining of how the 'late hours and fatigue' consequent from attending an endless stream of balls and card parties meant that she was plagued with the Vapours.[104] As Mrs Modish was so engrossed in her own amusement and ill health, she left little time for her daughters, hiring dancing-masters, music-masters, drawing-masters and French governesses to raise them in her absence. In response to Mrs Modish's lifestyle, the essay's faux narrator and moral commentator exclaimed, 'Your daughters must have been so educated as to fit them to be wives without conjugal affection, and mothers without material care'.[105]

In a similar vein, the Anglican clergyman James Hervey complained in his *Sermons and Miscellaneous Tracts* (1764) that modern ladies were neglecting their domestic responsibilities. As he lamented, contemporary women

> have no proper Employ for their delicate Capacities; but lose their Happiness, in Flights of Caprice, or Fits of the Vapour: lose their Time in the most insipid Chat, or the most whimsical Vagaries: While Thought is a Burthen, and Reflection is a Drudgery, Solitude fills them with Horror, and a serious Discourse makes them melancholy.[106]

Criticism of female susceptibility to nervous ailments fell neatly within what Colley has referred to as the 'renovated cult of female propriety and domesticity' in Britain in the second half of the eighteenth century.[107] The long-held notion that women were innately sensitive and vulnerable to nervous disease was complicated by the growing sense, particularly in the final quarter of the century, that nervous disease was the result of their luxurious and irresponsible living. Consequently, a disease that was once so symbolic of femininity and traditional female roles became symbolic of the female rejection of maternal duties and feminine morality. Women who compounded their innate nervous weakness through immoderate participation in modern commercial society had overstepped the bounds of fashionable refinement and entered a degenerative state.

Negative connotations surrounding nervous sufferers reached a particularly fevered pitch in the 1780s as the notion of hereditary nervousness gained acceptance among the medical faculty. The notion of hereditary disease was not new to the 1780s; as Sean Quinlan has shown, there were over thirty medical publications on the subject written between 1594 and 1748, explaining how even diseases like syphilis, gout, arthritis and insanity supposedly passed from generation to generation.[108] Likewise, Robert Burton's *Anatomy of Melancholy* hinted that melancholia could be hereditary, and Cheyne's *English Malady* specifically referred to the way in which such disorders could be 'original and hereditary'.[109] Still, inherited nervousness was not commonly discussed until the final quarter of the eighteenth century, when the concept of hereditary disease achieved widespread favour among leading physicians and medical academics.[110] By the nineteenth century, hereditary theories of nervous disease were commonplace, leading one member of the Edinburgh Royal Medical Society to remark in 1808 that 'among medical writers, no cause is more commonly assigned for these diseases than hereditary taint'.[111] Scientific theory regarding the hereditary nature of disordered nerves significantly affected popular opinion about the disease.

Indeed, the social implications of hereditary nervousness were enormously significant; no longer would the dangers of nervous debility be confined to one generation. One physician writing to Cullen on behalf of a patient in 1779 explained precisely this problem. His patient, he explained, a twenty-nine year old woman who was suffering from an incessant cough and back pain, had a compromised constitution on account of her mother's nervous disorder. Offering Cullen a brief introduction to the state of his patient's health he wrote,

> Her father [is] a healthy man, her mother tho not unhealthy has a delicacy of the nervous system (a family misfortune) that has often subjected her, as it does all of similar constitutions, to be hurt by what would give little disturbance to others more robust.[112]

Mothers who initiated their own nervous weakness through intemperate and luxurious living were doubly culpable for endangering their children's health as well as their own. Trotter expressed his particular disgust with unnatural, over-refined nervous females within the context of hereditary nervousness:

> From having injured her own frame by refinements in living, the mother thus sows the seeds of disease in the constitutions of her children: hence a weak body, delicate nerves, and their consequence, a sickly existence, become hereditary.[113]

Increasingly negative attitudes towards nervous women were also reflected in novels of the eighteenth century. Whereas the fainting heroines in the sentimental literature of the early part of the century were celebrated for the strength of their debilitating sensibility, the heroines of nineteenth-century novels exhibited stronger command of their deep feelings. For instance, in Jane Austen's *Sense and Sensibility* (1811) tempered emotions were valued over unbridled sensibility. Through this story, Austen instructed readers in the proper balance between indulging in sincere sentiments and functioning in a collected manner. Marianne, who through the majority of the novel suffers at the hands of her admirable yet life-threatening depth of feeling, learns to command her passions. Overcoming heartfelt despair after losing her first love, she prudently settles the seas of her tempestuous love life by embarking on a life with the slightly less dashing but far more practical Colonel Brandon. Alternatively, by the novel's end, the ever-sensible Elinor Dashwood embraces a healthy dose of her sister's romantic sensibility through her relationship with Edward Farrars. The perfect heroine clearly belonged somewhere between the initial over-sensibility of Marianne and the ultra-sensible nature of the early Elinor. While extreme depth of feeling was still venerable, the ability to contain this depth of feeling was a virtue. In this way, susceptibility to passion-induced nervous disorders was not, in itself, a flaw; indulging in these sufferings and becoming a useless 'emotional cripple' was.[114]

Austen's novels provide several examples of sufferers who exemplify these character flaws. In *Pride and Prejudice* (1813) and her unfinished novel *Sanditon* (1817), the nervous Mrs Bennet and the hypochondriac Parker sisters are surreptitiously ridiculed for their ceaseless and selfish attention to their personal health.[115] Unlike the lovesick Marianne, Austen exempts these characters from pity, cleverly displaying the artificial nature of their nervous sensibilities. Mrs Bennett is described by Austen as 'fancy[ing] herself nervous' while the 'invalid' Parker sisters indulge their supposed disorders, clinging to their poor health as a topic of conversation and a pleasurable source of personal attention.[116] In this way, Austen, like Wollstonecraft, displays disdain for the manipulative and affected behaviour of fake sufferers, and admiration for the personal resolve of true nervous sufferers who overcome their debilitating sensibility.

As Peter Logan has shown, the notion of 'overcoming' nervousness became a common theme in late eighteenth and early nineteenth-century novels, pertaining to heroes and heroines alike. William Godwin's *Caleb Williams* (1794) opens with Caleb 'riddled with the delicate "flutterings and palpitations" of his feminine sensibility', but concludes with his ability to overcome his nervousness and embrace more manly behaviour.[117] Mary Hays' *Memoirs of Emma Courtney* (1796) likewise tells the story of the Emma's transition from an overly-emotional, trembling, fainting, blushing and self-indulgent young lady to a 'socially useful' woman capable of rationally reflecting on her past, and gaining control over her once-debilitating passions.[118] Published two decades later, Maria Edgeworth's *Harrington* (1817) similarly praised the ability of its protagonist to overcome his incapacitating nervous fits by conquering his passions and taking control of his previously misguided sensibility.[119] The message of these novels was clear: a nervous body was a self-absorbed body.

By the end of the century, nervous weakness was greeted with far less congrat-
ulation than it was in Cheyne's day, although a natural and moderate feminine
weakness was still acceptable. As Walker noted in his *Observations*, 'together
with th[e] susceptibility of impression on the bodily organs, is connected that
sensibility of mind, which, when indulged in a proper degree, is a distinguishing
ornament of the female'.[120] Yet as doctors and moralists agreed by the late eighteenth century, nervous weakness and debility caused by artificial and luxurious
living only denoted the deterioration of society and a loss of female virtue.

As the novels of the period make clear, women were not the only ones
criticized for the escalating national threat posed by nervous disease late in
the century. Nervous males were also the frequent objects of derision from the
general public and the medical faculty late in the century. Depicted as weak
and effeminate, nervous males were chastised by moral and medical authors
for tipping the nation from its supposedly balanced pinnacle of civilization to
a weighty state of degenerative decay. As with women, the failing fashion for
overly-sensitive nervous males in the second half of the century was prompted
by both the period's medical theory and its cultural climate.

Well through the middle of the eighteenth century, nervous sensibility was
considered the mark of a refined and civilized man. Even as late as the 1770s,
enlightened authors heralded nervous sensibility and sympathy as the mark of
a modern gentleman. David Hume's essay 'Of the Delicacy of Taste and Passion' emphasized the particular importance of the arts for cultivating a modern
'elegance of sentiment', claiming that the contemplation of poetry, music and
painting would 'produce an agreeable melancholy, which, of all dispositions of
the mind, is the best suited to love and friendship'.[121] Delicacy and sensibility
were viewed as 'gentle virtues' capable of prompting moral and compassionate
behaviour.[122] As Silvia Sebastiani has shown, enlightenment writers like Hume,
Smith, Home and Adam Ferguson read history 'as a process of "feminization",
that is, as one of refinement and civility'. According to this view, man had progressed from an ancient rudimentary warrior-like state to one of sophisticated
compassion and sociability via his increased interaction with the softer sex.
Medical men frequently discussed this feminizing process in terms of the nerves
and nervous disease. Walker noted in his *Treatise on Nervous Diseases* that while
women were most prone to nervous diseases, 'next to them, those of the other
sex, who approach nearest to the temperament of females, are most liable to
them'.[123]

Towards the end of the century there was a growing sense that modern men
had surpassed the ideal state of feminized or softened manliness, becoming so
much like women that they had entered a state of effeminacy. Indulgence in
modern luxury and sedentary employments were believed to have a debilitating
effect on manly nerves. This fault was particularly devastating in times of mili-

tary conflict when men were in danger of becoming too effeminate to fight. The connections between luxury, effeminacy and military impotence were nothing new. They were standard tropes even in the seventeenth century, with Nicholas Barbon's *Discourse of Trade* (1690) complaining that trade had resulted in 'too much softening [of] the People by Ease and Luxury, which made their Bodies unfit to endure the Labour and Hardships of War'.[124] Similarly, Thomas Mun's early seventeenth-century pamphlet, *England's Treasure by Forreign Trade*, described how modern society was plagued by a 'general leprosie' of 'Piping, Potting, Feasting, Fashions, and mis-spending of our time In Idleness and Pleasure... [which] hath made us effeminate in our bodies, weak in our knowledg, poor in our Treasure, declined in our Valour, unfortunate in our Enterprises, and contemned by our Enemies'.[125] Yet eighteenth-century nerve theory presented a medical way of tracing societal degeneration and growing effeminacy. The unprecedented number of nervous sufferers reported by modern physicians, armed moralists with seemingly objective proof of modern effeminacy in the place of the seventeenth century's mere speculative warnings. Although these social commentators did not overtly express the medical origin of their ideas through citations of men like Whytt or Cullen, their tendency to buttress their ideas with references to nervous physiology betrays the medical foundations of their beliefs about femininity, masculinity and morality.

A Disease of the Nation

In light of the implications that a growing nervous population had for the nation's morals, manliness and military, it is not surprising to find that talk of the nerves frequently infiltrated political writings. While sources decrying weak nerves and effeminacy were most abundant in the final decades of the century as the medical profession became more involved in the regulation of the nation's moral as well as physical health, there was not a neatly traceable rise in this discourse. Rather, discussions of nervous effeminacy peaked and waned over the course of the period, with the highest peaks generally occurring in times of military conflict. Editions of the *Female Spectator* printed during the Seven Years' War decried the effeminacy of modern soldiers who cared more about the appearance of their uniforms than the outcome of battles.[126] Edinburgh's Select Society debated questions such as 'Whether a commercial and military spirit can subsist together in the same nation?' and Adam Ferguson, a professor of natural philosophy at the University of Edinburgh from 1759 to 1764, reminded his countrymen of the importance of mixing 'the military spirit with our civil and commercial policy'.[127] As Kathleen Wilson has explained, many Britons mid-century feared that an increasingly commercial society, and, in particular, the British penchant for fashionable French imports, was threatening Britain with 'national emasculation'. By adopting French styles and foppish behaviour, Britons were committing 'cultural treason' and were potentially sacrificing their stout English characters for French effeminacy in their insatiable quest for fashion.[128] Likewise, the Anglican cleric John Brown's *Estimate of the Manners and Principles of the Times* (1757) which went through seven editions in its first year in print could only warn his fellow commercial Englishmen of the disastrous effect which the increase of nervous disease would have on national defence claiming,

> Our effeminate and unmanly Life, working along with our Island-Climate, hath notoriously produced an Increase of *low Spirits* and *nervous Disorders*, whose natural and unalterable Character is that of *Fear.*[129]

In addition to compromising England's security against the French, Brown illustrated the way in which modern effeminacy had wreaked havoc in 1745, pitting the effeminate English against their more manly Scottish neighbours:

> How far this dastard Spirit of Effeminacy has crept upon us, and destroyed the national Spirit of Defence, may appear from the general *Panic* the Nation was thrown into, at the late *Rebellion.* When those of every Rank above a Constable, instead of arming themselves and encouraging the *People,* generally fled before the *Rebels*; while a Mob of ragged Highlanders marched unmolested to the Heart of a populous Kingdom.[130]

For most of the century, political concern over effeminately nervous males was typically expressed with regard to the military threat of the French. These discussions reached a fevered pitch by the time of the Revolution in 1789, remaining fairly constant through to the end of the Napoleonic Wars in 1815. The fear of a French invasion was very real. The French had attempted an invasion in Ireland in 1796 and 1798, and a small French force landed in Wales in 1797. The conquest of Britain was Napoleon's foremost military aim from 1798 to 1805.[131] Writing during the Napoleonic Wars, the social critic, nerve doctor and ex-naval physician Thomas Trotter expressed his particular fear of male nervousness and effeminacy with regard to national security. In the *View*, Trotter boldly expressed his fear that Britain would never retain her ascendancy among 'rival states' unless national mores were drastically altered:

> That is, by recurring to simplicity of living and manners, so as to check the increasing prevalence of nervous disorders; which, if not restrained soon, must inevitably sap our physical strength of constitution; make us an easy conquest to our invaders; and ultimately convert us into a nation of slaves and ideots.[132]

Fears of effeminacy, over-sensibility, and consequent nervous weakness amidst the heated political climate of the late eighteenth century prompted much national introspection, particularly amongst the English. Whereas in the middle of the century Englishmen complimented themselves on their well-balanced level of civilization, superior to the rustic Scots, and less effeminate than the nervously weak and over-refined French, by the turn of the century this self-reflection was not so congratulatory. In the face of unprecedented numbers of nervous and effeminate Englishmen, physicians at the turn of the century began to praise the healthiness of rustic Scottish living. In an article printed in an 1805 edition of the *London Medical and Physical Journal* titled 'temperament and diseases of the people inhabiting the Highlands of Aberdeenshire', the health of the Scots was openly praised:

> Few are the diseases that rage among inhabitants of the Highlands; I believe they enjoy a greater share of health than falls to the lot of those of any other nation. This can only be the effect of temperance and regular excitement; the want of effeminacy of manners; moderate exercise; a simple and regular regimen; a pure air, a certain serenity of mind, in being less agitated by the anxious cares of commercial life, which distract the thoughts, and dissipate the animal spirits...[133]

The difference between this and the relatively dissipated state of the English would not have gone unnoticed by readers of the *Journal*. In this context the Scots could also take pride in their less nervous and less effeminate, if less civilized, culture. As Wayne Wild has noted, the large number of medical prescriptions recommending the 'invigorating air' of the Highlands to nervous sufferers illustrated 'how Scottish Enlightenment medicine was able to offer a theory of environmentalism which gave direct scientific support to Scottish nationalism'.[134] The Scottish writer Henry Home exemplified this Scottish nationalism, noting in his *Sketches of the History of Man* (1775) that 'Luxury... renders the mind so effeminate, as to be subdued by every distress: the slightest pain, whether of mind or body, is a real evil: and any higher degree becomes severe torture. The French are far gone in that disease'. But, he noted, 'the British are gradually sinking into the same weakness of mind'. This decline was clearly due to the 'effeminacy' of the English. For, he continued, 'In Scotland, such refinement has not yet taken place'.[135]

Similarly, as Colin Kidd has explained, the argument that 'sturdy liberty-loving John Bulls' were turning into 'effeminate Frenchmen' also found expression in popular novels like Tobias Smollett's *Expedition of Humphry Clinker* (1771). This novel, Kidd notes, 'exploded conventional anti-Scottish prejudices and contrasted the manly virtues of North Britain – and rural Wales – with the corruption of the *beau monde* in Bath and London'.[136] In the face of growing number of nervous cases spurred on by luxury, immoderation and immorality, England was fast becoming a nation of un-motherly women and effeminate men, incapable of protecting national borders, destined to produce a new generation of nervous weaklings, and dragging the rest of Britain along with her down a slippery slope of degeneracy.

Aside from the potential inability of effeminate Britons to defend their borders, the very notion of medical sympathy became more threatening at the end of the century. Whytt noted the power of the sympathetic nervous system to promote similar action among spectators as early as 1751. In an effort to explain his meaning, Whytt used yawning as his example: 'Yawning is so catching as frequently to go round a whole company'. In 1764 Whytt further linked this contagious behaviour with the nervous system, marvelling at how there was such a strong 'sympathy between the nervous systems of different persons'.[137] Hysteria could be contagious, too. Whytt noted in his *Treatise* that 'it has frequently happened in the Royal Infirmary here [Edinburgh], that women have been seized with hysteric fits from seeing others attacked with them'.[138] As many believed, this hysteric contagion could have political consequences. After witnessing France's horrific Rein of Terror at the end of the century, many feared that Britons would sympathize with the politics of overly impassioned French revolutionaries, and spread contagious political hysteria at home. In response to these fears, politicians and philosophers began to stress the way in which citizens' ability to exercise self-control, restrain their passions and rationally govern their behaviour was crucial to the maintenance of a stable body politic.[139] William Godwin, the political philosopher, novelist and husband of Mary Wollstonecraft, noted in his *Enquiry Concerning Political Justice* (1793) that

> While the sympathy of opinion catches from man to man, especially in numerous meetings, and among persons whose passions have not been used to the curb of judgment, actions may be determined on, which solitary reflection would have rejected. There is nothing more barbarous, cruel, and blood-thirst, than the triumph of a mob. Sober thought should always prepare the way to the public assertion of truth. He, that would be the founder of a republic, should... be insensible to the energies of the most imperious passions of our nature.[140]

The Edinburgh-educated Scottish philosopher Dugald Stewart offered a similar sentiment in his study of the human mind, while lamenting the failure of so many citizens to engage in sober thought. The 'contagion of sympathetic imitation', Stewart feared, in which one person's behaviour prompted the same behaviour in onlookers, could have dire consequences for a passionate population unpractised in reason.[141] A man too easily moved was a man easily manipulated; the once-celebrated overly-sensitive man of feeling was now a fanatical fool.

Conclusion

The effect of negative modern views about nervous disease was a particular lack of sympathy towards sufferers. Instead of praise for their extreme sensibility and humanity, nervous sufferers in the second half of the century were increasingly portrayed as peevish, self-absorbed, immoral and artificial creatures. Rather than enriching society with their depth of feeling, nervous sufferers had become a national burden. In 1786 the Scottish physician and writer John Moore described a typically cowardly and self-absorbed hypochondriac in his *Medical Sketches*:

> Although in his brighter days he may have been a man of courage, he becomes preposterously afraid of death, now when he seems to have lost all relish for the enjoyments of life. Entirely occupied by his own uneasy thoughts and feelings, all other subjects of conversation appear impertinent, and are in reality as intolerable to him as the everlasting theme of his own complaints generally is to others.[142]

The poet William Cowper neatly captured popular negative sentiment towards nervous sufferers and hypochondriacs in his famous poem, 'The Task' (1785):

> In making known how oft they have been sick,
> And give us in recitals of disease
> A doctor's trouble, but without the fees:
> Relate how many weeks they kept their bed,
> How an emetic or cathartic sped,
> Nothing is slightly touched, much less forgot,
> Nose, ears and eyes seem present on the spot.
> Now the distemper spite of draught or pill
> Victorious seem'd, and now the doctor's skill;
> And now – alas for unforeseen mishaps!
> They put on a damp night-cap and relapse;
> They thought they must have died they were so bad,
> Their peevish hearers almost wish they had.[143]

Even in America nervous sufferers were objects of ridicule and criticism, as writers equated their over-delicacy with a loss of traditional virtue. According to one contributor to the *Columbian Magazine* in 1787, nervous sufferers even put religious virtue at risk:

> For persons of weak nerves, my friend thinks it will be necessary to provide a very modest preacher; one whose voice shall be soft and harmonious... He says, he has known some women have the *vapors* for two days, after hearing a sermon, filled with horrible images, delivered with thundering pulpit eloquence. Heaven will be tempting to such people, if they can be certain of lolling upon *sofas* when they get there.[144]

Trotter summarized modern sentiment towards nervous sufferers with his comment that 'if there is one disease more than another that is induced by indolence, by sloth, and want of active motion, it is that train of nervous weaknesses, which puts on the form of every other complaint, and becomes one of the greatest stings to human happiness'.[145]

Thus, nervous disease became less fashionable in Britain during the second half of the century as its supposed number of nervous sufferers increased in tandem with fears of national degeneracy. The severe national implications of nervous sufferings were further magnified by the heated political climate of the late eighteenth century, renewed emphasis on the connection between moral laxity and personal ill health, and by medical theories supporting the hereditary nature of nervous disease which threatened an ever-more degenerate population. Popular discussions of nervous disease extended beyond the fictional portrayals of fashionable sufferers in mid-century romantic novels; they also provided solid scientific evidence of Britain's collective moral and political decline by the century's end, demonstrating the seriousness with which nervous disease was taken by the general public. This earnest concern was encouraged by the growing body of scientific discourse about the nerves from 1764 onwards. The fact that so many patients were diagnosed with nervous disease even amidst this flurry of medical and social negativity towards nervous sufferers late in the century, proves that the diagnosis of nervous disease was not dependent on fashion. Rather, it was a genuine medical diagnosis that was, at the same time, often instigated by social causes and laden with cultural implications.

The co-operative nature of social and medical discussions about nervous disease further illustrates the strong link between medicine and society in the eighteenth century. While historians have most often explored the ways in which social factors influenced medical ideas about nervous disease, this chapter has shown that the interchange between medicine and society was far more reciprocal. Medical reports declaring unprecedented numbers of nervous sufferers fuelled popular anxiety over the spread of luxury and modern civilization, and scientific theories of hereditary nervousness convinced many Britons of their nation's degenerate future. The growing role of medical practitioners as moral guardians towards the end of the eighteenth century further fused medical and social matters, as doctors anxiously discussed the immoral causes and consequences of nervous disease.

Given the symbiotic nature of the relationship between medical and social ideas about the nerves, it is impossible to discover 'which came first'. Convincing arguments can be made for both sides. Christopher Lawrence has illustrated the way in which the nerve doctors composing nervous theories during the late eighteenth century were already steeped in the philosophical notions of people like Adam Smith, who discussed subjects like sympathy, sensibility and innate superiority of feeling at length.[146] Likewise, George Rousseau notes that Adam Smith's *Theory of Moral Sentiments* was a common addition to the personal libraries of late eighteenth-century medical men.[147] Yet it is also known that Smith was a close friend and a patient of Cullen's, the two men having met while teaching at the University of Glasgow before Smith ever committed his ideas about sensibility to paper.[148]

It is an impossible task to decide who influenced whom, or, even worse, who influenced whom first. Rather, it appears that the supposed divide between medicine and society was a porous one, allowing each side to influence the other. Nerve doctors, armed with the beliefs, anxieties and prejudices of their times, naturally subsumed their cultural beliefs into their medical theories and practices, believing, in light of national hysteria over degeneration and failing morals, that the number of nervous sufferers was far greater than suggested by their own case records. Yet just as significant is the way in which medical notions of healthy and unhealthy lifestyles allowed citizens to judge the status of individual and national morés on medical grounds. By the end of the eighteenth century, nervous disease was as much a disease of society as it was a legitimate disease of the body and mind. Far from glamorous, it was, as doctors and moralists feared, a physical punishment for over-civilization and a sign of Britain's failure to cope in a modern world ruled by fashion, temptation and lost virtue.

EPILOGUE

Published in serial between 1759 and 1767, Laurence Sterne's *Tristram Shandy* introduced an eccentric range of characters, several of whom suffered from some sort of nervous disorder resultant from excessive sensibility. 'The plan' of the novel, as Sterne wrote to a friend in 1759, was to take in 'not only the Weak part of the Sciences, in wch the true point of Ridicule lies – but every Thing else, which I find Laugh-at-able in my way –'.[1] Given the popularity of Sterne's work, it is clear that readers of *Tristram Shandy* did find the follies of its melancholic, hysteric and hypochondriac characters 'laugh-at-able'. Furthermore, given the popularity of medical tracts concerning nervous diseases mid-century, it is likely that this folly was particularly appreciated for its familiarity to Sterne's eighteenth-century readers. Yet it is precisely because Sterne's audience understood his joking portrayal of the nerves and nervous sufferers, that it cannot be dismissed as anecdotal. Discussions of nervous disorders permeated not only popular culture, but also the philosophical, medical and political culture of the eighteenth century. It is for this reason that nervous disease must be examined, not as a humorous example of 'science-gone-wrong' in the eighteenth century, but as a window through which we can better understand the complex relationship between medicine and society. For as Sterne's character Walter Shandy wisely declared, 'Every thing in this world ... is big with jest, – and has wit in it, and instruction too, – if we can but find it out'.[2]

The purpose of this study has been to 'find out' the true significance of nervous disease in late eighteenth-century Britain by balancing popular depictions of nervous ailments with an empirical exploration of the experience of living with, treating and coming to terms with disordered nerves. Popular discourse from the period frequently portrayed nervous disease as a purely fashionable phenomenon; nerve doctors were presented as mere pawns in the money-driven medical marketplace, and nervous patients flocking to the spas were painted as spurious attention-seekers, desperate for social recognition. Yet such portrayals were not representative of the majority of treating physicians or nervous patients. Nor did they give credit to the period's painstakingly crafted medical definitions of nervous disease. Nervous disease was taken seriously by the doctors that treated it, the patients that suffered from it, and ultimately, by an entire nation that feared the untimely demise of its collective nervous, and hence, moral and physical, strength.

By the turn of the century, the roar of popular discourse emphasizing the fashionable nature of nervous sufferings quieted to a murmur. As the physiological manifestations of nervous sensibility assumed newfound implications of affectation, effeminacy, moral laxity, unseemly excess and political degeneracy, disordered nerves gradually lost their estimable lustre. The Evangelical revivals of the late eighteenth and early nineteenth century further undermined the fashion for nervous complaints, through a heightened emphasis on self-control and useful action.[3] As Mark Micale has argued, the 'Evangelical ethos' decried the 'perceived excesses' of earlier years, offering instead an 'unrelenting emphasis on duty, earnestness, and will power' that valued 'discipline, productivity, and self-mastery'.[4] It also carried a stricter emphasis on proper gender roles, and a corresponding emphasis on masculine stoicism, which was highly incompatible with the eighteenth century's overly refined and emotional 'man of feeling'. Still, the nineteenth century did not mark a precise end to the disorder's fashionable implications, or to its symptomological existence.[5]

Melancholically gloomy art and literature composed in a 'nervous style' achieved unprecedented praise in the Romantic period. So too did the creators of these works. While considered tremendously susceptible to extreme sensibility and nervousness, they were often admired for their weakness, as the creative full nature of their artistic productions necessitated their ability to experience, indulge and convey an organic depth of feeling. Ivan Turgenev perfectly summarized this distinguishing trait in his novel, *Fathers and Sons* (1862), with one character's claim that the creative Romantics 'develop[ed] their nervous systems to the breaking point'.[6] In particular, the persona of the nervous Romantic poet was so common that a sickly and melancholic temperament seemed almost a necessary qualification for literary success. Samuel Taylor Coleridge was a raging hypochondriac diagnosed with a nervous disorder in 1796, which he attributed to anxiety.[7] The medically trained John Keats complained in his personal letters that he was 'very nervous', and acknowledged to his sister in 1820 that he was suffering from 'nervous irritability' and 'anxiety of mind' associated with 'the too great excitement of poetry'.[8] Likewise, grief stricken by the recent death of his mother and several close friends, Lord Byron confided to a correspondent in 1811, 'I am growing *nervous* ... really, wretchedly, ridiculously ... *nervous*'.[9] The link between poetic genius and nervous sufferings became so ingrained in the popular mind that the medical student William Gibbons felt it proper to compose several portions of his 1805 thesis on Hypochondria in verse. He described, for example, how the 'voluntary gloom' of many sufferers prompted them to 'request oblivion and demand the tomb'.[10]

The productive creativity inspired by the morbid sensibility of Romantic poets did not entirely exempt them from criticism. For example, William Hazlitt's 1822 essay 'On Effeminacy of Character' criticized Keats's poetry directly for exhibiting a 'deficiency in masculine energy of style'.[11] Yet in the eyes of most, the depth of feeling that inspired these poets' sufferings was also the key to their literary power. As the editor of Lord Byron's collected works explained in 1832, Byron's melancholy poems were

> the abstract spirit, as it were, of many griefs; – a confluence of sad thoughts from many sources of sorrow, refined and warmed in their passage through his fancy, and forming thus one deep reservoir of mournful feeling.[12]

The creative expression of Romantic poets allowed readers to dip their toes into this 'reservoir' of feeling, without becoming immersed in its dangerously enervating sentiment. Whereas the perceived value of nervous sensibility lay in its ability to promote sociable compassion and philanthropic behaviour, debilitating nervousness was incompatible with productive activity. By reading and enjoying the fruits of the poets' emotional excesses, Britons could, in turn, exercise and illustrate their capacity for depth and compassion without committing their own morbid indulgence. Romantic poets became self-sacrificing martyrs of sensibility, while ordinary British citizens were praised for having a similar capacity for debilitating feeling, but the self-command to avoid it.

An unrealized susceptibility to nervous disorders positively implied civilization and emotional depth. The surgeon and Royal Society fellow, Sir William Lawrence, neatly expressed this view in his *Lectures on Physiology* (1819). In terms highly reminiscent of Cheyne's *English Malady*, Lawrence explained the corporeal consequences of nineteenth-century civilized life:

> The accumulation of numbers in large cities, the noxious effects of impure air, sedentary habits, and unwholesome employments; – the excesses in diet, the luxurious food, the heating drinks ... and the pernicious seasonings, which stimulate and oppress the organs ... the delicacy and sensibility to external influences caused by our heated rooms, warm clothing, inactivity, and other indulgences, are so many fatal proofs that our most grievous ills are our own work, and might be obviated by a more simple and uniform way of life ...

Lawrence contrasted the ill health of civilized citizens with 'the mountain shepherd and his dog', a pair that he described as 'equally hardy'. There is little doubt that Lawrence was aware that his audience would prefer to be classified with the ranks of the over-refined than with a mountain mutt. In this way, self-congratulation for high levels of civilization and susceptibility to diseases of a civilized life were still praiseworthy to some degree. Yet Lawrence quickly qualified his surreptitious praise of civilization-induced illness, noting how a shepherd and dog could 'form an instructive contrast with a nervous and hysterical fine lady, and her lap-dog; the extreme point of degeneracy and imbecility of which each race is susceptible'.[13] Here, framed as a disease of civilization and sensibility, vulnerability to nervous disease was admirable, but nervous debility was not. Overly-sensitive or over-indulgent beings who fostered, cherished or feigned their nervous weakness were rendered useless in the name of the very fibres that were intended to incite an active civic spirit.[14]

Amidst the barrage of criticism allying profligate nervous sufferings with an amoral 'impotency of spirit', it is easy to understand why nineteenth-century patients plagued by typically 'nervous' symptoms, would have hoped to avoid this diagnosis.[15] Growing implications of effeminacy further underscored nervousness as an unwelcome diagnosis for men. A letter from the Edinburgh-educated physician Benjamin Vaughan to a patient in 1811 is suggestive of this newly undesirable nature of nervous diagnoses. Reiterating the symptoms of his patient's 'indisposition' involving weakness, indigestion, dizziness, low spirits and costiveness, Vaughan's list appears suspiciously identical to those 'denominated nervous' by Whytt over fifty years before. Nevertheless, the surviving draft of Vaughan's letter suggests an interesting discomfort in providing his patient with a nervous diagnosis. In his recommendation for treatment, Vaughan tip-toed around the precise diagnosis, suggesting instead that his medical advice would 'not materially differ from Dr Cullen's system for nervous diseases noticed by him under the head of neuroses or nervous diseases'. Vaughan also included in this letter a summary of a female patient 'of delicate habit' who suffered from similar symptoms. After describing his successful treatment of this patient in detail, Vaughan subtly hinted, 'The same plan has benefited others'.[16] Vaughan's effort to tactfully deliver his medical advice suggests that cultural judgements could alter a formal diagnosis, but not its objectively experienced symptoms.

Indeed, the symptoms of nervous disease continued long after its reign as a fashionable disorder had ended. Physicians continued to decry a perceived growth in nervous sufferers in the nineteenth century, with Dr John Reid's *Essays on Hypochondriacal and Other Nervous Affections* declaring in 1817 that the number of nervous sufferers was 'daily increasing'.[17] Publications on nervous disorders also continued in the first quarter of the century, although they were not as numerous as in the century before.[18] While they had a more subtle presence in the social and medical worlds than they did previously, the symptoms of disordered nerves also maintained a steady presence in medical casebooks and hospital registers.

By the second half of the nineteenth century, nervous symptoms were contextualized in a wholly different way than they were one hundred years earlier. Medical theory still subscribed to the Brunonian notion that human body was equipped with a finite amount of nervous energy, and that taxing the body's supply through over-stimulation could have permanently debilitating consequences. Yet instead of being weakened by luxury, laziness or over-sensibility which had become so odious to late eighteenth- and early nineteenth-century citizens, nervous patients were now deemed 'guilty' of draining their nerve force through more active and admirable factors including prolonged concentration, hard work and keeping up in a fast-paced world. The fashion for disordered nerves had returned.

The revival of fashionable nervous weakness was strongest in America in the late nineteenth century. Echoing Cheyne's *English Malady* from nearly 150 years before, the American electrotherapist George Beard referred to nervous disease as a specifically American disorder, even titling his book on the subject *American Nervousness* (1881). As he proudly proclaimed in his introduction,

> A new crop of diseases has sprung up in America, of which Great Britain until lately knew nothing or but little. A class of functional diseases of the nervous system, now beginning to be known everywhere in civilization, seem to have first taken root under an American sky, whence their seed is being distributed. All this is modern, and originally American; and no age, no country, and no form of civilization, not Greece, nor Rome, nor Spain, nor the Netherlands, in the days of their glory, possessed such maladies.[19]

According to Beard, modern civilization was the greatest culprit for American nervousness, which he termed 'Neurasthenia'. In an industrial world of railways, telegraphs, canals, steam-ships and even the growing popularity of wristwatches, American businessmen drained their nerve-force in a frantic attempt to keep up.[20] Americans also had the added stress of living in a more socially mobile, and thus more highly competitive society than Europeans. The ambition required to survive in this Darwinian society was a significant drain on Americans' nervous energy.

Beard's *American Nervousness* was intended for citizens in the upper echelons of society – the intellectual and professional businessmen who supposedly bore the greatest stresses in the nation's gilded age.[21] Thus, suffering from such a disorder denoted a person's active participation in a fashionably fast-paced world. By the early twentieth century, after this supposedly American disease had spread to Europe, the French physician Paul Dubois reflected that, like nervous disorders almost two hundred years before, this 'new' nervous disease had become a fashionable ailment:

> Since the works of George Beard, a new nervous disease has been imported from America, and seems to be propagated like an epidemic. The name of neurasthenia is on everybody's lips; it is the fashionable new disease.[22]

The symptoms of this 'new disease' were identical to those discussed by nerve doctors in the eighteenth century, prompting many British physicians to challenge its novelty. For instance, the physician Sir Andrew Clark of the London Hospital insisted in 1889 that the symptoms of neurasthenia had 'been more or less fully recognized and described by every competent observer and writer from the days of Cheyne and Whytt until now'.[23] Thus, while the observed symptoms remained constant over time, it was the medical theory and explanatory diagnoses that had changed.

Neurasthenia further echoed eighteenth-century nervousness in its supposed spread to the lower classes. A quarter of a century after Beard's introduction of the diagnosis, the physician Sir Thomas Clifford Allbutt declared that neurasthenia was no longer exclusive to wealthy businessmen. As he claimed,

> [It] is common enough also in the wage-earning classes of England ... The truth is that neurasthenia is found no more in the market-place than in the rectory or in the workhouse.[24]

As in the eighteenth century, the acknowledged spread of neurasthenia to the lower classes preceded its demise as a 'fashionable diagnosis'. Suddenly the increasing number of neurasthenic sufferers was robbing the nation of valuable brainpower, manpower and money. People who heedlessly taxed their nervous resources through immoderate work and stress were irresponsibly endangering their long-term productivity and economic contribution to society.[25] Like 'nervousness', 'neurasthenia' concluded its fashionable reign as an alleged threat to national moral and medical health.

Factors such as consumer society, fashion, wealth, sensibility, gender and morals remained important frameworks for contextualizing nervous weakness throughout the eighteenth and nineteenth centuries. While these frameworks often helped the public to make sense of disordered nerves, they also created impossibly tidy explanations for a disease that was notoriously varied and resistant to definition. In reality, the experience of treating and suffering from a nervous disorder consistently defied culturally imposed explanations and simple stereotypes. Often portrayed as an imaginary condition invented by quack doctors to take advantage of lucrative consumers, medical theory behind disordered nervous systems were studied seriously by a wealth of dedicated physicians. Understood as a fashionable disorder, typical nervous symptoms were decidedly not. Regarded as a disease of the wealthy and over-refined, poor sufferers maintained a constant presence in medical records. An assumed consequence of refined sensibility, many patients believed that they suffered as a result of vulgar indiscretion. Mocked as an excuse for sociable cures and trips to the spa, nervous disease often required unpleasant treatments like siphons and sickening medications. A presumed disorder of delicate females, men regularly sought treatment for their ailing nerves. Believed to be a specifically 'English malady', it was, in fact, an international diagnosis. Thus, while explanatory contexts may have helped patients, practitioners and the general public to make sense of disordered nerves, they offer only a shallow and singular representation of the true depth and multi-faceted nature of the nervous experience. This investigation of the experience of nervous patients and their practitioners reminds historians that this broadly defined 'disease of civilization' was only the sum of its parts.

Appendix 1: First-Tier Nerve Doctors

Appendix   183

Appendix 1: First-Tier Nerve Doctors

First Tier Nerve Doctors

Name	Education	Career	Honours/Societies	Relevant Publications
Cooke, John (1756–1838)	Studied in London and Edinburgh; MD, Leiden, 1781	Physician: practised in London; Physician to Royal General Dispensary, London; Physician to London Hospital, 1784; Lecturer, London hospital	Fellow, RCPL, 1807; Fellow, Royal Society, 1817; Fellow, Antiquarian Society; President, Medico-Chirurgical Society, 1822-1823	Treatise on Nervous Diseases (1823)
Cullen, William (1710–1790)	Studied at Glasgow and Edinburgh; Apprenticed to Glasgow surgeon apothecary; Ship's surgeon for 6 mos. in West Indies; Worked in London apothecary shop; MD, Glasgow, 1740	Physician and Professor: practised in Hamilton, Glasgow and Edinburgh; Professor of the practice of medicine at Edinburgh; Physician, Edinburgh Royal Infirmary	Founding member of Edinburgh's RMS; Royal Society of Edinburgh and London; Member of several debating and dining clubs; Fellow, RCPE; president, 1773-1775	Nosology (1769); Materia Medica (1772); First Lines of the Practice of Physic (1777–1784)
Falconer, William (1744–1824)	MD, Edinburgh, 1766; 2nd MD, Leiden, 1767	Physician: practised in Bath; Physician, Chester Infirmary, 1767; Physician, Bath General Hospital, 1784	Extra-Licentiate of RCP in 1767; Fellow, Royal Society, London, 1773; Bath and West of England Society; Manchester Literary and Philosophical Society; Dissertation won the Fothergill Medal in 1796; Silver medal from Medical Society of London in 1805	Dissertation: Influence of the Passions upon Disorders of the Body (1788)
Gilchrist, Ebenezer (1708–1774)	Studied at Edinburgh, London and Paris; MD, Rheims, 1732	Physician: practised in Dumfries		The Use of Sea Voyages in Medicine (1756)
Gregory, John (1724–1773)	Studied at Edinburgh and Leiden; MD, Aberdeen, 1746	Physician and Professor: practised in Aberdeen, London and Edinburgh; First physician in Scotland to George III; Physician, Edinburgh Royal Infirmary; Lecturer, King's College, Aberdeen, 1746	Fellow, Royal Society, 1756; Fellow, RCPE in 1765; Edinburgh Medical Society; Aberdeen Philosophical Society	Lectures on the Duties and Qualifications of a Physician (1772); Elements of the Practice of Physic (1772); A Father's Legacy to his Daughters (1774)

First Tier

Nerve Doctors Name	Education	Career	Honours/Societies	Relevant Publications
Halford, Sir Henry (1766–1844)	Studied at Edinburgh MD, Oxford, 1791	Physician: practised in London Physician to Middlesex hospital, 17?3 Physician-extraordinary to George III, 1793.	Gordon Mills Society for agricultural Improvement in Aberdeen Fellow, RCPL, 1794; president, 1820 Fellow, Royal Society, 1810 Fellow, Antiquaries Society	Private/unpublished writings about nervous disease including papers delivered to RCPL.
Heberden, William (1710–1801)	MD, Cambridge, 1738	Physician: practised in London	Fellow, RCPL, 1746 Royal Society, 1749 Society of Antiquaries, 1770 Honorary member, Royal Society of Medicine, Paris, 1778	Commentaries on the History and Cure of Diseases (Written in 1782, published posthumously in 1802).
Lettsom, John Coakley (1744–1815)	Apprenticed to Yorkshire surgeon and apothecary, 1761 Surgeon's dresser, St. Thomas' Hospital, London, 1766 Studied medicine at Edinburgh, 1768 MD, Leiden, 1769	Physician: practised in London Co-founder and physician, General Dispensary in London Co-founder, Royal sea-bathing Infirmary at Margate, 1791	Licentiate, RCPL, 1770 Fellow, Royal Society, 1773 Co-founder, London Medical Society, 1773 Co-founder, Royal Humane Society, 1774 President, London Philosophical Society, 1812	Dissertation: The Natural History of the Tea Tree (1772) Hints Designed to Promote Beneficence, Temperance, and Medical Science (1802)
Oliver, William (1695–1764)	Studied at Leiden MD, Cambridge, 1725	Physician: practised in Plymouth and Bath Instigator of Bath Mineral Hospital and physician to hospital, 1740	Fellow, Royal Society, 1730	A Practical Dissertation on Bath Waters (1707) Cases of Persons Admitted into the Infirmary at Bath under the Care of Doctor Oliver (1760) Cases also reprinted in Rice Charleton's Three Tracts on Bath Water (1774)
Parry, Caleb Hillier (1755–1822)	Studied in London and Edinburgh MD, Edinburgh, 1778	Physician: practised in Bath Physician, Bath Pauper Charity and ... Hospital, Licentiate, RCPL, 1778	President Royal Medical Society, 1777	Collections from the Unpublished Medical Writings of the Late Caleb Hillier Parry (1825)

First Tier
Nerve Doctors

Name	Education	Career	Honours/Societies	Relevant Publications
Walker, Sayer (1748–1826)	Studied in Montpellier and Edinburgh MD, Aberdeen, 1791	Physician, Bath General Hospital, 1799 Physician and Presbyterian Minister: practised in London Physician in Ordinary to London Lying-in Hosital, 1794	Bath and West Agricultural Society President, Fleece Medical Society Bath Philosophical Society Fellow, Royal Society, 1800 Licentiate, RCPL, 1792 Treasurer, Medical Society of London	Treatise on Nervous Diseases (1796) Observations on the Constitution of Women (1803)
Whytt, Robert (1714–1766)	Studied in Edinburgh, London, Paris and Leiden MD, Rheims, 1736 MD, St. Andrews, 1737	Physician and Professor: practised in Edinburgh Professor of the Practice of Medicine in Edinburgh, 1747 Lectured at Edinburgh Royal Infirmary, 1760 Physician to King of Scotland	Fellow, RCPE, 1738; president, 1763 Fellow, Royal Society, 1752 Select Society	An Enquiry into the Causes which Promote the Circulation of Fluids in the Small Vessels of Animals (1745/46) Essay on the Vital and other Involuntary Motions of Animals (1751) Observations on the Nature, Causes, and Cure of those Disorders... Nervous, Hyp, Hysteric (1764)
Wilson, Andrew (1718–1792)	MD, Edinburgh, 1749	Physician: practised in Newcastle upon Tyne and London Physician, London Medical Asylum	Licentiate, RCPL, 1764	Medical Researches, being an enquiry into the nature and origin of hysterics in the female constitution (1776) Short remarks upon autumnal disorders of the bowels (1765)

Appendix 2 Second-Tier Nerve Doctors

Second Tier Nerve Doctors Name	Education	Career	Honours/Societies	Relevant Publications
Adair, James Makittrick (1728–1801)	MD, Edinburgh, 1766	Physician: practised in Antigua, Andover, G▉ford and Bath		Medical Cautions for the Consideration of Invalids (1786) Essays on Fashionable Diseases (1790)
Beddoes, Thomas (1760–1808)	Studied in London MD, Oxford, 1786	Physician: practised in Bristol Established Pneumatic Institute in Bristol He▉ells		Hygeia (1802-1803) The Manual of Health (1806)
Hill, John (1714–1775)	Apprenticed in London MD, St. Andrews, 1751	Apothecary: practised in London	Failed attempt to join the Royal Society, 1747 Knighted in Sweden, 1774	The Construction of the Nerves (1758) Hypochondriasis: A Practical Treatise (1766)
Neale, Adam (c. 1778–1832)	MD, Edinburgh, 1802	Physician: practised in Exeter and Chelten▉a and military Unsuccessful candidate for office of physican▉ Devon and Exeter Hospital Physician to the forces, 1808 Physician-extraordinary to the duke of Kent, ▉08 Physician to the British Embassy at Constanti▉ple, 1808	Licentiate, RCPL, 1806 Fellow, Linnean Society	Practical Dissertations on Nervous Complaints and other Diseases Incident to the Human Body, 3rd edn. (1796) Letter to a professor of medicine in the University of Edinburgh respecting the nature and properties of the mineral waters of Cheltenham (1820)
Perfect, William (1731–1809)	Apprenticed to London surgeon, 1749 MD, St. Andrews, 1783	Physician and Surgeon: practised in Kent Ran lunatic asylum in Kent	Freemason, 1765 Held office of provincial grand orator, 1787 Provincial grand master of the county of Kent, 1795 London Medical Society	Cases of Insanity, the Epilepsy... and Nervous Disoders, Successfully Treated (1778)

Second Tier Nerve Doctors

Name	Education	Career	Honours/Societies	Relevant Publications
Rymer, James (unknown–1842)	Apprenticed to surgeon and apothecary; Studied at Edinburgh	Surgeon: practised in Reigate, Ramsgate, and navy	Contributed to General Magazine of Arts and Sciences, Political Chronicle and Westminster Journal.	A Sketch of Great Yarmouth, with some Reflections on Cold Bathing (1777); A Tract Upon Indigestion and the Hypochondriac Disease (1785); A Treatise on Diet and Regimen (1828)
Scot, John (Dates unknown)	MD, location unknown	Physician: practised in London		Remarkable Cures of Gouty, Bilious, and Nervous Cases (1780); An Enquiry into the origin of the gout wherein its various symptoms... and those of all... nervous disorders are traced (1783)
Smith, Hugh (1735–1789)	MD, Leiden, 1755	Physician: practised in London		The Family Physician (1760); Letters to Married Women (1774); The Use and Abuse of Mineral Waters (1776); An Essay on the Nerves - to which is added an essay on foreign tea (1795)
Thomson, Alexander (1767–c. 1801)	MD, location unknown	Physician: practised in London		An Enquiry into the Nature, Causes, and Method of Cure, of Nervous Disorders in a Letter to a Friend (1781); The Family Physician; or, Domestic Medical Friend (1801)
Trotter, Thomas (1760–1832)	MD, Edinburgh, 1788	Physician and Surgeon: practised in Navy and Newcastle upon Tyne; Physician, Royal Naval Hospital at Haslar	Literary and Philosophical Society; Composed and published plays and poetry	Medicina Nautica (1797); Essay on Drunkenness (1804); View of the Nervous Temperament (1807)

Appendix 3: Quack Doctors

Quack Doctors Name	Education	Career	Honours/Societies	Relevant Publications
Brodum, William (1767–1824)	Purchased MD from Aberdeen, 1791	Physician and vendor of nervous cordial: practised in London		A Guide to Old Age or a Cure for the Indescretions of Youth (1795)
		Had lawsuit with Lettsom over his legitimacy as a physician		By his Majesty's Royal Letters Patent: Dr. Brodum's Nervous Cordial, and Botanical Syrup (1808)
Graham, James (1745–1794)	Studied at Edinburgh	Practised in New York, Philadelphia, Bristol, Bath and London		The Guardian Goddess of Health (1780)
	Never attained degree, but called himself an MD			
Knight, W. D. (dates unknown)				Hint to Valetudinarians (1796)
Lowther, William (dates unknown)		Practised in Bath		Published advertisements in Bath regarding his nervous powders and drops
Rowley, William (1742–1806)	Trained in London	Man-midwife and surgeon: practised in London	Licentiate, RCPL, 1784	A Treatise on Female, Nervous, Hysterical, Hypochondriacal, Bilious, Convulsive Diseases etc. (1788)
	MD, St. Andrews, 1774	Physician at the Marylebone Infirmary, London		
Solomon, Samuel (1768–1819)	Purchased MD from Aberdeen, 1796 (Registrar suspected his supporting certificates were forged)	Patent medicine manufacturer: practised in Liverpool		An Account of that most excellent medicine the cordial balm of Gilead (1799)
Webster, Joshua (1709–1801)	Claims an MD, but is cited as a surgeon in the Corporation of Surgeons of London membership list (1777)	Surgeon: practised in London and Bath		Published advertisements in London such as his True and Brief Account of the Celebrated English Diet Drink (1799)

NOTES

Introduction

1. J. Gregory, *Lectures on the Duties and Qualifications of a Physician*, 2nd edn (London, 1772), pp. 88, 91.
2. J. Gregory, *A Comparative View of the State and Faculties of Man with Those of the Animal World*, 7th edn (London, 1777), p. 270.
3. While some eighteenth-century medical texts included disorders like epilepsy and palsy in their categorization of nervous disease, the vast majority of practitioners and laymen used the diagnosis to refer only to diseases 'more particularly denominated nervous' including melancholia, hysteria and hypochondria. This study employs this more common categorization of nervous disease, limiting its discussion to these particular ailments.
4. G. Cheyne as quoted in R. Porter, *George Cheyne: The English Malady* (London: Routledge, 1991), p. xxx.
5. Ibid., p. xxx.
6. Ibid., p. xi.
7. Ibid., p. xxvi.
8. T. Beddoes, 'Extracts from Dr Beddoes's Common-place books', *Edinburgh Medical and Surgical Journal*, 7 (1811), pp. 185, 187.
9. See in particular N. Jewson, 'Medical Knowledge and the Patronage System in Eighteenth-Century England', *Sociology*, 8:3 (1974), pp. 369–85.
10. For instance, G. J. Barker-Benfield, *The Culture of Sensibility: Sex and Society in Eighteenth-Century Britain* (Chicago, IL: Chicago University Press, 1992); B. Taylor and S. Knott, (eds), *Women, Gender and Enlightenment* (London: Palgrave Macmillan, 2007); M. Micale, *Hysterical Men: The Hidden History of Male Nervous Illness* (Boston, MA: Harvard University Press, 2008).
11. For example, see: C. Lawrence, 'Medicine as Culture: Edinburgh and the Scottish Enlightenment' (PhD Dissertation, UCL, 1984); C. Lawrence, 'The Nervous System and Society in the Scottish Enlightenment', in B. Barnes and S. Shapin, (eds), *Natural Order: Historical Studies of Scientific Culture* (Beverley Hills, CA: Sage Publications, 1979), pp. 19–40; A. Vila, *Enlightenment and Pathology: Sensibility in the Literature and Medicine of Eighteenth-Century France* (Baltimore, MD: Johns Hopkins University Press, 1998); C. Withers and P. Wood, (eds), *Science and Medicine in the Scottish Enlightenment* (East Linton: Tuckwell Press, 2002).

12. A few such studies include: J. Mullan, *Sentiment and Sociability: The Language of Feeling in the Eighteenth Century* (Oxford: Oxford University Press, 1988); J. Brewer, 'Sentiment and Sensibility' in James Chandler, (ed.), *The Cambridge History of English Romantic Literature* (Cambridge: Cambridge University Press, 2009); M. Ellis, *The Politics of Sensibility: Race, Gender and Commerce in the Sentimental Novel* (Cambridge: Cambridge University Press, 1996); A. J. Van Sant, *Eighteenth-Century Sensibility and the Novel: the Senses in Social Context* (Cambridge: Cambridge University Press, 1993); S. Knott, *Sensibility and the American Revolution* (Chapel Hill, NC: University of North Carolina Press, 2009); P. Logan, *Nerves and Narratives* (Berkeley, CA: University of California Press, 1997); R. Stephanson, 'Richardson's "Nerves": The Physiology of Sensibility in Clarissa', *Journal of the History of Ideas*, 49:2 (1998), pp. 267–85.

13. The experiences of these men are related in several studies, including: A. Ingram, *Boswell's Creative Gloom: A Study of Imagery and Melancholy in the Writings of James Boswell* (New Jersey: Barnes and Noble Books, 1982); G. Rousseau, 'Coleridge's Dreaming Gut: Digestion, Genius, Hypochondria', in C. Forth and A. Carden-Coyne (eds), *Cultures of the Abdomen: Diet, Digestion, and Fat in the Modern World* (New York: Palgrave Macmillan, 2005), pp. 105–26; R. Porter, '"The Hunger of Imagination": Approaching Samuel Johnson's Melancholy', in W. F. Bynum, R. Porter, and M. Shepherd (eds), *The Anatomy of Madness: Essays in the History of Psychiatry*, 2 vols (London: Tavistock Publications, 1985), vol. 1, pp. 63–88; J. Wiltshire, *Samuel Johnson in the Medical World* (Cambridge: Cambridge University Press, 1991).

14. F. Albritton Jonsson has also claimed that historians 'do not yet have a clear understanding of how hypochondria was experienced by the majority of its victims'. Jonsson, 'The Physiology of Hypochondria in Eighteenth-Century Britain' in Forth and Carden Coyne, (eds), *Cultures of the Abdomen*, p. 14.

15. Wayne Wild also examines this body of letters, with a particular emphasis on the language of sensibility employed by Cullen and his patients in *Medicine-by-Post: The Changing Voice of Illness in Eighteenth-Century British Consultation Letters and Literature* (Amsterdam: Rodopi Press, 2006).

16. See J. Todd, *Sensibility: An Introduction* (London: Methuen, 1986).

17. Logan also notes that nervous disease 'enjoyed its clearest moment of cultural ascendancy in the late Georgian period, before its 'cultural status changed' in the early Victorian years', in *Nerves and Narratives*, p. 5.

18. Sydenham as quoted in R. Whytt, *Observations on the Nature, Causes, and Cure of those Disorders which have been Commonly Called Nervous, Hypochondriac, or Hysteric*, 2nd edn (Edinburgh, 1765), p. 96.

19. While some historians have described nervous disease as the precursor to contemporary diagnoses such as heartburn, irritable bowel syndrome, chronic fatigue and severe depression, I would argue that there is no modern diagnosis capable of encompassing the confused conglomeration of mental and physical symptoms entailed in a nervous diagnosis of the eighteenth century.

1 Defining Nervous Disease in Eighteenth-Century Britain

1. Whytt, *Observations*.

2. J. Hill, *Hypochondriasis: A Practical Treatise on the Nature and Cure of that Disorder* (London, 1766), p. 1.

3. The varying and often contradictory theories about nervous disease over time make it impossible to chart an all-inclusive or neatly linear history of the subject. This chapter provides only a general overview of some of the most popular and widely discussed opinions on nervous disease.
4. Whytt, *Observations,* p. iv.
5. See R. Porter, 'The Body and the Mind, the Doctor and the Patient: Negotiating Hysteria', in S. Gilman, *Hysteria Beyond Freud* (Berkeley, CA: University of California Press, 1993), pp. 225–86; J. Boss, 'The Seventeenth-Century Transformation of the Hysteric Affection, and Sydenham's Baconian Medicine', *Psychological Medicine,* 9 (1979), pp. 221–34; S. W. Jackson, 'Melancholia and Mechanical Explanation in Eighteenth-Century Medicine', *Journal of the History of Medicine and Allied Sciences,* 38 (1983), p. 298.
6. This is not to argue that the cultural and pathological definitions are separate. Rather, they were mutually supportive and sustaining. See Van Sant, *Eighteenth-Century Sensibility,* pp. 3–4.
7. In this chapter, as in the rest of the book, the 'public' refers to a literate, non-medical laity, which was nonetheless aware of medical arguments, and capable of judging and expressing opinions on medical subjects through conversation, informal writings or publications. This 'public' is in opposition to the 'private' medical profession. I use the word 'popular' to describe general sentiments of the 'public'.
8. G. E. Berrios, 'Hypochondriasis: History of the Concept', in V. Starcevic and D. R. Lipsitt (eds), *Hypochondriasis: Modern Perspectives on an Ancient Malady* (Oxford: Oxford University Press, 2001), p. 5.
9. T. M. Brown, 'Descartes, Dualism, and Psychosomatic Medicine' in Bynum and Porter (eds), *The Anatomy of Madness,* vol. 1, pp. 40–62, on p. 41.
10. Boss, 'The Seventeenth-Century', p. 222.
11. R. Peirce, *History and Memoirs of the Bath: Containing Observations on what Cures have been there Wrought* (London, 1713), pp. 190–1.
12. Burton also failed to explain whether black bile was the cause or effect of the disorder.
13. R. Burton, *Anatomy of Melancholy,* ed. T. C. Faulkner, N. K. Kiessling and R. L. Blair, 6 vols (1621; Oxford: Clarendon Press, 1989), vol. 1, p. 162.
14. Ibid., pp. 246–7.
15. Ibid., p. 120.
16. Ibid., p. 302.
17. Aristotle, as quoted in H. Deutsch, 'Symptomatic Correspondences: The Author's Case in Eighteenth-Century Britain', *Cultural Critique,* 42 (Spring, 1999), p. 37.
18. Burton, *Anatomy* (1800 edition), p. 264.
19. Burton as quoted in Berrios, *Hypochondriasis,* p. 6.
20. G. S. Rousseau, *Nervous Acts: Essays on Literature, Culture and Sensibility* (New York: Palgrave Macmillan, 2004), pp. 164–5.
21. T. Willis, *London Practice of Physick* (London, 1685), p. 307.
22. Ibid., p. 311.
23. Rousseau, *Nervous Acts,* p. 166. As Logan has explained, even for those that denied that the brain was the 'somatic site for the mind, it was generally acknowledged that the nervous system represented an interface between the material and psychic realms'. See Logan, *Nerves and Narratives,* p. 7.
24. Willis as quoted in Berrios, *Hypochondriasis,* p. 8.
25. Rousseau, *Nervous Acts,* p. 11.
26. Rousseau, 'Originated Neurology', p. 24.

27. Sydenham as quoted in Boss, 'The Seventeenth-Century Transformation', p. 230.
28. T. Sydenham, *Dr Sydenham's Compleat Method of Curing Almost all Diseases, and Description of Their Symptoms,* 4th edn (London, 1710), p. 6.
29. Sydenham, as quoted in Berrios, *Hypochondriasis,* p. 8.
30. Locke as quoted in Barker-Benfield, *The Culture of Sensibility,* p. 4.
31. P. Miller, 'What Effects have the Powers of the Mind in the Production & Cure of Disease?', Dissertations Read to the Royal Medical Society at the Royal Medical Society, Edinburgh (hereafter DRRMS), 50 (1803–4), p. 371.
32. R. Schofield, *Mechanism and Materialism: British Natural Philosophy in an Age of Reason* (Princeton, NJ: Princeton University Press, 1970), p. 13.
33. Newton as quoted in Baker-Benfield, *Culture,* p. 5.
34. Jackson, 'Melancholia', p. 307.
35. Ibid., p. 299.
36. Ibid., p. 301.
37. A. Cunningham, 'Medicine to Calm the Mind: Boerhaave's medical system, and why it was adopted in Edinburgh', in A. Cunningham and R. French (eds), *The Medical Enlightenment of the Eighteenth Century* (Cambridge: Cambridge University Press, 1990), p. 43.
38. H. Steinke, *Irritating Experiments: Haller's Concept and the European Controversy on Irritability and Sensibility, 1750–90* (Amsterdam: Rodopi, 2005), p. 212.
39. Ibid., p. 20.
40. Schofield, *Mechanism and Materialism,* p. 103.
41. While intriguing to many medical men, there was significant confusion regarding the aether's precise operation and function, even by Newton. See A. Thackray, *Atoms and Powers* (Cambridge, MA: Harvard University Press, 1970), p. 26.
42. J. Rocca, 'William Cullen (1710–90) and Robert Whytt (1714–66) on the Nervous System', in H. Whitaker, C. U. M. Smith, and S. Finger (eds), *Brain, Mind and Medicine: Essays in Eighteenth-Century Neuroscience* (New York: Springer, 2007), pp. 85–98, p. 85.
43. Ibid., p. 86.
44. Ibid., pp. 90–1.
45. E. Clarke and C. D. O'Malley, *The Human Brain and Spinal Cord: A Historical Study Illustrated by Writings from Antiquity* 2nd edn (San Francisco, CA: Norman Publishing, 1996), p. 339. Whytt's beliefs were largely a halfway house between the mechanist and animist positions. As Whytt's colleague explained, 'It appears that both parties have erred, – the mechanicians [*sic*], in attempting to define all things from their art, without being sufficiently acquainted with the structure of the parts ... and those who, hating the very name of mechanics, have declared that our body is independent of those very laws by which all bodies ... are governed'. Cullen as quoted in J. Thompson, *An Account of the Life, Lectures and Writings of William Cullen, M.D.* (London, 1832), pp. 209–10.
46. R. French, 'Sickness and the Soul: Stahl, Hoffman and Sauvages on Pathology', in Cunningham and French (eds), *The Medical Enlightenment,* pp. 000–000 p. 92.
47. Pickstone argues that neither the RCP nor the professors at the University of Edinburgh in the mid-eighteenth century held any sort of uniform religious belief. See J. Pickstone, 'Establishment and Dissent in Nineteenth-Century Medicine: An Exploration of Some Correspondence and Connections between Religious and Medical Belief Systems in Early Industrial England', in W. J. Shiels (ed.), *The Church and Healing* (Oxford: Basil Blackwell, 1982), p. 172.

48. F. Di Trocchio, 'The Vital Principle in Therapy: Barthez and the Theory of Fluxions' in Guido Cimino and Francois Duchesneau (eds), *Vitalisms from Haller to the Cell Theory* (Firenze: Leo S. Olshki Editore, 1997), pp. 88, 92.

49. R. K. French, 'Ether and Physiology', in G. N. Cantor and M. J. S. Hodge (eds), *Conceptions of Ether: Studies in the History of Ether Theories, 1740–1900* (Cambridge: Cambridge University Press, 1981), p. 131.

50. Cullen as quoted in Rocca, 'William Cullen', p. 94.

51. Schofield, *Mechanism and Materialism*, p. 207.

52. R. Rey, 'Vitalism, Disease and Society' in R. Porter (ed.), *Medicine in the Enlightenment* (Amsterdam: Rodopi, 1995), p. 274.

53. E. Williams, *A Cultural History of Medical Vitalism in Enlightenment Montpellier* (Aldershot: Ashgate Publishing Ltd, 2003), pp. 3–4.

54. Blackmore as quoted in Berrios, *Hypochondriasis*, p. 9.

55. B. Mandeville, *Treatise of the Hypochondriack and Hysterick Diseases* (London, 1730), p. 90.

56. Ibid., pp. iv–v.

57. Ibid., p. 124.

58. M. Flemyng, *The Nature of the Nervous Fluid, or Animal Spirits, Demonstrated: With an Introductory Preface* (London, 1751), pp. vi–vii.

59. Ibid., pp. 1, 24.

60. Ibid., p. 9.

61. D. Kinneir, *A New Essay on the Nerves and the Doctrine of the Animal Spirits Rationally Considered* (London, 1737), p. 13.

62. By 1750 an estimated 'sixty per cent of men and forty per cent of women could read'. G. J. Barker Benfield, 'Sensibility', in I. McCalman, *An Oxford Companion to the Romantic Age* (Oxford: Oxford University Press, 1993), pp. 102–13, p. 106.

63. R. Porter, 'Addicted to Modernity: Nervousness in the Early Consumer Society', in J. Melling and J. Barr, *Culture in History: Production, Consumption and Values in Historical Perspective* (Exeter: University of Exeter Press, 1992); R. Porter. 'Lay Medical Knowledge in the Eighteenth Century: the Evidence of the Gentleman's Magazine', *Medical History*, 29 (1985), pp. 138–68; G. S. Rousseau, 'Science Books and Their Readers in the Eighteenth Century', in I. Rivers (ed.), *Books and Their Readers in Eighteenth-Century England* (Leicester: Leicester University Press, 1982), pp. 197–255.

64. R. J. Thornton, *The Philosophy of Medicine*, 4th edn (London, 1799), vol. 1, p. i.

65. J. Thomson, *The Seasons, A Hymn* (London, 1731), pp. 57–69. Also cited in Barker-Benfield, *The Culture of Sensibility*, p. 6.

66. F. Algarotti, *Sir Isaac Newton's Philosophy Explain'd for the Use of Ladies*, 2 vols (London, 1739), vol. 1, p. 17.

67. Mandeville, *A Treatise*, p. 182.

68. G. Cheyne, *English Malady* (London, 1733), p. 52.

69. A. Guerrini, *Obesity and Depression in the Enlightenment: The Life and Times of George Cheyne* (Oklahoma City: University of Oklahoma Press, 1999), p. 153.

70. Cheyne, *English Malady*, p. 46.

71. Ibid., p. 260.

72. Ibid., p. 180.

73. Ibid., pp. 98, 134.

74. Ibid., p. 52.

75. Ibid., p. 46.

76. Mandeville, *A Treatise*, p. 106.
77. Cheyne, *English Malady*, p. 47.
78. For example, according to the bill for 1665, twenty-three people died of fright and forty-six people died of grief. See 'A Generall Bill for this Present Year', in J. Graunt, *London's Dreadfull Visitation: or, a Collection of all the Bills of Mortality for this Present Year* (London, 1665).
79. E. Baynard, *Health: A Poem Shewing how to Procure, Preserve, and Restore it*, 4th edn (London, 1716), pp. 1–2.
80. G. Cheyne, *An Essay of Health and Long Life* (London, 1724), p. 171.
81. Porter, *George Cheyne*, p. ix.
82. Johnson as quoted in Porter, *George Cheyne*, p. xi.
83. For more on Cheyne and Richardson see D. Shuttleton, '"Pamela's Library": Samuel Richardson and Dr Cheyne's "Universal Cure"', *Eighteenth Century Life*, 23:1 (1999), pp. 59–79.
84. *The Letters of Doctor George Cheyne to Samuel Richardson (1733–1743)*, C. F. Mullett (ed.) (Columbia, MO: University of Missouri, 1943), pp. 54, 61.
85. Cheyne as quoted in Mullett, *Letters*, p. 69. For more on Cheyne's willingness to discuss his own ailments see A. Guerrini, 'Case History as Spiritual Autobiography: George Cheyne's "Case of the Author"', *Eighteenth-Century Life*, 19 (1995), pp. 17–27.
86. Richardson as quoted in Stephanson, 'Richardson's "Nerves"', p. 271.
87. J. Mullan, 'Sentimental Novels', in John Richetti (ed.), *The Cambridge Companion to the Eighteenth-Century Novel* (Cambridge: Cambridge University Press, 1996), p. 249, and Sterne as quoted in Van Sant, *Eighteenth-Century Sensibility*, p. 104.
88. C. Lawlor and A. Suzuki (eds), *Science of Body and Mind, Literature and Science, 1660–1834*, vol. 2 (London: Pickering and Chatto, 2003), p. xvii, Mullan, 'Sentimental Novels', p. 250 and M. Cecil as quoted in A. Vrettos, *Somatic Fictions: Imagining Illness in Victorian Culture* (Stanford, CA: Stanford University Press, 1995), p. 59.
89. The reading public spanned all classes, ranging from domestic servants to aristocrats. J. P. Hunter, 'The Novel and Social/Cultural History', in Richetti, *Cambridge Companion*, p. 23, 19.
90. Micale argues that this sensibility was only equated with effeminacy later in the century in *Hysterical Men*.
91. Richardson as quoted in Wild, *Medicine-by-Post*, p. 248.
92. Stephanson, 'Richardson's "Nerves"', p. 272.
93. Lawlor, *Consumption and Literature*, p. 77.
94. C. Lawlor and A. Suzuki, *Science of Body and Mind: Literature and Science, 1600–1843*, vol. 2: *Sciences of Body and Mind* (London: Pickering and Chatto, 2003), p. xiii.
95. Wild also argues that the use of nervous disease in these novels served a 'metaphorical' purpose to illustrate a character's 'morality and individual strength of character'. Wild, *Medicine-by-Post*, p. 247.
96. Micale, *Hysterical Men*, p. 27.
97. Lady Bradshaigh to Richardson as quoted in Mullan, 'Sentimental Novels', p. 247.
98. Mullan, 'Sentimental Novels', p. 247. For more on Richardson and women's self-fashioning through reading, see S. Whyman, 'Letter Writing and the Rise of the Novel: The Epistolary Literacy of Jane Johnson and Samuel Richardson', *Huntington Library Quarterly*, 70:4 (2007), pp. 577–606. Van Sant also explains how eighteenth-century audiences read for sensation 'in order to be thrilled or to have their fibres shaken'. See Van Sant, *Eighteenth-Century Sensibility*, p. 117.

99. J. Dwyer, *Virtuous Discourse: Sensibility and Community in Late Eighteenth-Century Scotland* (Edinburgh: John Donald Publishers, 1987), p. 142.
100. Mackenzie as quoted in Ellis, *The Politics of Sensibility*, p. 16.
101. Guerrini, *Obesity*, p. 165.
102. G. Cheyne, *Essay on Regimen* (London, 1740), p. ii.
103. J. Schmidt, *Melancholy and the Care of the Soul: Religion, Moral Philosophy and Madness in Early Modern England* (Aldershot: Ashgate, 2007), p. 35.
104. Ellis discusses the wide-ranging domain of eighteenth-century sensibility, illustrating its significance to philosophy, theology, politics and medicine. See Ellis, *Politics of Sensibility*, pp. 20, 22.
105. Albrecht von Haller as quoted in Van Sant, *Eighteenth-Century Sensibility*, p. 57.
106. Van Sant, *Eighteenth-Century Sensibility*, p. 57.
107. D. Hume, *A Treatise of Human Nature*, vol. 2 (London, 1739), pp. 72–3.
108. Dwyer, *Virtuous Discourse*, p. 52.
109. Ibid., pp. 39, 54.
110. Whytt, *Observations*, p. 212.
111. Van Sant, *Eighteenth-Century Sensibility*, p. 96.
112. T. Lutz, *American Nervousness: An Anecdotal History* (Ithaca, NY: Cornell University Press, 1991), p. 2.
113. W. Buchan, *Domestic Medicine*, 2nd edn (London, 1772), p. 532.
114. 'Hypochondriack', and 'Melancholy' in Johnson, *Dictionary*.
115. Cheyne, in R. Warner (ed.), *Original Letters from Richard Baxter, Matthew Prior, etc.* (Bath, 1817), pp. 78–9.
116. A. Neale, *Practical Dissertations on Nervous Complaints and other Diseases Incident to the Human Body* 3rd edn (London, 1796), pp. 49–50.
117. For example, Buchan's list of 'nervous diseases', in *Domestic Medicine* (1769) included palsy and epilepsy.
118. Whytt, *Observations*, p. iii.
119. Ibid., p. 97.
120. Ibid., p. 93.
121. Ibid., p. 93.
122. Ibid., p. iv.
123. Ibid., p. 2.
124. R. Whytt, 'Clinical Lectures' (1762–4), p. 179: Royal College of Physicians, Edinburgh.
125. Whytt, *Observations*, pp. 102–3.
126. Ibid., 103.
127. Ibid., pp. 103–4.
128. Ibid., p. 118.
129. Ibid., p. 96.
130. W. F. Bynum, 'Cullen and the Nervous System', in A. Doig *et al.* (eds), *William Cullen and the Eighteenth-Century Medical World* (Edinburgh: Edinburgh University Press, 1993), p. 159.
131. Bynum, 'Cullen and the Nervous System', p. 159.
132. J. Oppenheim, *'Shattered Nerves: Doctors, Patients, and Depression in Victorian England* (Oxford: Oxford University Press, 1991), pp. 8, 13.
133. Cullen in J. Thompson (ed.), *The Works of William Cullen*, vol. 2 (Edinburgh, 1827), p. 330.

134. Letters to Cullen at the Royal College of Physicians, Edinburgh (hereafter LTC), vol. 2 (1775), no. 101: Prescription 'For Mr Halkerston', n.d.
135. LTC, vol. 7 (1780), no. 138: Physician to Cullen regarding 'G.D'. n.d.
136. LTC, vol. 8 (1781), no. 26: John Mudie to Cullen, 13 March 1781.
137. LTC, vol. 5 (1778), no. 138: James Mill to Cullen, n.d.
138. R.G. Munro, 'A Case of Hypochondriasis', DRRMS, 17 (1785), p. 501.
139. A. Thompson, *An Enquiry into the Nature, Causes, and Method of Cure, of Nervous Disorders: In a Letter to a Friend* (London, 1781), pp. 1, 2.
140. B. Rush, *Essays Literary, Moral and Philosophical* (Philadelphia, 1798), p. 326.
141. Ibid., p. 339.
142. Brown became an enemy to Cullen after concluding that Cullen thwarted his attempt to become Professor of Medicine at the University of Edinburgh in 1776. See Thornton, *Philosophy of Medicine*; T. Beddoes, 'Biographical Preface', in J. Brown, *Elements of Medicine* (London, 1795); W. F. Bynum and R. Porter (eds), *Brunonianism in Britain and Europe* (London: Wellcome Institute for the History of Medicine, 1988) and G. Risse, *New Medical Challenges During the Scottish Enlightenment* (Amsterdam: Rodopi Press, 2005), pp. 105–32.
143. McCalman, *Oxford Companion*, pp. 5, 6, and Brown, *Elements,* p. lxiv.
144. Anon., 'Lectures on the Elements of Medicine by Dr Brown' (1785): Royal College of Physicians, Edinburgh.
145. Anon., 'Lectures'.
146. Thornton, *The Philosophy of Medicine*, p. 320.
147. 'Extracts from Dr Beddoes's Common-Place Books' *Edinburgh Medical and Surgical Journal*, 7 (1811), p. 189. In Greek mythology Procrustes is the supposed son of Poseidon who lured strangers into his home, tied them to his iron bed, and either stretched or cut them to fit its length.
148. Thornton, *The Philosophy of Medicine*, p. 136.
149. M. Barfoot, 'Brunonianism Under the Bed: An Alternative to University Medicine in Edinburgh in the 1780s', in Bynum and Porter, *Brunonianism*, p. 25.
150. Brown as quoted in G. Risse, 'The Brunonian System of Medicine: Its Theoretical and Practical Implications', *Clio Medica*, 5 (Oxford: Pergamon Press, 1970), p. 49.
151. Lawlor, *Literature and Science,* p. xviii and C. Lawrence, 'Cullen, Brown, and the Poverty of Essentialism', in Bynum and Porter (ed.), *Brunonianism*, p. 14.
152. G. Risse, 'Brunonian Therapeutics: New Wine in Old Bottles?', in Bynum and Porter, *Brunonianism*, p. 61.
153. S. Walker, *A Treatise on Nervous Diseases* (London, 1796), p. 13.
154. T. Trotter, *A View of the Nervous Temperament* (London, 1807), p. xvi.
155. Whytt, *Observations*, p. iv.
156. This is not to suggest that science is entirely 'objective', or that physicians were able to divorce themselves from their cultural context. Nonetheless, furtive efforts were made by these physicians to observe and diagnose patients with as little prejudice as possible.

2 Quacks, Social Climbers, Social Critics and Gentlemen Physicians: the Nerve Doctors of Late Eighteenth-Century Britain

1. An earlier edition of this chapter appeared in G. Colburn (ed.), *The English Malady: Enabling and Disabling Fictions* (Cambridge: Cambridge Scholars Press, 2008), pp. 67–94. It is published here with the permission of Cambridge Scholars Publishing.
2. T. Beddoes, preface to J. Brown, *The Elements of Medicine* (London, 1795), pp. cxvi, cxvii.
3. Beddoes in Brown, *Elements*, pp. cxviii, cxix, cxx, cxxi.
4. For more on these professional divisions see H. Dingwall, *Physicians, Surgeons and Apothecaries: Medical Practice in Seventeenth-Century Edinburgh* (East Linton: Tuckwell Press, 1995).
5. The term 'nerve doctor' refers to medical practitioners who regarded themselves as experts on nervous disease, leading them to publish on the subject and to commonly diagnose such complaints. Corfield has also addressed the need for further classification of medical practitioners while claiming that 'by the nineteenth century, a hierarchy of esteem differentiated the grand consultants from the rank-and-file general practitioners, who in turn ranked above the multitude of medical "irregulars"'. See P. Corfield, *Power and the Professions* (London: Routledge, 1995), p. 226.
6. L. Rosner also refers to the elite of the medical profession as 'gentlemen physicians' in *Medical Education in the Age of Improvement: Edinburgh Students and Apprentices, 1760–1826* (Edinburgh: Edinburgh University Press, 1991).
7. See appendix for further details of the nerve doctors included in this study. For another good example of the social and professional profiling of eighteenth-century medical practitioners, see R. L. Emerson and P. Wood, 'Science and Enlightenment in Glasgow, 1690–1802', in Withers and Wood (eds), *Science and Medicine in the Scottish Enlightenment*, pp. 79–142.
8. G. S. Rousseau (ed.), 'Originated Neurology: Nerves, Spirits and Fibres', in G. S. Rousseau (ed.), *Nervous Acts: Essays on Literature, Culture and Sensibility* (New York: Palgrave Macmillan, 2004), p. 27.
9. See R. Porter, 'The Sexual Politics of James Graham', *British Journal of Eighteenth-Century Studies*, 5 (1982), pp. 199–206; Porter, 'Addicted to Modernity'; R. Porter, *Doctor of Society: Thomas Beddoes and the Sick Trade in Late-Enlightenment England* (London: Routledge, 1992). Predating the confines of this study are several other influential publications on nerve doctors such as G. Rousseau (ed.), *The Letters and Papers of Sir John Hill, 1714–1775* (New York: American Medical Society, 1982), G. S. Rousseau, 'John Hill, Universal Genius Manqué: Remarks on his Life and Times, with a Checklist of his Works', in J. A. Leo and G. S. Rousseau, *The Renaissance Man in the Eighteenth Century* (Los Angeles, CA: Clark Memorial Library, 1978), pp. 45–129, and Porter (ed.), *George Cheyne*.
10. Neale, *Practical Dissertations on Nervous Complaints*, p. 18.
11. W. Heberden, *Commentaries on the History and Cure of Diseases* (London, 1802), p. 226. Published in 1802, *Commentaries* was completed in 1782.
12. Whytt, 'Casebook', p. 18: Royal College of Physicians, Edinburgh.
13. R. Campbell, *The London Tradesman* (London, 1747), p. 43.
14. Campbell, *The London Tradesman*, p. 64. Patrick Wallis demonstrates the shallow nature of this stereotype in his research detailing the close professional relationships fostered between physicians and apothecaries. See P. Wallis, 'Medicines for London: The Trade,

Regulation and Lifecycle of London Apothecaries, *c.* 1610–*c.*1670' (D.Phil. thesis, University of Oxford, 2002), pp. 241–80.

15. LTC, vol. 1 (1755–74), no. 56: Griffith Stewart to Cullen, 29 April 1767.
16. Of the thirty medical practitioners reviewed in this study, thirteen are identified as 'first tier' physicians.
17. Members of the Royal College of Physicians, London had to be Anglican and hold degrees from either Oxford or Cambridge. The majority of members came from wealthy families. I. Loudon has determined the status and occupation of the fathers of eighteenth-century members of the RCP. See I. Loudon, *Medical Care and the General Practitioner, 1750–1850* (Oxford: Clarendon Press, 1986), p. 33. For more on the privileged membership of London's Royal College of Physicians, see Bynum, *Science and the Practice of Medicine*, p. 3. Networking, nepotism and patronage among academic physicians are discussed in R. Emerson, *Professors, Patronage and Politics: The Aberdeen Universities in the Eighteenth Century* (Aberdeen: Aberdeen University Press, 1992).
18. Prior to the Medical Act of 1858, practitioners in possession of enough money could purchase medical degrees at such institutions as Aberdeen and St Andrews. None of the elite nerve doctors purchased their degrees.
19. Rosner, *Medical Education,* pp. 63, 53, 62.
20. For more on the credibility which academic posts lent to medical practitioners, see L. S. Jacyna, *Philosophic Whigs: Medicine, Science and Citizenship in Edinburgh, 1789–1848* (London: Routledge, 1994), pp. 113–15.
21. W. Cullen, *Nosology* (Edinburgh, 1800), p. 97.
22. Corfield, *Power,* p. 21. For more on the importance of technical language to the creation of an elite tier of medical professionals see S. Lawrence, 'Anatomy and Address: Creating Medical Gentlemen in Eighteenth-Century London', in V. Nutton and R. Porter (eds), *The History of Medical Education in Britain* (Amsterdam: Rodopl Press, 1995), pp. 199–228.
23. W. Falconer, *Remarks on the Influence of Climate, Situation, Nature of Country, Population, Nature of Food, and Way of Life on the Disposition and Temper, Manners and Behaviour, Intellects, Laws and Customs, Form of Government, and Religion of Mankind* (London, 1781), p. 254, and Walker, *A Treatise on Nervous Diseases*, p. xi.
24. L. Vaughan discusses the importance of club and society memberships to the development of physicians' professional networks in '"Improvements in the Art of Healing": William Heberden (1710–1801) and the Emergence of Modern Medicine in Eighteenth-Century England' (D.Phil, University of Oxford, 2005), pp. 195–208.
25. A. Fothergill, Letterbook (1789–1813) Mss.B.F823, pp. 23, 33, 54, 151, 184, and Benjamin Smith Barton Papers, B. B284d (Series II, Subject Files, Miscellaneous), 'Publications', 1 June 1799, American Philosophical Society.
26. F. Winslow, *Physic and Physicians: A Medical Sketch Book, Exhibiting the Public and Private Life of the Most Celebrated Medical Men of Former Days*, 2 vols (London, 1839), vol. 1, p. 145.
27. Thornton, *The Philosophy of Medicine*, vol. 1, p. 125.
28. Winslow, *Physic and Physicians*, vol. 1, p. 145.
29. Heberden, *William Heberden*, p. 89.
30. For more on the prestige of working in voluntary hospitals, see Lawrence, *Charitable Knowledge* and M. Fissell, *Patients, Power, and the Poor in Eighteenth-Century Bristol* (Cambridge: Cambridge University Press, 1991), p. 144.
31. Walker, *A Treatise on Nervous Diseases*, p. 144.

32. From available biographical information, it appears that of my thirty nerve doctors, four first-tier physicians, four second-tier physicians, and one third-tier physician were educated by Cullen.
33. The first six faculty members of the Medical School of the College of Philadelphia were educated at Edinburgh, with six of the twelve senior fellows having been under the direct tutelage of Cullen. Even after the establishment of the medical school in Pennsylvania in 1765, over 100 Americans received medical degrees from the University of Edinburgh in the second half of the eighteenth century. See M. O'Donnell, 'Cullen's Influence on American Medicine', in A. Doig, J. P. S. Ferguson, I. A. Milne and R. Passmore (eds), *William Cullen and the Eighteenth Century Medical World* (Edinburgh: Edinburgh University Press, 1993), pp. 234–46. For more on the prestige of Edinburgh's medical school in the eighteenth century see Rosner, *Medical Education.*
34. M. Hutt, 'Medical Biography and Autobiography in Britain, 1780–1920' (D.Phil, University of Oxford, 1995), p. 4.
35. W. Falconer, 'Robert Whytt's Clinical Lectures, 1762–1764', MS Whytt/2, p. 15: Royal College of Physicians, Edinburgh. Falconer's notebook also includes notes on lectures delivered by Cullen.
36. W. Cullen, 'A Course of Lectures on the Institutions of Medicine', 28 October 1772, MS D298, p. 159: Bodleian Library, Oxford.
37. Bynum, *Science and the Practice of Medicine*, p. 14.
38. Risse, *New Medical Challenges*, p. 7.
39. DRRMS, vol. 5 (1772), p. 228, vol. 12 (1780–1), p. 19. For examples of dissertations on hypochondria and hysteria see vol. 3 (1770), p. 189, vol. 5 (1772), p. 299, vol. 16 (1784–5), p. 46, vol. 24 (1789–90), pp. 1, 428.
40. F. Claxton, 'Whether Have Nervous Diseases Increased Since the Introduction of Tea and Coffee and in what Respects are they Useful?' DRRMS, vol. 5 (1772), pp. 229, 228.
41. Uroscopists diagnosed and prescribed for patients based on the appearance and taste of their patients' urine. Common since ancient times, uroscopy was increasingly associated with quackery towards the end of the seventeenth century.
42. J. C. Lettsom, 'Fugitive Pieces', vol. 1 MS 3246, p. 46: Wellcome Library Archives, London.
43. Ibid., 'Fugitive Pieces', p. 46–7.
44. R. Porter, 'I Think ye Both Quacks: The Controversy between Dr Theodor Myersbach and Dr John Coakley Lettsom', in W.F. Bynum and R. Porter (eds), *Medical Fringe and Medical Orthodoxy 1750–1850* (London: Croom Helm, 1987), pp. 56–78, on p. 63; Anon., *The Impostor Detected; or, the Physician the Greater Cheat* (London, 1776), p. 41.
45. Anon., *Impostor Detected,* pp. 49–50.
46. LTC, vol. 7 (1780), no. 154: George Walide to Cullen, 28 October 1780.
47. G. Logan as quoted in S. Knott, 'A Cultural History of Sensibility in the Era of the American Revolution' (D.Phil thesis, Oxford University, 1999), p. 77. Knott's work has since appeared as *Sensibility and the American Revolution* (Chapel Hill, NC: University of North Carolina Press, 2009). While this quotation did not appear in Knott's publication, all subsequent references to this study pertain to her published book.
48. LTC, vol. 1 (1755–74), no. 176: Turner to Cullen, n.d.
49. LTC, vol. 1 (1755–1774), no. 181: Edward Watson to Cullen, 24 October 1774.
50. LTC, vol. 1 (1755–1774), no. 173: Stark to Cullen, 26 September 1774.
51. Letter from James Jay to John Coakley Lettsom, 21 March 1812, MS 5370/47: Wellcome Library Archives, London.

52. Letter to Collyns from Matthew Baillie, September 18, 1808, MS 226: Royal College of Physicians, London.

53. G. T. Bettany, *Eminent Doctors: Their Lives and Their Work,* vol. 2 (London, 1885), p. 53.

54. Porter also recognizes Beddoes's role as a social critic, referring to him as a 'Doctor of Society'. See Porter, *Doctor of Society.*

55. W. Perfect, *Cases of Insanity, the Epilepsy... and Nervous Disorders, Successfully Treated,* 2nd edn (Rochester, 1785), p. 101.

56. De La Roche to William Cullen, 11 July 1772, MS Cullen 147, University of Glasgow Special Collections.

57. Anon., 'Review of Thomas Trotter's *View of the Nervous Temperament', Edinburgh Medical and Surgical Journal: Exhibiting a Concise View of the Latest and Most Important Discoveries in Medicine, Surgery, and Pharmacy,* vol. 3 (1807), p. 473.

58. J. M. Adair, *Medical Cautions for the Consideration of Invalids* (Bath, 1785), p. xi–xii.

59. J. M. Adair, *Unanswerable Arguments against the Abolition of the Slave Trade* (London, 1790), p. xiii.

60. C. Lawrence, *Medicine in the Making of Modern Britain, 1700–1920* (London: Routledge, 1994), p. 29.

61. T. Beddoes, *Hygeia: or Essays Moral and Medical, on the Causes Affecting the Personal State of our Middling and Affluent Classes,* vol. 1 (Bristol, 1802), p. 11.

62. Beddoes, *Hygeia,* vol. 1, p. 84.

63. Ibid., vol. 3, p. 205.

64. Trotter, *A View of the Nervous Temperament,* p. xii.

65. Ibid., p. 144.

66. Anon., 'Review of Thomas Trotter', *Edinburgh Medical and Surgical Journal,* 1 (1805) p. 473.

67. Letter from Thomas Beddoes to Frank Darwin, 16 March 1800, J91797 MD Douce d. 21, folio 158, Bodleian Library, Oxford.

68. Among Trotter's many reform efforts were campaigns to appoint a Physician General for the Navy, improve military discipline and naval hospitals and end military impressments. I. A. Porter, 'Thomas Trotter, M.D., Naval Physician' in *Medical History,* vol. 7, no. 2 (1963), pp. 154–64.

69. Cheyne, *Essay of Health,* p. 134.

70. J. Rymer, *A Tract Upon Indigestion and the Hypochondriac Disease* (London, 1785), p. 11.

71. Ibid., pp. 11–12.

72. Some first-tier physicians like Lettsom and Gregory did mention the greater number of upper-class sufferers in their writings. Although not to the same extent as second-tier physicians, the presence of social observations in their publications illustrates the difficulty of imposing a strict classificatory system on eighteenth-century nerve doctors. Despite this fact, the educations, social connections and medical recommendations of these physicians still qualifies them, in my view, as physicians of the first tier.

73. Falconer, 'Robert Whytt's Clinical Lectures', p. 181.

74. Walker, *A Treatise on Nervous Diseases,* p. 97.

75. For a discussion on the presence of hypochondriacs, hysterics and melancholics at the Edinburgh Royal Infirmary, see G. B. Risse, *Hospital Life in Enlightenment Scotland: Care and Teaching at the Royal Infirmary of Edinburgh* (Cambridge: Cambridge University Press, 1986).

76. Trotter, *A View of the Nervous Temperament,* p. xvii.

77. Ibid., p. xvii.

78. Ibid., p. viii.
79. T. Trotter, *Medicina Nautica: An Essay on the Diseases of Seamen* (London, 1803), p. 15.
80. Trotter, *A View of the Nervous Temperament,* p. ii.
81. T. Trotter, *An Essay Medical, Philosophical, and Chemical on Drunkenness and its Effects on the Human Body* (London: Routledge, 1988), pp. ix, viii.
82. Gregory, *Lectures,* pp. i, 22–3.
83. LTC, vol. 2 (1775), no. 1: Hugh Downman to Cullen, 5 January 1775. Acknowledging his intention to publish the poem in his letter to Cullen, the poet/physician consummated this threat in his later publication, *Infancy: or, the Management of Children* (Edinburgh, 1776), pp. 68–70. This medical book was written in verse.
84. B. Rush, as quoted in Knott, *Sensibility,* p. 100.
85. T. J. Pettigrew, *Eulogy on John Coakley Lettsom* (London, 1816), p. 10.
86. Hill, *Hypochondriasis,* p. 21.
87. Perfect, *Cases of Insanity,* pp. 115, 116, 110.
88. Ibid., pp. 129, 130–1.
89. Neale, *Practical Dissertations on Nervous Complaints,* p. 29.
90. T. Percival, *Medical Ethics* (Manchester, 1803), p. 46. This is not to suggest that contention did not exist among well-established physicians. D. Harley's work on professional disputes among eighteenth-century medical men reveals how physicians whose abilities were publicly challenged frequently responded with 'dignified silence' in print, while committing reputational warfare in private conversations. See D. Harley, 'Honour and Property: the Structure of Professional Disputes in Eighteenth-Century English Medicine', in Cunningham and French (eds), *The Medical Enlightenment,* pp. 146–8.
91. B. Rush, 'Unpublished journal commencing August 31st 1766', p. 57. Microfilm, University of Edinburgh Special Collections.
92. *Edinburgh Advertiser,* 24 September 1771 as quoted in Dingwall, 'To Be Insert in the Mercury', p. 35.
93. LTC, vol. 1 (1755–74), no. 168: Joseph Sanderson to Cullen, n.d. See also LTC, vol. 11 (1784), no. 102: Thomas Egon to Cullen, 25 July 1784.
94. W. Rowley, *A Treatise on Female, Nervous, Hysterical, Hypochondriacal, Bilious, Convulsive Diseases; Apoplexy and Palsy; with thoughts on Madness, Suicide, &c.* (London, 1788), p. 87, 95, 197.
95. Anon., 'Dr Rowley on Cow-pox Inoculation' *Medical and Physical Journal,* 14 (1805), p. 566.
96. 'C. R.' in Rowley, *A Treatise,* front inscription of copy at Wellcome Library, London.
97. Munk's Roll was a biographical reference of all members of the Royal College of Physicians. W. Munk, *Roll of the Royal College of Physicians of London,* vol. 2 (London, 1878), p. 341.
98. In this study of thirty nerve doctors, seven were identified as quacks. The precise proportion of quack doctors treating nervous disease compared to first and second-tier practitioners is difficult to judge given the haphazard nature of quack publications.
99. R. Porter, *Quacks: Fakers and Charlatans in English Medicine* (Stroud: Tempus Publishing, 2000), p. 11.
100. *Medical Spectator,* 2:43 (23 February 1793), p. 324.
101. Porter, *Quacks,* p. 33.
102. J. Paris as quoted in P. S. Brown, 'Medicines Advertised in Eighteenth-Century Bath Newspapers', *Medical History,* 20:2 (1976), p. 164.

103. J. Graham, *Health! Soundness! Strength! and Happiness! to the People!* (Manchester, 1784), pp. 9–10.

104. While networking with other medical professionals was unnecessary for doctors selling proprietary medicines, work on the manufacture of Anthony Daffy's Elixir has revealed the importance of networking with merchants and businessmen. See D. B. Haycock and P. Wallis, eds., *Quackery and Commerce in Seventeenth-Century London: The Proprietary Medicine Business of Anthony Daffy* (London: Wellcome Trust, 2005).

105. D. Porter and R. Porter (eds), *Patient's Progress: Doctors and Doctoring in Eighteenth-Century England* (Oxford: Basil Blackwell Ltd, 1989), p. 96, R. Porter, 'Graham, James (1745–1794)', *ODNB*, Oxford University Press, Sept 2004; online edn, Jan 2006 [http://www.oxforddnb.com/view/article/11199, accessed 26 July 2007]

106. J. Lane, *A Social History of Medicine: Health, Healing and Disease in England, 1750–1950* (London: Routledge, 2001), p. 8.

107. Brown, 'Medicines Advertised', p. 162.

108. Graham, *Health!*, p. 9.

109. W. D. Knight, *A Hint to Valetudinarians* (London, 1796), p. 38.

110. *Pope's Bath Chronicle*, 9 January 1766, p. 7.

111. *Pope's Bath Chronicle*, 16 January 1766, p. 12, and 30 January 1766, p. 18.

112. Brown, 'Medicines Advertised', pp. 152, 158.

113. Beddoes in Brown, *Elements*, p. cxxv.

3 'Fester'd with Nonsense': Nervous Patients in Late Eighteenth-Century Britain

1. For the importance of patient letters and diaries to medical historians, see J. Lane, "'The Doctor Scolds Me": The Diaries and Correspondence of Patients in the Eighteenth Century', in R. Porter (ed.), *Patients and Practitioners: Lay Perceptions of Medicine in Pre-Industrial Society* (Cambridge: Cambridge University Press, 1985), pp. 205–48, W. Ruberg, 'The Letter as Medicine: Studying Health and Illness in Dutch Daily Correspondence, 1770–1850', *Social History of Medicine*, 23:3 (2010), pp. 492–508, L. W. Smith, "'An Account of an Unaccountable Distemper": The Experience of Pain in Early Eighteenth-Century England and France', *Eighteenth-Century Studies*, 41:4 (2008), pp. 459–80, W. de Blecourt and C. Usborne (eds), *Cultural Approaches to the History of Medicine* (London: Palgrave Macmillan, 2004), and Wild, *Medicine-By-Post*. For more on the importance of the patient's perspective, see G. Risse and J. H. Warner, 'Reconstructing Clinical Activities: Patient Records in Medical History', *Social History of Medicine*, 5 (1992), pp. 183–205.

2. R. Porter, 'The Rise of the Physical Examination', in Bynum and Porter (eds), *Medicine and the Five Senses*, p. 180.

3. Porter and Porter (eds), *Patients Progress*, p. 74.

4. LTC, vol. 11 (1784), no. 3: G. Watts to Cullen, 1 January 1784.

5. Cullen usually responded to his patients' letters within a day. G. Risse, 'Cullen as Clinician: Organisation and Strategies of an Eighteenth-Century Medical Practice', in Doig et al., pp. 133–51, p. 136.

6. LTC, vol. 12 (1785), no. 168: J. Nicholson to Cullen, 30 October 1785.

7. LTC, vol. 6 (1779), no. 27: Colonel Clark to Cullen, February 1779.

8. LTC, vol. 4 (1777), no. 92: George Rae to Cullen, 21 July 1777.

9. LTC, vol. 1 (1755–1774), no. 102: Anon. to Cullen, March 1773.
10. Jewson, 'Medical Knowledge', p. 379.
11. Cullen typically charged two guineas for a postal consultation. Wild, *Medicine-by-Post*, p. 17.
12. P. Slack, 'Mirrors of Health and Treasures of Poor Men: the use of vernacular medical literature in Tudor England' in C. Webster (ed.), *Health, Medicine and Mortality in the Sixteenth Century* (Cambridge: Cambridge University Press, 1979), pp. 239–40. G. Smith, 'Prescribing the Rules of Health: Self-Help and Advice in the Late Eighteenth Century', in Roy Porter (ed.), *Patients and Practitioners*, pp. 251, 262.
13. H. Newdigate-Newdegate, *The Cheverels of Cheverel Manor* (London: Longmans, Green and Co., 1898), pp. 131, 135.
14. LTC, vol. 2 (1775), no. 48: Ann Ormston to Cullen, June 1775.
15. LTC, vol. 2 (1775), no. 62: Ann Ormston to Cullen, July 1775.
16. LTC, vol. 17 (1789–1790), no. 34: Surteer to Cullen, 9 December 1789.
17. LTC, vol. 12 (1785), no. 119: J. Nicholson to Cullen, 27 July 1785,
18. LTC, vol. 1 (1755–1774), no. 101: Anon. to Cullen, 20 March 1773.
19. LTC, vol. 9 (1782), no. 94: James Burnett to Cullen, 15 May 1782.
20. LTC, vol. 1 (1755–1774), no. 101: Thomas Christie to Cullen, 20 March 1773.
21. The concluding pages of this letter are catalogued separately under MS no. 123.
22. Anon. to Cullen, March 20, 1773 #101 in Letters to Cullen, vol. 1 (1755–1774).
23. Whytt, *Observations*, pp. iv, 203.
24. LTC, vol. 17 (1789–90), no. 22: Bradley Smith to Cullen, 24 October 1789.
25. This problem will soon be alleviated thanks to D. Shuttleton's efforts to digitize the collection at the University of Glasgow.
26. LTC, vol. 12 (1785), no. 109: Charles Charleton to Cullen, 14 July 1785.
27. For example, see R. Porter, 'Introduction', in *George Cheyne*, and G. S Rousseau (ed.), *Nervous Acts: Essays on Literature, Culture and Sensibility* (New York: Palgrave Macmillan, 2004), pp. 255–6.
28. Porter, '"The Hunger of Imagination"', p. 79.
29. Porter, 'Introduction', p. xxxviii.
30. George Lyttleton to Mrs Montagu, Montagu Papers, box 57, MS 1265, Huntington Library. Hulse (1682–1759) was a fashionable physician in London and a member of the Royal College of Physicians.
31. Gregory acknowledges receipt of this poem on 11 August, 1767, MO box 62, Huntington Library.
32. N. R. Needham, 'Maxwell , Darcy, Lady Maxwell of Pollok (1742/3–1810)', *ODNB*, Oxford University Press, 2004 [http://www.oxforddnb.com/view/article/63479, accessed 7 March 2011]
33. J. Lancaster, *The Life of Darcy, Lady Maxwell of Pollock*, 2 vols (London, 1821), vol. 1, pp. vi, i.
34. Ibid., p. i.
35. Ibid., pp. 133, 277, 192.
36. Ibid., p. 26.
37. Ibid., p. 293.
38. Early modern Protestants frequently regarded illness as an opportunity to 'exhibit grace' and the acceptance of God's will. M. Fissell, 'The Disappearance of the Patient's Narrative and the Invention of Hospital Medicine', in R. French and A. Wear, *British Medicine in an Age of Reform* (London: Routledge, 1991), p. 98.

39. Porter, 'Hunger of Imagination', p. 79.
40. Micale, *Hysterical Men*, pp. 21, 27, 26.
41. Porter, 'Hunger of Imagination', p. 65.
42. Ibid., p. 79.
43. R. Porter, *Flesh in the Age of Reason* (London: Allen Lane, 2003), p. 173; S. Johnson as quoted in Porter, 'Hunger of Imagination', p. 66.
44. Wiltshire, *Samuel Johnson*, pp. 12–13.
45. J. Boswell as quoted in Wiltshire, *Samuel Johnson*, p. 22.
46. Newdigate-Newdegate, *Cheverels*, p. 131.
47. A. Lewer, 'Newdigate, Sir Roger, fifth baronet (1719–1806)', *ODNB*, Oxford University Press, 2004 [http://www.oxforddnb.com/view/article/20003, accessed 31 March 2011].
48. J. Lucas, 'An Account of a Singular Case', *Medical Observations and Inquiries*, vol. 5 (London, 1776), p. 73.
49. 'Case of Mrs Wynn', LTC, vol. 14 (1787–1788), no. 25: Anon. to Cullen, 1787.
50. John Mitchell to James Innes, 11 October 1803, GD113/5/459/1: National Archives of Scotland.
51. LTC, vol. 11 (1784), no. 3: Watts to Cullen, 1 January 1784.
52. LTC, vol. 3 (1776), no. 80: 'Mr. Shields' Case', 22 June 1776.
53. Mr. Cowmeadow to Cullen as quoted in Wild, *Medicine-by-Post*, p. 221.
54. LTC, vol. 7 (1785), no. 120: Ralph Ogle to Cullen, 28 July 1785.
55. 'Case of Miss Betty Ogilvie', LTC, vol. 9 (1782), no. 135: Anon. to Cullen, June 1782.
56. Wild's review of Cullen's correspondence similarly concluded that women were willing to describe their symptoms in 'utilitarian' terms, and were 'not gagged by the conventions of sensibility'. Wild, *Medicine-by-Post*, p. 201.
57. LTC, vol. 8 (1781), no. 47: Robert Ligertwood to Cullen, 30 April 1781.
58. LTC, vol. 8 (1781), no. 95: Robert Ligertwood to Cullen, 31 August 1781. Unfortunately, I have not been able to locate a copy of this treatise.
59. LTC, vol. 4 (1777), no. 24: Robert Ligertwood to Cullen, 6 February 1777.
60. LTC, vol. 4 (1777), no. 133: Robert Ligertwood to Cullen, n.d; this appears to be the concluding fragment of the 6 February letter.
61. LTC, vol. 5 (1778), MS 63–65, June 1778.
62. LTC, vol. 4 (1777), MS 103: Lord Gardenstone to Cullen, August 1777.
63. F. Garden, *Travelling memorandums,* vol. 1 (Edinburgh, 1791), pp. 58–59.
64. Garden, *Travelling memorandums,* vol. II, pp. 60–61.
65. LTC, vol. 1 (1755–1774), no. 186: Anon. Letter from Geneva to Cullen, November 1774.
66. A. Vila, 'The Philosophe's Stomach: Hedonism, Hypochondria, and the Intellectual in Enlightenment France', in Forth and Carden-Coyne (eds), *Cultures of the Abdomen*, p. 90.
67. Vila, 'Philosophe's Stomach', p. 97.
68. Hume to G. Cheyne, in *The Letters of David Hume*, J. Y. T., Greig (ed.) (Oxford: Oxford Clarendon Press, 1932), pp. 14–15.
69. Hume as quoted in Micale, *Hysterical Men*, p. 34.
70. Smith, 'An Account', p. 461.
71. LTC, vol. 12 (1785), no. 110: John Warrandice to Cullen, 14 July 1785.
72. LTC, vol. 3 (1776), no. 73: John Henderson to Cullen, 15 June 1776.
73. LTC, vol. 3 (1776), nos. 55–56: Thomas Christie to Cullen, 4 May 1776.

74. This is in contrast to Schmidt's suggestion that hypochondriac patients 'declined from discussing their mental "trouble of mind" with their physicians'. See Schmidt, *Melancholy*, p. 155.
75. Boswell as quoted in Ingram, *Boswell's Creative Gloom*, p. 18.
76. LTC, vol. 1 (1755–1774), no. 101: Anon. to Cullen, 20 March 1773.
77. LTC, vol. 17 (1789–1790), no. 32: Sandilands to Cullen, 23 November 1789.
78. LTC, vol. 14 (1787), no. 13: William Stewart to Cullen, 15 January 1787.
79. LTC, vol. 7 (1780), no. 154: George Walide to Cullen, 28 October 1780.
80. LTC, vol. 5 (1778), MS 140: Elliot to Cullen, 11 December 1778.
81. LTC, vol. 1 (1755–1774), no. 143: Patrick Scott to Cullen, 5 March 1774.
82. LTC, vol. 17 (1789–1790), no. 125: Anon. to Cullen, n.d.
83. LTC, vol. 5 (1778), no. 60: Thomas Bushby to Cullen, 23 June 1778.
84. LTC, vol. 12 (1985), no. 110: John Warrandice to Cullen, 14 July 1785.
85. LTC, vol. 12 (1985), no. 110: John Warrandice to Cullen, 14 July 1785.
86. LTC, vol. 12 (1785), no. 110: John Warrandice to Cullen, 14 July 1785.
87. Following the publication of the Swiss physician, S. Tissot's treatise, *Onanism: Or a Treatise Upon the Disorders Produced by Masturbation: Or, the Dangerous Effects of Secret and Excessive Venery* (1760), England saw the flurried publication of several other like-minded medical treatises threatening offenders with mental instability and a general loss of manly vigour. These fears were magnified in the nineteenth century as doctors argued that unnecessary sexual activity could deplete the body's finite supply of nerve force. For more on this, see B. Barker-Benfield, 'The Spermatic Economy: A Nineteenth Century View of Sexuality', *Feminist Studies*, 1:1 (1972), pp. 45–74.
88. LTC, vol. 8 (1781), no. 48: 'Mr Pinkerton's Case', Anon. to Cullen, April 1781.
89. LTC, vol. 12 (1785), no. 119: J. Nicholson to Cullen, 27 July 1785.
90. LTC, vol. 12 (1785), no. 109: Reverend C. Charleton to Cullen, 14 July 1785.
91. Cullen complied with this request.
92. LTC, vol. 5 (1778), no. 136: Anon. to Cullen, November 1778.
93. LTC, vol. 17 (1789–1790), no. 125: Anon. to Cullen, n.d.
94. LTC, vol. 17 (1789–1790), no. 34: Reverend Surteer to Cullen, 9 December 1789.
95. LTC, vol. 12 (1785), no 171: Letter from Alexander Douglass to Cullen, n.d.
96. LTC, vol. 17 (1789–1790), no. 93: Letter from Cullen to anon. physician, n.d.
97. LTC, vol. 12 (1785), no. 110: John Warrandice to Cullen, 14 July 1785.
98. LTC, vol. 17 (1789–1790), no. 83: 'Case sent to Dr. Raymond', n.d.
99. LTC, vol. 1 (1755–1774), no. 48: Finny to Cullen, May 1766.
100. LTC, vol. 3 (1776), no. 80: 'Shields's Case', Anon. to Cullen, 22 June 1776.
101. LTC, vol. 12 (1785), no. 120: Ralph Ogle to Cullen, 28 July 1785.
102. LTC, vol. 1 (1755–1774), no. 101: Thomas Christie to Cullen, 20 March 1773.
103. LTC, vol. 17 (1789–1790), no. 25: Smith to Cullen, 29 October 1789.
104. LTC, vol. 14 (1787), no. 13: William Stewart to Cullen, 15 January 1787.
105. LTC, vol. 12 (1785), no. 191: Robert Dow to Cullen, 29 October 1785.
106. P. Thicknesse, *The Valetudinarians Bath Guide* (London, 1780), p. 9.
107. LTC, vol. 12 (1785), no. 163: Alexander Douglas to Cullen, 21 September 1785.
108. LTC, vol. 12 (1785), no. 113: John Warrandice to Cullen, 19 July 1785.
109. Beddoes, *Hygeia*, vol. 1, p. 97.
110. LTC, vol. 3 (1776), no. 17: W.R. Wilson to Cullen, 22 January 1776.
111. Winslow, *Physic and Physicians*, vol. 1, p. 42.

112. J. Moore as quoted in R. Porter and D. Porter (eds), *In Sickness and in Health: The British Experience, 1650–1850* (London: Fourth Estate,1988), p. 203.
113. J. Wiltshire, *Jane Austen and the Body: 'The Picture of Health'* (Cambridge: Cambridge University Press, 1992), p. 126.
114. Recent efforts to investigate these issues include G. Risse's *New Medical Challenges*, highlighting the average number, age and sex of hypochondriac and hysteric patients admitted to the Edinburgh Royal Infirmary, and Micale's work on the surprising significance of male sufferers in *Hysterical Men*.
115. Sir Henry Halford's case books (1787–1791), MS 2915D – MS 3000D: Royal College of Physicians, London.
116. J. C. Lettsom, *Medical Memoirs of the General Dispensary in London for Part of the Years 1773 and 1774* (London, 1774).
117. 'Report of Diseases in the Public and Private Practice of One of the Physicians of the Finsbury Dispensary from the 20th of July to the 20th of August', *London Medical and Physical Journal*, 14 (1805), p. 275.
118. R. Willan, *Reports on the Diseases in London, particularly During the Years 1796, 97, 98, 99, and 1800* (London, 1801), p. 52; Whytt, *Observations*, p. iv.
119. De La Roche to William Cullen, 11 July 1772, MS Cullen #147, University of Glasgow Special Collections.
120. 'Dr Clarke's Medical Report from Nottingham', *Edinburgh Medical and Surgical Journal*, 4 (1808), pp. 440–1.
121. Whytt, *Observations*, p. 105.
122. 'Dr Clarke's Medical Report', pp. 440–1.
123. Risse, *New Medical Challenges,* pp. 321, 322.
124. E. Johnston, 'Case of Hypochondriasis', DRRMS, vol. 5 (1772), p. 299.
125. T. Clotnies, 'Case of L H', DRRMS, vol. 16 (1784–5), p. 105
126. Anon., 'A Woman Aged 64: Case of Hypochondriasis', DRRMS, 13 (1780), p. 138.
127. Bath General Hospital Admission Register (1742): Bath and North East Somerset Record Office.
128. Most eighteenth-century charity hospitals published statistics for their subscribers, revealing whether patients were dismissed as cured, incurable, poorly behaved, or dead. Because incurable or dead patients reflected poorly on the abilities of the hospital's treating physicians, it was in the self-interest of hospital physicians and governors to admit patients selectively. For more on hospital admissions procedures, see Risse, *Hospital Life in Enlightenment Scotland*, G. Risse, *Mending Bodies, Saving Souls: A History of Hospitals* (Oxford: Oxford University Press, 1999), and Lawrence, *Charitable Knowledge.*
129. Risse, 'Cullen as Clinician', p. 136.
130. LTC, vol. 5 (1778), no. 138: John Mill to Cullen, 1778.
131. LTC, vol. 6 (1779), no. 25: Thomas Mack to Cullen, 27 February 1779.
132. P. Earle provides a useful discussion of blurry class divisions in eighteenth-century Britain, defining the 'middling sort' as above the labouring class, but below people of 'independent means' in *The Making of the English Middle Class: Business, Society and Family Life in London 1660–1730* (Berkeley, CA: University of California Press, 1989).
133. J. Boswell, 'The Hypochondriac', *London Magazine*, 47:47 (February 1778), p. 58.
134. W. Heberden, *Commentaries on the History and Cure of Diseases* (London, 1802), p. 224.
135. Trotter, *A View of the Nervous Temperament* (London, 1807), pp. 40–1.
136. LTC, vol. 1 (1774–1774), 56: Griffith Stewart to Cullen, 29 April 1767.

137. Trotter, *Medicina Nautica: An Essay on the Diseases of Seamen,* vol. 3, p. 360.

138. Ibid., pp. 369, 367, 369, 366, 371, 367.

139. LTC, vol. 7 (1780), MS 20: David Watson to Cullen, 1 February 1780.

140. LTC, vol. 7 (1780), no. 116: anonymous physician to Cullen, August 1780.

141. LTC vol. 2 (1775), no 135: 'The Case of Captain Wilson', n.d.

142. LTC, vol. 2 (1775), no 25: Captain Ferguson to Cullen, 26 February 1775.

143. James Dallas as quoted in Wild, *Medicine-by-Post*, p. 217.

144. For more on the effect of narrative paradigms on disease experience, see Vrettos, *Somatic Fictions*.

145. LTC, vol. 5 (1778), no. 19: Nicholas Ryzack to Cullen, 11 February 1778.

146. Smith, 'An Account', p. 472.

147. Patients and practitioners employed a mixture of humoural and nervous theories in their disease explanations throughout the eighteenth century. See Ruberg, 'The Letter as Medicine', p. 504. Cullen's correspondence includes multiple letters from nervous patients describing their disorders in this manner, such as one who claimed that his originated from 'some original quality on the Blood, scorbutick or otherwise acrimonious and discordant to the nerves'. LTC, vol. 1 (1755–1774), no. 123: Thomas Christie to Cullen, 20 March 1773.

148. Lawlor, *Consumption and Literature*, p. 5.

4 The Pursuit of Health: The Treatment of Nervous Disease

1. Buchan, *Domestic Medicine,* 2nd edn, p. 532.

2. Whytt, *Observations*, p. 329.

3. LTC, vol. 2 (1775), no. 103: 'For Mrs Oswald', n.d.

4. The term 'natural' refers to the manipulation of the non-naturals as opposed to 'artificial treatments' like store-bought medicines.

5. Whytt, *Observations*, p. 334.

6. Ibid., p. 332.

7. Ibid.

8. LTC, vol. 3 (1776), no. 12 and 16: Whyte to Cullen, and no. 5: Cullen to Whyte, 7 January 1776.

9. A. Emch-Deriaz, 'The non-naturals made easy' in R. Porter (ed.), *The Popularization of Medicine, 1650–1850* (London: Routledge, 1992), p. 135.

10. Buchan, *Domestic Medicine*, p. 184.

11. G. Cheyne, *Essay of Health and Long Life*, 6th edn (London, 1725), p. 45.

12. J. Wesley, *Primitive Physic*, 20th edn (London, 1781), p. xiv. After reading Cheyne's *Natural Method of Curing Diseases* in 1724, Wesley wrote to his mother, 'I cannot but observe it is one of the most ingenious books which I ever saw'. W. Plasha, 'The Social Construction of Melancholia in the Eighteenth-Century: Medical and Religious Approaches to the Life and Work of Samuel Johnson and John Wesley' (Oxford University DPhil, 1993), p. 93.

13. CCL, vol. 1: Cullen to Naven's physician, 26 May 1768, p. 3.

14. CCL, vol. 1: Cullen to Cochran, 13 July 1768, p. 30.

15. LTC, vol. 12 (1785), no. 199: John Heysham to Cullen, 7 November 1785.

16. Baynard, *Health*, p. 16.

17. For more on the relationship between the stomach and nervous disorders see Vila, 'The Philosophe's Stomach'. See also E. Williams, 'Stomach and Psyche: Eating, Digestion, and Mental Illness in the Medicine of Philippe Pinel', *Bulletin of the History of Medicine*, 84:3 (Oxford, 2010), pp. 358–86.

18. Trotter, *A View of the Nervous Temperament*, p. 69.

19. LTC, vol. 2 (1775), no 103: 'For Mrs Oswald', n.d.

20. Risse, *New Medical Challenges*, p. 150.

21. LTC, vol. 17 (1789–90), no. 83: 'Dr Raymond's Opinion', n.d.

22. Benjamin Bell, 'prescription for Miss Grant', 30 April 1788, GD248/369/7/10: National Archives of Scotland.

23. Falconer, *Remarks*, p. 232, p. 519.

24. Kinneir, *A New Essay on the Nerves*, p. 92.

25. John Wynter, in R. Warner (ed.), *Original Letters for Richard Baxter, Matthew Prior, etc.* (Bath, 1817), p. 62. To this Cheyne wrote an equally fiery reply, concluding with the verse, 'I cannot your prescription *try*, But heartily *'forgive'*; ''Tis nat'ral you should bid *me* die, That you yourself may *live!*' Cheyne, in Warner, *Original Letters*, p. 63.

26. A. Guerrini, 'A Diet for a Sensitive Soul: Vegetarianism in Eighteenth-Century Britain', *Eighteenth Century Life*, 23:2 (1999), p. 37, and G. S. Rousseau, 'Science Books and Their Readers in the Eighteenth Century', in I. Rivers (ed.), *Books and Their Readers in Eighteenth-Century England* (Leicester: Leicester University Press, 1982), p. 249.

27. Whytt, *Observations*, pp. 412–13.

28. Ibid., p. 417.

29. Risse, *New Medical Challenges*, p. 151.

30. J. C. Lettsom, *The Natural History of the Tea-Tree with Observations on the Medical Qualities of Tea, and on the Effects of Tea-Drinking*, 2nd edn (London, 1799), p. 79.

31. Falconer, *Observations on the History and Cure of Diseases*, p. 230.

32. Buchan, *Domestic Medicine*, p. 535.

33. CCL, vol. 1: Cullen to Cochran, 13 July 1768, p. 29.

34. Cheyne, *The English Malady*, p. 120.

35. A. Sutherland, *An Attempt to Ascertain and Extend the Virtues of Bath and Bristol Waters*, 2nd edn (London, 1764), p. 302.

36. Ibid., p. 302.

37. LTC, vol. 1 (1755–74), no. 42: Cullen to Lord Moray, March 1766.

38. Vaughan to anon., 11 June 1811, Benjamin Vaughan Papers, No. 2, Medicine: BC46p, American Philosophical Society.

39. LTC, vol. 17 (1789–90), no. 22: Bradley Smith to Cullen, 24 October 1789.

40. F. Fuller, *Medicina Gymnastica* (London, 1705), p. 250.

41. Whytt, *Observations*, p. 436.

42. Buchan, *Domestic Medicine*, p. 536.

43. Whytt, *Observations*, p. 357.

44. 'Dr Rutherford's Clinical Lectures' (1751), Western Manuscript no. 86, p. 147: Wellcome Library Archives, London.

45. LTC, vol. 2 (1775), no. 103: 'For Mrs Oswald', n.d.

46. Cheyne, *The English Malady*, p. 180.

47. Benjamin Bell to Miss Grant, 30 April 1788, GD248/369/7/10: National Archives of Scotland.

48. LTC, vol. 14 (1787), no. 38: Wood to Cullen, 25 February 1787.

49. E. Gilchrist, *Sea Voyages, The Use of Sea Voyages in Medicine,* 2nd edn (London, 1757), p. 85.
50. Ibid., p. 66.
51. Ibid., p. 13.
52. Ibid., pp. 47–8.
53. Ibid., p. 91.
54. Ibid., p. ix–x.
55. Friendly Traveller, *The Ensign of Peace* (London, 1775), p. 89.
56. Gilchrist, *Voyages,* pp. 11–12.
57. *The Letters of Doctor George Cheyne to Samuel Richardson (1733–1743),* ed. C. F. Mullett (Columbia: University of Missouri, 1943), p. 61.
58. London Society of Cabinet-Makers, *The Cabinet-Makers London Book of Prices* (London, 1788), p. 141.
59. R. Mead, *Medical Precepts and Cautions* (London, 1751), p. 267.
60. Sutherland, *An Attempt,* p. 303.
61. Whytt, *Observations,* p. 355.
62. Trotter, *A View of the Nervous Temperament,* p. 258.
63. T. Clotnies, 'Case of I.H', DRRMS, vol. 16 (1784–5), p. 187.
64. W. Falconer, *A Practical Dissertation on the Medicinal Effects of the Bath Waters* (Bath, 1790), p. 164–5.
65. Gilchrist, *Voyages,* p. 76.
66. J. Anderson, *Institutes of Physics,* 4th edn (Glasgow, 1786), p. 334.
67. J. Gregory quoted in P. Gouk, 'Music's Pathological and Therapeutic Effects on the Body Politic: Doctor John Gregory's Views' in P. Gouk and H. Hills, *Representing Emotions: New Connections in the Histories of Art, Music and Medicine* (Aldershot: Ashgate, 2005), p. 101.
68. Gregory, *Lectures,* p. 25.
69. J. Boswell, 'The Hypochondriack', *London Magazine,* 6 (March 1778).
70. *The Letters of Samuel Johnson,* ed. B. Redford, 3 vols, vol. 1, 1731–72 (Oxford: Clarendon Press, 1992), p. 242.
71. Letter from Samuel Johnson to Elizabeth Aston, November 1767, in *The Letters of Samuel Johnson,* ed. Redford, p. 292.
72. LTC, vol. 11 (1784), no. 68: Anon. to Cullen, n.d.
73. LTC, vol. 4 (1777), no. 73: Saunders to Cullen, 22 May 1777.
74. LTC vol. 4 (1774), no. 76: 28 May 1777.
75. Trotter, *Medicina Nautica,* vol. 3, pp. 374–5.
76. A. Duncan as quoted in S. Baur, *Hypochondria: Woeful Imaginings* (Berkeley, CA: University of California Press, 1988), p. 27.
77. Risse, *New Medical Challenges,* p. 333.
78. Cullen as quoted in J. Andrews, 'Letting Madness Range: Travel and Mental Disorder, c. 1700–1900', in R. Wrigley and G. Revill (eds), *Pathologies of Travel* (Amsterdam: Rodopi Press, 2000), p. 32.
79. Andrews, 'Letting Madness Range', p. 28.
80. Buchan, *Domestic Medicine,* p. 536.
81. A. Borsay, *Medicine and Charity in Georgian Bath: A Social History of the General Infirmary, c. 1739–1830* (Aldershot: Ashgate Publishing Ltd., 1999), p. 8.
82. H. Walpole as quoted in E. S. Turner, *Taking the Cure* (London: Michael Joseph Ltd, 1967), p. 9.

83. J. Byng as quoted in Porter and Porter, *In Sickness and in Health*, p. 197.

84. *The Correspondence of Adam Smith*, ed. E. C. Mossner (Oxford: Clarendon Press, 1977), p. 204.

85. Miller, 'What Effects', pp. 372–3.

86. Ibid., p. 372.

87. T. Thompson, MD, *Medical Consultations on Various Diseases; published from the Letters of Thomas Thompson* (London, 1773), p. 36.

88. Heberden, *Commentaries on the History and Cure of Diseases*, pp. 78–79.

89. LTC, vol. 17 (1789–90), 44: Cullen to Miller, n.d.

90. W. Heberden, 'Preliminary Observations', *c.* 1782, MS 344, p. 3: Royal College of Physicians, London.

91. J. C. Lettsom, 'Miscellaneous Essays', MS 3248: Wellcome Library Archives, London.

92. Cheyne, *Essay of Health*, p. 6.

93. P. Borsay, *The Image of Georgian Bath, 1700–2000* (Oxford: Oxford University Press, 2000), pp. 27–29.

94. See Jewson, 'Medical Knowledge'.

95. J. Walton, *The English Seaside Resort: A Social History 1750–1914* (Leicester: Leicester University Press, 1983), p. 11.

96. John Anderson to Mr Pridden, 3 May 1792, MS 6118 Margate Sea-Bathing Infirmary #67615: Wellcome Library Archives, London.

97. Gilchrist, *Voyages*, p. 53.

98. Falconer, *Remarks*, p. 21.

99. Trotter, *A View of the Nervous Temperament*, p. 282.

100. Risse, *New Medical Challenges*, p. 322.

101. LTC, vol. 8 (1781), no. 47: Robert Ligertwood to Cullen, 30 April 1781.

102. LTC, vol. 17 (1789–1790), no. 94: Shireff to Cullen, 8 December 1791 and 'Case sent to Dr Raymond to be laid before Cullen', LTC vol. 17 (1789–1790), no. 83: Anon., n.d.

103. LTC, vol. 3 (1776), no. 55: Thomas Christie to Cullen, 4 May 1776.

104. LTC, vol. 1 (1755–1774), no. 101: Thomas Christie to Cullen, March 1773.

105. Buchan, *Domestic Medicine*, p. 539.

106. Trotter, *A View of the Nervous Temperament*, p. 230.

107. LTC, vol. 17 (1789–1790), no. 22: Bradley Smith to Cullen, 24 October 1789.

108. Sir Henry Halford's case notes, MS 2915D–3000D: Royal College of Physicians, London.

109. Buchan, *Domestic Medicine*, p. 562.

110. LTC, vol. 3 (1776), no. 51: Alexander Dunlop to Cullen, 21 April 1776.

111. Rowley, *A Treatise*, p. 118.

112. J. Ball, *A New Compendious Dispensatory* (London, 1769), pp. 21, 111, 224.

113. W. Lewis, *Experimental History of the Materia Medica,* 3rd edn (London, 1784), p. 488.

114. Whytt, *Observations*, p. 338 and Buchan, *Domestic Medicine*, p. 538.

115. A. Duncan, *Annals of Medicine for the Year 1796* (Edinburgh, 1796), p. 67.

116. Lewis, *Experimental*, pp. 485, 491.

117. Whytt, *Observations*, p. 337 and Bath and Co., *A Description of the Names and Qualities of those Medicinal Compositions contained in the Domestic Medicine Chests* (London, 1775), p. 5.

118. T. Skeete, *Experiments and Observations on Quilled and Red Peruvian Bark* (London, 1786), pp. 11–12; Lewis, *Experimental*, p. 492; Whytt, *Observations*, p. 338.

119. Whytt, *Observations*, pp. 336, 337.

120. Skeete, *Experiments*, p. 275.

121. Whytt, *Observations*, p. 342.

122. Lewis, *Experimental,* pp. 295, 296.

123. Whytt, *Observations*, p. 343, Lewis, *Experimental*, p. 296.

124. Lewis, *Experimental*, p. 295.

125. Whytt, *Observations*, p. 344.

126. A. Thompson, 'An Inquiry into the Natural History and Medical Uses of Several Mineral Steel Waters', *Medical Essays and Observations*, 5th edn, 2 vols (Edinburgh, 1771), vol. 2, p. 52.

127. Smith to Hume, 16 June 1776 in Mossner, *Correspondence,* p. 201.

128. C. Anstey, *The New Bath Guide* (Bath, 1784), p. 14.

129. W. Oliver, *A Practical Dissertation on Bath-Waters* (London, 1719), p. 45.

130. P. Thicknesse, *The New Prose Bath Guide* (London, 1778), p. 25.

131. W. Alexander, *Plain and Easy Directions for the use of the Harrowgate Waters* (Edinburgh, 1773), pp. 9–10.

132. Alexander, *Plain and Easy Directions*, p. 10.

133. G. Milligen, 'An Account of the Virtues and Use of the mineral waters near Moffatt', *Medical Essays and Observations*, 5th edn, 2 vols (Edinburgh, 1771), vol. 1, p. 56.

134. T. Fawcett, 'Selling the Bath Waters: Medical Propaganda at an Eighteenth-Century Spa', *Somerset Archaeology and Natural History*, 134 (Taunton: John and Josephine Pentney, 1990), p. 198.

135. S. McIntyre, 'The Mineral Water Trade in the Eighteenth Century', *Journal of Transport History*, 2:1 (1973), pp. 1–19, on pp. 8, 11.

136. LTC, vol. 1 (1755–1774), no. 193: Joseph Sanderson to Cullen, 8 November 1774.

137. LTC, vol. 2 (1775), nos. 101, 102: 'For Mr Halkerston', n.d.

138. C. M. Foust, *Rhubarb: The Wondrous Drug* (Princeton, NJ: Princeton University Press, 1992), pp. 145–6.

139. LTC, vol. 12 (1785), no. 207: John Warrandice to Cullen, 21 November 1785.

140. J. W. Estes, *Dictionary of Protopharmacology: Therapeutic Practices, 1700–1850* (Canton: Science History Publications, 1990), p. 205.

141. Buchan, *Domestic Medicine*, pp. 538, 539.

142. J. Quincy, *Pharmacopia Officinalis & Extemporanea: or, a Complete English Dispensatory*, 14th edn. (London, 1769), p. 452., p. 434.

143. Buchan, *Domestic Medicine,* pp. 538–9.

144. J. Jones as quoted in A. H. Maehle, 'Pharmacological Experimentation with Opium in the Eighteenth Century', in R. Porter (ed.), *Drugs and Narcotics in History* (Cambridge: Cambridge University Press, 1995), pp. 66–7.

145. Lewis, *Experimental,* p. 461, 462.

146. Ibid., p. 462.

147. Ibid., p. 463.

148. Trotter, *A View of the Nervous Temperament*, p. 138.

149. Ibid., p. 312.

150. Ambrose Godfrey, 'receipt book', *c.* 1730, Godfrey, Ince & Greenish Manuscripts, IRA1997.143: Royal Pharmaceutical Society, London.

151. Lewis, *Experimental*, pp. 465, 466.

152. Ibid., pp. 180, 182.

153. D. Cox, *Directions for Medicine Chests* (Gloucester, 1799), p. 28 and Lewis, *Experimental*, p. 182.

212 Notes to pages 124–9

154. Cox, *Directions*, p. 28.
155. Lewis, *Experimental*, pp. 429, 427.
156. Ibid., p. 428.
157. Ibid., p. 429.
158. Whytt, *Observations*, p. 370.
159. Quincy, *Pharmacopia*, p. 612.
160. N. McKendrick discusses the unprecedented number of advertisements in newspapers in the eighteenth century and Porter discusses the particular growth of medical advertisements. See N. McKendrick, J. Brewer and J. H. Plumb (eds), *The Birth of a Consumer Society: The Commercialization of Eighteenth-Century England* (London, Europa Publications Ltd., 1982), p. 11 and Porter, *Quacks*, pp. 54–5.
161. P. S. Brown, 'Medicines Advertised in Eighteenth-Century Bath Newspapers', *Medical History*, 20:2 (April 1976), p. 158.
162. Trotter, *A View of the Nervous Temperament*, p. 104.
163. *Bath Chronicle*, 21 February 1782 4.b and 12 January 1792, 4.d.
164. Brown, 'Medicines Advertised', p. 162.
165. J. Trusler, *The London Adviser and Guide* (London, 1786), p. 175.
166. Anon. physician as quoted in Brown, 'Medicines Advertised', p. 163.
167. S. Solomon, *An Account of That Most Excellent Medicine the Cordial Balm of Gilead* (Chester, 1799), p. 1.
168. J. Webster, *A True and Brief Account (With Directions for the Use) of the CEREVISIA ANGLICANA* (London, n.d.), p. 16.
169. Solomon, *An Account*, p. 3.
170. J. C. Lettsom, *Hints Designed to Promote Beneficence, Temperance, and Medical Science*, vol. 1 (London, 1797), p. 181.
171. W. Chamberlaine, *The ... Treatment ... (London, 1795)*, p. 12.
172. Ibid., p. 14.
173. D. Cox, *Family Medical Compendium* (London, 1790), p. 12.
174. M. A. Stewart, 'Berkeley, George (1685–1753)', *ODNB*, Oxford University Press, 2004; online edn, May 2005 [http://www.oxforddnb.com/view/article/2211, accessed 23 July 2007]
175. John Rutty to William Clark, October 1748, American Philosophical Society, MSS. film.488.
176. Cox, *Medical Compendium*, p. 63.
177. Ibid., p. 64.
178. Wesley, *Primitive Physic*, p. 81.
179. Ibid., p. viii.
180. D. Armstrong, *Herbs that Work: The Scientific Evidence of their Healing Powers* (Berkeley, CA: Ulysses Press, 2001), pp. 85, 153, 128.
181. LTC, vol. 1 (1755–74), no. 177: William Nevin to Cullen, 10 October 1774.
182. LTC, vol. 4 (1777), no. 92: Rae to Cullen, 21 July 1777.
183. LTC, vol. 6 (1779), no. 25: Thomas Mack to Cullen, 27 February 1779.
184. CCL, vol. 11: Letter from Cullen to Weetwood's physician, p. 158.
185. LTC, vol. 17 (1789–90), no. 83: Raymond to Cullen, n.d.
186. T. Clotnies, 'Case of I.H', DRRMS, vol. 16, p. 185.
187. LTC, vol. 1 (1755–1774), no. 102: Anon. to Cullen, March 1773.
188. Perfect, *Cases of Insanity*, p. 61.
189. LTC, vol. 1 (1755–1774), no. 141: John Andrew to Cullen, 23 February 1774.

190. LTC, vol. 17 (1789–1790), no. 25: Smith to Cullen, 29 October 1789.
191. Rowley, *A Treatise*, p. 124.
192. Gregory, *Lectures*, p. 62.
193. J. Haygarth, *Of the Imagination as a Cure and as a Cure of Disorders of the Body* (Bath, 1800), pp. 29, 28, 29.
194. Haygarth, *Of the Imagination*, p. 30.
195. LTC, vol. 1 (1755–74), no. 14: Rachel Cuthbert to Cullen, n.d.
196. LTC, vol. 1 (1755–74), no. 71: 'James' to Cullen, 4 September 1775.
197. Haygarth, *Of the Imagination*, p. 32.
198. Whytt, *Observations*, p. 438.
199. W. Gibbons, *Inaugural Essay on Hypochondriasis* (Philadelphia, 1805), 610 Diss. Vol. 13, 'Collection of Medical Dissertations', p. 23, American Philosophical Society.
200. Risse, 'Cullen as Clinician', p. 146. Wild also discusses the more 'robust' therapies endured by infirmary patients in *Medicine-by-Post*, p. 206.
201. Risse, *New Medical Challenges*, p. 327.
202. Risse, 'Cullen as Clinician', p. 146.
203. LTC, vol. 12 (1785), no. 207: John Warrandice to Cullen, 21 November 1785.
204. LTC, vol. 10 (1783): William Ingham to Cullen, 2 June 1783.
205. LTC, vol. 10 (1783): William Ingham to Cullen, 8 December 1783.
206. Risse, *New Medical Challenges*, p. 333.
207. J. H. Schoenheider, 'Remarks on the Hypochondriacal Disease and on the use of Leeches in it', *London Medical Journal*, 1 (1781), pp. 398–9.
208. R. King, *An Inaugural Essay on Blisters* (Philadelphia, PA, 1799), p. 30.
209. LTC, vol. 12 (1785), no. 171: Alexander Douglas to Cullen, 5 October 1785.
210. King, *An Inaugural Essay*, p. 35.
211. Risse, *New Medical Challenges*, p. 332.
212. For example, see LTC, vol. 3 (1776), no. 5: Prescription from Cullen to Reddie, 7 January 1776.
213. LTC, vol. 2 (1775), no. 139: Cullen to anon., n.d.
214. LTC, vol. 12 (1785), no. 200: Alexander Browne to Cullen, 6 November 1785.
215. J. I. Wand-Tetley, 'Historical Methods of Counter-Irritation' in *Rheumatology*, 3 (1956), pp. 91–2 and Wiltshire, *Samuel Johnson*, p. 15.
216. LTC, vol. 3 (1776), no. 5: 'For Mr Reddie', 7 January 1776.
217. LTC, vol. 3 (1776), no. 55: Thomas Christie to Cullen, 4 May 1776.
218. P. Fara, *Sympathetic Attractions: Magnetic Practices, Beliefs, and Symbolism in Eighteenth-Century England* (Princeton, NJ: Princeton University Press, 1996), p. 18.
219. Risse, *New Medical Challenges*, pp. 332–3.
220. J. Wesley, *The Desideratum: or, Electricity Made Plain and Useful* (London, 1760), p. vii.
221. A. von Haller first demonstrated his theory of irritability mid-century, using electricity to stimulate the nerves and muscles of dead frogs. M. Bresadola, 'Early Galvanism as Technique and Medical Practice', in P. Bertucci and G. Pancaldi (eds), *Electric Bodies: Episodes in the History of Medical Electricity* (Bologna: Universita di Bologna, 2001), pp. 161–2.
222. M. Rowbottom and C. Susskind, *Electricity and Medicine: History of Their Interaction* (San Francisco: San Francisco Press, Inc., 1984), p. 25.
223. Anonymous patient as quoted by Cadwallader Evans in 'A Relation of a Cure Performed by Electricity', *Medical Observations and Inquiries*, 1 (London, 1757), pp. 85–86.
224. LTC, vol. 12 (1785), no. 172: 'J.M' to Cullen, 7 October 1785.

225. Howell, 'Electricity', p. 429.

226. Howell, 'Electricity', p. 425.

227. E. Nairne, *The Description and use of Nairne's patent Electrical Machine*, 4th edn. (London, 1793), p. 62.

228. Bertucci, 'Electrical Body of Knowledge', p. 66.

229. P. Bertucci, 'Revealing Sparks: John Wesley and the Religious Utility of Electrical Healing', *British Journal of the History of Science* vol. 39, part 3 (2006), p. 345; Nairne, *The Description*, p. 73.

230. LTC, vol 17 (1789–90), no. 83: "Dr Raymond's Opinion", n.d.

231. LTC, vol. 1 (1755–1774), no. 66: Alexander Henry to Cullen, 27 December 1769.

232. LTC, vol. 10 (1783), no. 10: William Ingham to Cullen, 2 June 1783.

233. LTC, vol. 8 (1781), no. 25: Robert Redpath to Cullen, 13 March 1781.

234. LTC, vol. 5 (1778), no. 67: Thomas Hephen to Cullen, 4 July 1778.

235. LTC, vol. 6 (1779), no. 142: Buchan to Cullen, 18 September 1779.

5 A Disease of the Body and of the Times

1. F. Jonsson and M. Micale also identify Trotter's work in 1807 as a pivotal publication, marking a shift away from eighteenth-century discourse regarding the fashionable implications of nervous disease. See Jonsson, 'The Physiology of Hypochondria in Eighteenth-Century Britain' in Forth and Carden-Coyne (eds), *Cultures of the Abdomen*, p. 25 and Micale, *Hysterical Men*, p. 81.

2. M. Cohen explores how mid-eighteenth-century Britons equated 'French politeness' with effeminacy and English politeness with 'manliness and liberty', in *Fashioning Masculinity: National Identity and Language in the Eighteenth Century* (London: Routledge, 1996), pp. 42–53.

3. Lawrence, 'Medicine as Culture'.

4. J. M. Adair, *Essays on Fashionable Diseases* (London, 1790) and S. Tissot, *An Essay on Disorders of the People of Fashion* (London, 1771).

5. Dingwall, 'To Be Insert in the Mercury'.

6. W. Temple and Sydenham as quoted in Schmidt, *Melancholy*, p. 152.

7. Cheyne, *The English Malady*, p. ii.

8. Anon., 'Review of Tissot's *Traite des Nerfs et de leurs maladies*', *London Medical Journal*, vol. 1 (1781), p. 33.

9. Trotter, *A View of the Nervous Temperament*, p. xvii.

10. G. S. Rousseau, as quoted in Barker-Benfield, *The Culture of Sensibility*, p. 3.

11. Cheyne, *The English Malady*, p. 34.

12. Anon., *The Prosperity of Britain Proved from the Degeneracy of its People* (London, 1757), pp. 18, 17.

13. J. Raven, *Judging New Wealth: Popular Publishing and Responses to Commerce in England, 1750–1800* (Oxford: Clarendon Press, 1992), p. 169.

14. J. Boswell, *Boswell's Column: Being his Seventy Contributions to the London Magazine under the Pseudonym The Hypochondriac from 1777 to 1783*, ed. M. Bailey (London: William Kimber, 1951), p. 251.

15. Gregory, *Comparative View*, pp. 91–2.

16. E. Gibbon, *The History of the Decline and Fall of the Roman Empire*, vol II, 4th edn. (Dublin, 1777), p. 378.

17. E. Haywood (ed.), *The Female Spectator*, 5th edn (London, 1755), vol. 3, p. 191. Raven argues that 'warnings based on alleged classical precedent for the fall of empires' increased from the mid-1750s. See Raven, *Judging New Wealth*, p. 171.
18. Haywood (ed.), *Female Spectator*, vol. 1, pp. 277–8.
19. Gregory, *Comparative View*, vol. 2, p. 117 and Beddoes, *Hygeia*, p. 92.
20. Trotter, *A View of the Nervous Temperament*, p. 89.
21. Beddoes openly lamented the tendency of Britons to 'overlook the inseparable connection between moral and medical topics'. See Beddoes, *Hygeia*, p. 83. For more on his social reforms see Porter, *Doctor of Society*, pp. 154–92.
22. Beddoes, *Hygeia*, p. 207.
23. For evidence of Lettsom's emphasis on moral medicine, see his 'Moral and Physical Thermometer' (1780), which equated particular vices with corresponding diseases. For example, perjury was a suggested cause of epilepsy, while swearing could result in jaundice.
24. A. Wilson, *Rational Advice to the Military, When Exposed to the Inclemency of Hot Climates and Seasons* (London, 1780), p. 11.
25. Gregory, *Comparative View*, pp. 33, xvi.
26. H. Home, *Sketches of the History of Man*, 4 vols (Dublin, 1775), vol. 2, p. 133.
27. Catherine Powys, 'Journal from 1795', Add. 42161, p. 8: British Library.
28. Cheyne, *The English Malady*, p. ii.
29. Gregory as quoted in C. Lawrence, 'The Nervous System and Society in the Scottish Enlightenment', in Barnes and Shapin (eds), *Natural Order*, pp. 29–30.
30. B. Rush as quoted in Baur, *Hypochondria*, p. 27.
31. Walker, *A Treatise on Nervous Diseases*, p. 96.
32. Trotter, *A View of the Nervous Temperament*, p. xvii.
33. Boswell, *Boswell's Column*, p. 43.
34. Lettsom, *Hints*, vol. 1, p. 11.
35. W. Heberden, 'Collection of Essays', MS 345, pp. 169, 163: Royal College of Physicians, London.
36. Sutherland, *An Attempt*, p 288.
37. J. C. Lettsom, *The Natural History of the Tea-Tree with Observations on the Medical Qualities of Tea, and on the Effects of Tea-Drinking*, 2nd edn (London, 1799), p. 67.
38. Lettsom, *The Natural History*, p. 69.
39. A. Thompson, *An Enquiry into the Nature, Causes, and Method of Cure, of Nervous Disorders* (London, 1781), p. 3.
40. E. Johnstone, 'Case of Hypochondriasis', DRRMS, vol. 5 (1772), p. 301.
41. Lettsom, *The Natural History*, p. 101.
42. McKendrick, Brewer and Plumb (eds), *The Birth of a Consumer Society*, p. 29.
43. Wild, *Medicine-By-Post*, p. 116.
44. Bynum, *Science and the Practice of Medicine*, p. 17.
45. S. Quinlan, 'Sensibility and Human Science in the Enlightenment', *Eighteenth Century Studies*, 37:2 (2004), pp. 299–300.
46. Cullen referred to contagion as 'human miasm', thereby proving the fluidity of contagionist and anti-contagionist thought in the late eighteenth-century. C. Hamlin, 'Predisposing Causes and Public Health in Early Nineteenth-Century Medical Thought', *Social History of Medicine*, 5 (1992), p. 47.
47. W. Cullen, *First Lines of the Practice of Physic* (Edinburgh, 1777), pp. 72, 74.
48. J. Pringle, *Observations on the Diseases of the Army* (London, 1752), p. 96.

49. Cullen's *Nosology* was published in seventeen editions from 1769–1831.
50. E. Chadwick as quoted in Logan, *Nerves and Narratives*, p. 151.
51. Melville, *Nerves and Narratives*, pp. 146–7.
52. J. A. Mangan and J. Walvin, *Manliness and Morality: Middle-Class Masculinity in Britain and America, 1800–1940* (Manchester: Manchester University Press, 1987).
53. G. Grinnell, *The Age of Hypochondria: Interpreting Romantic Health and Illness* (New York: Palgrave Macmillan, 2010), p. 5.
54. Haywood, *Female Spectator,* vol. 1, p. 284.
55. Ibid., p. 285.
56. Ibid., p. 284.
57. Boswell, *Boswell's Column,* p. 44.
58. T. Thompson, *Medical Consultations on Various Diseases* (London, 1773), p. 34.
59. Thompson, *Medical Consultations,* p. 35.
60. R. J. Thornton, *The Philosophy of Medicine,* 4th edn, 5 vols (London, 1799), vol. 2, p. 294.
61. Heberden, *Commentaries on the History and Cure of Diseases,* p. 235.
62. LTC, vol. 6 (1779), no. 181: John McKie to Cullen, 9 December 1779.
63. W. Falconer, *A Dissertation on the Influence of the Passions Upon Disorders of the Body,* 3rd edn. (London, 1796), p. 112–13.
64. 'Blue devils' were a common visual metaphor for depression. J. Woodforde to Anthony Fothergill, 10 June 1792 in 'Anthony Fothergill Letterbook, 1789–1813', pp. 94–95, Mss.B.F823, American Philosophical Society.
65. C. H. Parry, *Collections from the Unpublished Medical Writings of the Late Caleb Hillier Parry* (London, 1825), p. 369.
66. Falconer, *A Dissertation,* p. 129.
67. Parry, *Collections,* pp. 368, 369.
68. Ibid., pp. 346, 347.
69. Heberden, *Commentaries on the History and Cure of Diseases,* pp. 235–6.
70. Johnson to Elizabeth Langton, 17 April, 1771, in *The Letters of Samuel Johnson,* ed. Redford, vol. 1 1731–72, p. 359.
71. *The Letters of Samuel Johnson,* ed. R. W. Chapman, 3 vols (Oxford: Clarendon Press, 1952), vol. 3, pp. 71, 123.
72. *The Letters of Johnson,* ed. Redford, vol. 1, pp. 394–5.
73. For more on Smith's hypochondria see Barfoot, 'On William Cullen'.
74. David Hume to Adam Smith, 28 January 1772, in E. C. Mossner (ed.), *The Correspondence of Adam Smith* (Oxford: Clarendon Press, 1977), p. 160.
75. *Edward Gibbon: Memoirs of my Life,* ed. G. A. Bonnard (London: Thomas Nelson and Sons Ltd., 1966), p. 29. Cardinal Quirini was a cardinal of the Roman Catholic Church, and Vatican librarian.
76. *Edward Gibbon,* ed. Bonnard, p. 40.
77. LTC, vol. 17 (1789–90), no. 30: Sandilands to Cullen, 6 November 1789.
78. Peirce, *History and Memoirs of the Bath,* p. 191.
79. Barker-Benfield, *Culture of Sensibility,* p. 24.
80. S. Walker, *Observations on the Constitution of Women and on some of the diseases to which they are more especially liable* (London, 1803), pp. 13, 14.
81. R. Shoemaker, *Gender in English Society, 1650–1850: The Emergence of Separate Spheres?* (London: Longman Ltd, 1998), p. 22.
82. J. Fordyce, *Sermons to Young Women,* 8th edn, 2 vols (London, 1775), vol. 1, pp. 88, 8.
83. Ibid., p. 236.

84. M. C. Moran, 'Between the Savage and the Civil: Dr John Gregory's Natural History of Femininity' in Knott and Taylor (eds), *Women, Gender and Enlightenment*, p. 8.
85. J. Gregory, *A Father's Legacy to His Daughters* (Edinburgh, 1793), p. 12.
86. Ibid., p. 23.
87. Ibid., p. 31.
88. Ibid., p. 38.
89. M. Wollstonecraft, *A Vindication of the Rights of Woman* (London, 1792), p. 53.
90. Ibid., p. 38.
91. Ibid., p. 55.
92. Ibid., pp. 220, 5.
93. Ibid., p. 5.
94. H. Chapone, *Letters on the Improvement of the Mind, addressed to a Young Lady,* 7th edn (London, 1777), pp. 66–7.
95. J. Burton, *Lectures on Female Education and Manners*, 3rd edn (Dublin, 1794), p. 337.
96. H. More, *Strictures on the Modern System of Female Education*, 4th edn (Dublin, 1799), p. 51.
97. Beddoes, *Hygeia*, vol. 1, p. 62.
98. Walker, *Observations*, p. 4.
99. Ibid., p. 11.
100. Trotter, *A View of the Nervous Temperament*, p. 49.
101. Ibid., p. 49.
102. Ibid., p. 51.
103. L. Colley, *Britons: Forging the Nation, 1707–1837* (London: Vintage, 1992), p. 240.
104. Anon., *Dialogues of the Dead* (London, 1760), p. 302.
105. Ibid., p. 305.
106. J. Hervey, *Sermons and Miscellaneous Tracts* (London, 1764), pp. 18–19.
107. Colley, *Britons*, p. 262.
108. S. M. Quinlan, 'Inheriting Vice, Acquiring Virtue: Hereditary Disease and Moral Hygiene in Eighteenth-Century France', *Bulletin of the History of Medicine*, 80:4 (2006), p. 654.
109. Cheyne, *The English Malady*, p. 5.
110. Quinlan, 'Inheriting Vice', p. 651.
111. J. Barron, 'What States of the Constitution Chiefly Predispose to Melancholic and Hypochondriacal Affections?', DRRMS, 52 (1804–5), p. 383.
112. LTC, vol. 6 (1779), no. 17a: Anonymous to Cullen, 1 March 1779.
113. Trotter, *A View of the Nervous Temperament*, pp. 52–3.
114. M. Gaul, *English Romanticism: The Human Context* (London: W.W. Norton, 1988), p. 231.
115. Published in 1813, *Pride and Prejudice* was written in 1796–7. *Sanditon* was published after Austen's death, in 1817.
116. For a discussion of illness in Austen's novels see Wiltshire, *Jane Austen and the Body*.
117. Logan, *Nerves and Narratives*, p. 50.
118. Ibid., p. 67.
119. Ibid., pp. 109–10.
120. Walker, *Observations*, p. 11.
121. D. Hume, *Essays Moral Political and Literary* (Oxford: Oxford University Press, 1963), p. 6.
122. Risse, *New Medical Challenges*, p. 29.

123. Walker, *A Treatise on Nervous Diseases*, pp. 91–2.
124. N. Barbon as quoted in C. J. Berry, *The Idea of Luxury: A Conceptual and Historical Investigation* (Cambridge: Cambridge University Press, 1994), pp. 109–10.
125. T. Mun as quoted in ibid., p. 104.
126. Haywood, *Female Spectator*, vol. 1, p. 89.
127. J. Robertson, *The Scottish Enlightenment and the Militia Issue* (Edinburgh: John Donald Publishers Ltd., 1985), pp. 86, 205.
128. K. Wilson, *The Sense of the People: Politics, Culture and Imperialism in England, 1715–1785* (Cambridge: Cambridge University Press, 1998), pp. 191, 189. Also see M. Cohen, 'Manliness, Effeminacy and the French: Gender and the Construction of National Character in Eighteenth-Century England', in T. Hitchcock and M. Cohen (eds), *English Masculinities, 1660–1800* (London: Longman Ltd., 1999), pp. 44–62.
129. J. Brown, *An Estimate of the Manners and Principles of the Times* (London, 1757), pp. 89–90.
130. Brown, *An Estimate*, p. 91.
131. Colley, *Britons*, p. 286.
132. Trotter, *A View of the Nervous Temperament*, p. xi.
133. T. Peaal, 'Observations on the Temperament and Diseases of the People Inhabiting the Highlands of Aberdeenshire', *London Medical and Physical Journal*, 13 (1805), p. 28. Highlanders commonly represented all Scotsmen in English publications. See S. Conway, *War and National Identity in the Mid-Eighteenth-Century British Isles* (Oxford: Oxford University Press, 2001), p. 873.
134. Wild, *Medicine-By-Post*, p. 192.
135. Home, *Sketches*, vol. 2, p. 136.
136. C. Kidd, 'Integration: Patriotism and Nationalism' in H. T. Dickinson (ed.), *A Companion to Eighteenth-Century Britain* (Oxford: Basil Blackwell Publishers Ltd, 2002) p. 372
137. Whytt as quoted in F. Schiller, 'Yawning?' *Journal of the History of the Neurosciences*, vol. 11 (2002), p. 392.
138. Whytt, *Observations*, p. 215.
139. T. Dixon, 'Patients and Passions: Languages of Medicine and Emotion, 1789–1850', in F. B. Alberiti (ed.), *Medicine, Emotion and Disease, 1700–1950* (London: Palgrave Macmillan, 2006), pp. 35–6.
140. W. Godwin, *An Enquiry Concerning Political Justice*, 2 vols (Dublin, 1793), vol. 1, p. 191.
141. D. Stewart, *Elements of the Philosophy of the Human Mind*, 3 vols (London: 1827), vol. 3, p. 210. Volumes 1 and 2 were published in 1792 and 1814, respectively.
142. J. Moore, *Medical Sketches* (London, 1786), p. 253.
143. W. Cowper as quoted in Porter and Porter, *In Sickness and in Health*, pp. 229–30.
144. *Columbian Magazine* as quoted in Knott, 'A Cultural History of Sensibility', p. 92. This quotation was not included in Knott's revised publication, *Sensibility and the American Revolution* (Chapel Hill, NC: University of North Carolina Press, 2009).
145. Trotter, *A View of the Nervous Temperament*, p. 68.
146. Lawrence, 'Medicine as Culture', pp. 312–86.
147. G. S. Rousseau, 'Psychology', in G. S. Rousseau and R. Porter (eds), *The Ferment of Knowledge: Studies in the Historiography of Eighteenth-Century Science* (Cambridge: Cambridge University Press, 1980), p. 177.
148. A. L. Donovan, *Philosophical Chemistry in the Scottish Enlightenment* (Edinburgh: Edinburgh University Press, 1975), p. 72.

Epilogue

1. L. Sterne as quoted in A. B. Howes (ed.), *Sterne: The Critical Heritage* (London: Routledge & Kegan Paul, 1974), p. 39.
2. Howes (ed.), *Sterne*, p. 136.
3. Oppenheim, *'Shattered Nerves'*, p. 14.
4. Micale, *Hysterical Men*, pp. 53, 54, 55.
5. For a brief overview of sources indicating the continued fashionable implications of nervous disease in the nineteenth century see G. S. Rousseau, 'Culture Viewed in Geological Time', in Rousseau (ed.), *Nervous Acts* (Basingstoke: Palgrave Macmillan, 2004), pp. 272–4.
6. I. Turgenev, *Fathers and Sons*, trans. R. Matlaw (New York: W.W. Norton & Company, 1966), p. 13.
7. G. S. Rousseau, 'Coleridge's Dreaming Gut', in C. Forth and A. Carden-Coyne (eds), *Cultures of the Abdomen: Diet, Digestion, and Fat in the Modern World* (New York: Palgrave Macmillan, 2005), p. 112. See also G. C. Grinnell, 'A Portrait of the Artist as a Dead Man: Coleridge's Hypochondria', in Colburn (ed.), *The English Malady*, pp. 177–99.
8. Keats as quoted in Lawlor, *Consumption and Literature*, p. 136.
9. J. Moore, *The Works of Lord Byron*, 14 vols (London, 1832), vol. 2, p. 77.
10. W. Gibbon, *An Inaugural Essay on Hypochondriasis* (1805), p. 7 in 'Collection of Medical Dissertations', 610 Diss. Vol. 13, American Philosophical Society. Although an American medical student, Gibbon's research relied overwhelmingly upon British sources.
11. Hazlitt as quoted in A. K. Mellor, 'Keats and the Complexities of Gender', in S. J. Wolfson (ed.), *The Cambridge Companion to Keats* (Cambridge: Cambridge University Press, 2001), p. 214.
12. Moore, *The Works,* pp. 75–6.
13. W. Lawrence, *Lectures on Physiology, Zoology and the Natural History of Man* (London, 1819), p. 239.
14. Dwyer, *Virtuous Discourse*, p. 64.
15. Anon., *Edinburgh Medical and Surgical Journal*, vol. 12 (1816), p. 469.
16. Vaughan to anon., 18 June 1811, Benjamin Vaughan Papers, no. 2, Medicine: BV46p, American Philosophical Society.
17. J. Reid, *Essays on Hypochondriacal and Other Nervous Affections* (Philadelphia, 1817), p. 9.
18. Micale, *Hysterical Men,* p. 59.
19. G. M. Beard, *American Nervousness: Its Causes and Consequences* (New York, 1881), pp. vii–vii.
20. Ibid., p. 164.
21. R. Porter, 'Nervousness, Eighteenth and Nineteenth Century Style: From Luxury to Labour', in M. Gijswijt-Hofstra and R. Porter (eds), *Cultures of Neurasthenia from Beard to the First World War* (Amsterdam: Rodopi, 2001), p. 39.
22. P. Dubois as quoted in E. Shorter, *From Paralysis to Fatigue: A History of Psychosomatic Illness in the Modern Era* (New York: The Free Press, 1992), p. 221.
23. A. Clark as quoted in Porter, 'Nervousness', p. 41.
24. T. Clifford Allbutt as quoted in C. Sengoopta, '"A Mob of Incoherent Symptoms"? Neurasthenia in British Medical Discourse, 1860–1920', in Gijswijt-Hofstra (ed.), *Cultures*, p. 98.
25. Porter, 'Nervousness', p. 38.

WORKS CITED

Manuscript Sources

American Philosophical Society, Philadelphia

> Fothergill, Anthony, Letterbook, 1789–1813, Mss.B.F823.

> Smith Barton, Benjamin, Papers (Series II: Subject Files, Miscellaneous, 'Publications', 1 June 1799, B B284.d.

Bath and North East Somerset Record Office

> Bath General Hospital Admissions Register, 1742–52.

Bodleian Library, Oxford

> Beddoes, Thomas, Correspondence, 39197 MS douce d. 21 fols 158–159.

> Cullen, William, 'A Course of Lectures on the Institutions of Medicine', 1772, MS D298.

British Library, London

> Powys, Catherine, Journal from 1795, Add. 42161.

Huntington Library, San Marino

> Montagu Papers, box 57 and 62.

National Archives of Scotland, Edinburgh

> Grant Correspondence, 1784–1794, GD248/189/4.

> Innes, James, Correspondence,1796–1806, GD113/5/459/1.

> Miscellaneous Letters to Jane Grant, wife of Sir James Grant of Grant, 1767–1800, GD248/369.

Royal College of Physicians Archives, Edinburgh

> Anon., 'An Essay on the Hypochondriac Disease in a Letter', c. 1775–1800.

> Cullen, William, Consultation Correspondence, 21 vols (1755–1790).

> Falconer, William, Robert Whytt's Clinical Lectures, 1762–1764, MS Whytt/2.

> Letters to Cullen, 1755–1790, MS Cullen.

> Whytt, Robert, Casebook, MS Whytt.

Royal College of Physicians Archives, London

    Burges, John, 'Pharmacopoeia', MS 180.

    Halford, Sir Henry, Casebooks, 1787–1791, MS 2915D - MS 3000D.

    Heberden, William, 'Collection of Essays', MS 345.

    —, 'Preliminary Observations', *c.* 1782, MS 344.

    Miscellaneous Letters, MS 226.

Royal Medical Society, Edinburgh

    Dissertations Read at the Royal Medical Society of Edinburgh, vol. 1 (1751), vol. 52 (1804–5).

Royal Pharmaceutical Society, London

    Godfrey, Ambrose, receipt book, *c.* 1730, Godfrey, Ince and Greenish Manuscripts, IRA1997.143.

University of Edinburgh Special Collections

    Rush, Benjamin, 'Unpublished Journal Commencing August 31st 1766', Microfilm.

University of Glasgow Special Collections

    Cullen, William, 'Essay on Custom', MS Cullen 342.

    De La Roche, Letter to Cullen, 11 July 1772, MS Cullen 147.

Wellcome Library, London

    Lettsom, John Coakley, Correspondence, MS.5370.

    —, 'Fugitive Pieces', MS. 3248–4240.

    —, 'Miscellaneous Essays', MS 3248.

    Dr Rutherford's Clinical Lectures, 1751, Western Manuscripts no. 86.

    Letters relating to the Margate Sea-Bathing Infirmary, MS 6118.

Printed Primary Sources

Adair, J. M., *Medical Cautions for the Consideration of Invalids* (Bath, 1785).

—, *Essays on Fashionable Diseases* (London, 1790).

—, *Unanswerable Arguments against the Abolition of the Slave Trade* (London, 1790).

Alexander, W., *Plain and Easy Directions for the Use of the Harrowgate Waters* (Edinburgh, 1773).

Algarotti, F., *Sir Isaac Newton's Philosophy Explain'd for the Use of the Ladies*, 2 vols (London, 1739).

Anderson, J., *Institutes of Physics*, 4th edn (Glasgow, 1786).

Anstey, C., *The New Bath Guide*, 12th edn (Bath, 1784).

Ball, J., *A New Compendious Dispensatory* (London, 1769).

Bath and Co., A Description of the Names and Qualities of those Medicinal Compositions Contained in the Domestic Medicine Chests (London, 1775).

Baynard, E., *Health: A Poem Shewing how to Procure, Preserve, and Restore it,* 4th edn (London, 1716).

Beard, G., *American Nervousness: Its Causes and Consequences* (New York, 1881).

Beddoes, T., 'Biographical Preface, in J. Brown, *Elements of Medicine* (London, 1795).

—, *Hygeia: or Essays Moral and Medical, on the Causes Affecting the Personal State of our Middling and Affluent Classes,* 3 vols (Bristol, 1802).

Boswell, J., *Boswell's Column: Being his Seventy Contributions to the London Magazine under the Pseudonym The Hypochondriac from 1777 to 1783,* ed. M. Bailey (London: William Kimber, 1951).

Brown, J., *An Estimate of the Manners and Principles of the Times* (London, 1757).

Brown, J., *The Elements of Medicine* (London, 1795).

Buchan, W., *Domestic Medicine,* 2nd edn (London, 1772).

Burton, J., *Lectures on Female Education and Manners,* 3rd edn (Dublin, 1794).

Burton, R., *Anatomy of Melancholy* (1621) (Oxford, Clarendon Press, 1989).

Campbell, R., *The London Tradesman* (London, 1747).

Chamberlaine, W., *The West-India Seaman's Medical Dictionary* (London, 1785).

Chapone, H., *Letters on the Improvement of the Mind, addressed to a Young Lady,* 7th edn (London, 1777).

Cheyne, G., *An Essay of Health and Long Life* (London, 1724).

—, *The English Malady* (London, 1733).

—, *Essay on Regimen* (London, 1740).

—, *The Letters of Dr. George Cheyne to the Countess of Huntingdon,* ed. C. Mullett (San Marino: Huntington Library, 1940).

—, *The Letters of Doctor George Cheyne to Samuel Richardson (1733–1743),* ed. C. Mullett (Columbia, MO: University of Missouri, 1943).

Cox, D., *Family Medical Compendium* (London, 1790).

—, *Directions for Medicine Chests* (Gloucester, 1799).

Cullen, W., *Nosology* (1769; Edinburgh, 1800).

—, *First Lines of the Practice of Physic* (Edinburgh, 1777).

Dialogues of the Dead (London, 1760).

Downman, H., *Infancy: or, the Management of Children* (Edinburgh, 1776).

Duncan, A., *Annals of Medicine for the Year 1796* (Edinburgh, 1796).

Edinburgh Medical and Surgical Journal (Edinburgh, 1805–7).

Elements of the Practice of Physic, for the use of those Students who Attend the Lectures Read on this Subject at Guy's Hospital (London, 1798).

Falconer, W., *Remarks on the Influence of Climate, Situation, Nature of Country, Population, Nature of Food, and Way of Life on the Disposition and Temper, Manners and Behaviour, Intellects, Laws and Customs, Form of Government, and Religion of Mankind* (London, 1781).

—, *A Practical Dissertation on the Medicinal Effects of the Bath Waters* (Bath, 1790).

—, *A Dissertation on the Influence of the Passions Upon Disorders of the Body,* 3rd edn (London, 1796).

Flemyng, M., *The Nature of the Nervous Fluid, or Animal Spirits Demonstrated: With an Introductory Preface* (London, 1751).

Fordyce, J., *Sermons to Young Women,* 8th edn (London, 1775).

Friendly Traveller, *The Ensign of Peace* (London, 1775).

Fuller, F., *Medicina Gymnastica: Or, A Treatise Concerning the Power of Exercise* (London, 1705).

Garden, F., *Travelling memorandums, made in a tour upon the continent of Europe, in the years 1786, 87 &88,* 3 vols (Edinburgh, 1791).

Gibbon, E., *The History of the Decline and Fall of the Roman Empire,* 4th edn, 2 vols (Dublin, 1777).

—, *Edward Gibbon: Memoirs of My Life,* ed. G. Bonnard (London: Thomas Nelson and Sons, 1966).

Gilchrist, E., *The Use of Sea Voyages in Medicine,* 2nd edn (London, 1757).

Gisborne, T., *An Enquiry into the Duties of Men in the Higher and Middle Classes of Society in Great Britain Resulting from their Respective Stations, Professions and Employments,* 2 vols (London, 1795).

Godwin, W., *An Enquiry Concerning Political Justice,* 2 vols (Dublin, 1793).

Graham, J., *Health! Soundness! Strength! And Happiness! To the People!* (Manchester, 1784).

Graunt, J., *London's Dreadfull Visitation: or, a Collection of all the Bills of Mortality for this Present Year* (London, 1665).

Gregory, J., *Lectures on the Duties and Qualifications of a Physician,* 2nd edn (London, 1772).

—, *A Comparative View of the State and Faculties of Man with Those of the Animal World,* 7th edn (London, 1777).

—, *A Father's Legacy to His Daughters* (Edinburgh, 1793).

Haygarth, J., *Of the Imagination as a Cure and as a Cure of the Disorders of the Body* (Bath, 1800).

Haywood, E. (ed.), *The Female Spectator,* 5th edn, 4 vols (London, 1755).

Heberden, W., *Commentaries on the History and Cure of Diseases* (London, 1802).

Hervey, J., *Sermons and Miscellaneous Tracts* (London, 1764).

Hill, J., *Hypochondriasis: A Practical Treatise on the Nature and Cure of that Disorder* (London, 1766).

Home, H., *Sketches of the History of Man,* 4 vols (Dublin, 1775).

Hume, D., *A Treatise of Human Nature*, vol. 2 (London, 1739).

—, *The Letters of David Hume*, ed. J. Greig (Oxford: Clarendon Press, 1932).

—, *Essays Moral, Political and Literary* (Oxford: Oxford University Press, 1963).

Johnson, S., *A Dictionary of the English Language* (1755; London: Longman, 1979).

—, *The Letters of Samuel Johnson With Mrs Thrale's Genuine Letters to Him*, ed. R. W. Chapman, 3 vols (Oxford: Clarendon Press, 1952).

—, *The Letters of Samuel Johnson, 1731–1772*, ed. B. Redford (Oxford: Clarendon Press, 1992).

King, R., *An Inaugural Essay on Blisters* (Philadelphia, 1799).

Kinneir, D., *A New Essay on the Nerves and the Doctrine of the Animal Spirits Rationally Considered* (London, 1737).

Knight, W. D., *A Hint to Valetudinarians* (London, 1796).

Lancaster, J., *The Life of Darcy, Lady Maxwell of Pollock; Late of Edinburgh: Compiled from her Voluminous Diary and Correspondence* (London, 1821).

Lawrence, W., *Lectures on Physiology, Zoology and the Natural History of Man* (London, 1819).

Lettsom, J. C., *Medical Memoirs of the General Dispensary in London, for Part of the Years 1773 and 1774* (London, 1774).

—, *Moral and Physical Thermometer* (London, 1780).

—, *Hints Designed to Promote Beneficence, Temperance, and Medical Science* (London, 1797).

—, *The Natural History of the Tea-Tree with Observations on the Medical Qualities of Tea, and on the Effects of Tea-Drinking*, 2nd edn (London, 1799).

Lewis, W., *Experimental History of the Materia Medica*, 3rd edn (London, 1784).

Locke, J., *Essay Concerning Human Understanding*, 2nd edn (London, 1690).

London Medical and Physical Journal, 1799–1807.

London Society of Cabinet Makers, *The Cabinet-Makers London Book of Prices* (London, 1788).

Mandeville, B., *A Treatise of the Hypochondriack and Hysterick Diseases*, 3rd edn (London, 1730).

Mead, R., *Medical Precepts and Cautions* (London, 1751).

Medical Observations and Inquiries, 6 vols (London, 1757–84).

Milligen, G., 'An Account of the Virtues and Use of the Mineral Waters near Moffatt', *Medical Essays and Observations*, 5th edn, 2 vols (Edinburgh, 1771).

Moore, J., *Medical Sketches* (London, 1786).

Moore, T., *The Works of Lord Byron*, 14 vols (London, 1832).

More, H., *Strictures on the Modern System of Female Education*, 4th edn (Dublin, 1799).

Munk, W., *Roll of the Royal College of Physicians of London*, 2nd edn, 3 vols (London, 1878).

Nairne, E., *The Description and use of Nairne's Patent Electrical Machine*, 4th edn (London, 1793).

Neale, A., *Practical Dissertations on Nervous Complaints and other Diseases Incident to the Human Body*, 3rd edn (London, 1796).

Newdigate-Newdegate, H., *The Cheverels of Cheverel Manor* (London, 1898).

Oliver, W., *A Practical Dissertation on Bath-Waters* (London, 1719).

Parry, C. H., *Collections from the Unpublished Medical Writings of the Late Caleb Hillier Parry* (London, 1825).

Peirce, R., *History and Memoirs of the Bath: Containing Observations on What Cures have been there Wrought* (London, 1713).

Percival, T., *Medical Ethics* (Manchester, 1803).

Perfect, W., *Cases of Insanity, the Epilepsy ... and Nervous Disorders, Successfully Treated*, 2nd edn (Rochester, 1785).

Pettigrew, T. J., *An Eulogy on John Coakley Lettsom* (London, 1816).

Pringle, J., *Observations on the Diseases of the Army* (London, 1752).

The Prosperity of Britain Proved from the Degeneracy of its People (London, 1757).

Quincy, J., *Pharmacopia Officinalis and Extemporanea: or, a Complete English Dispensatory*, 14th edn (London, 1769).

Reid, J., *Essays on Hypochondriacal and Other Nervous Affections* (Philadelphia, 1817).

Rowley, W., *A Treatise on Female Nervous, Hysterical, Hypochondriacal, Bilious, Convulsive Diseases, Apoplexy and Palsy; with thoughts on Madness, Suicide, &c.* (London, 1788).

Rush, B., *Essays Literary, Moral and Philosophical* (Philadelphia, 1798).

Rymer, J., *A Tract Upon Indigestion and the Hypochondriac Disease* (London, 1785).

Schoenheider, J. H., 'Remarks on the Hypochondriacal Disease and on the use of Leeches in it', *London Medical Journal*, 1 (1781), pp. 398–9

Simmons, S., *The Medical Register* (London, 1779, 1780, 1783).

Skeete, T., *Experiments and Observations on Quilled and Red Peruvian Bark* (London, 1786).

Smellie, A., *Literary and Characteristical Lives of John Gregory, MD, Henry Home, Lord Kames, David Hume, Esq., and Adam Smith* (Edinburgh, 1800).

Smith, A., *The Correspondence of Adam Smith*, ed. E. C. Mossner (Oxford: Clarendon Press, 1977).

Solomon, S., *An Account of that Most Excellent Medicine the Cordial Balm of Gilead* (Chester, 1799).

Stewart, D., *Elements of the Philosophy of the Human Mind*, vol. 3 (London, 1827).

Sutherland, A., *An Attempt to Ascertain and Extend the Virtues of Bath and Bristol Waters*, 2nd edn (London, 1764).

Sydenham, T., *Dr. Sydenham's Compleat Method of Curing Almost all Diseases*, 4th edn (London, 1710).

Thicknesse, P., *The New Prose Bath Guide* (London, 1778).

—, *The Valetudinarians Bath Guide: or, the Means of Obtaining Long Life and Health* (London, 1780).

Thompson, A., 'An Inquiry into the Natural History and Medical Uses of Several Mineral Steel Waters', *Medical Essays and Observations*, 5th edn, 2 vols (Edinburgh, 1771).

—, *An Inquiry into the Nature, Causes, and Method of Cure, of Nervous Disorders: In a Letter to a Friend* (London, 1781).

Thompson, J. (ed.), *The Works of William Cullen* (Edinburgh, 1827).

—, *An Account of the Life, Lectures and Writings of William Cullen, MD* (Edinburgh, 1832).

Thompson, T., *Medical Consultations on Various Diseases; published from the Letters of Thomas Thompson* (London, 1773).

Thomson, J., *The Seasons: A Hymn* (London, 1731).

Thornton, R. J., *The Philosophy of Medicine*, 4th edn, 5 vols (London, 1799).

Tissot, S., *Onanism: Or a Treatise Upon the Disorders Produced by Masturbation: Or, the Dangerous Effects of Secret and Excessive Venery* (1760).

—, *An Essay on Disorders of the People of Fashion* (London, 1771).

Trotter, T., *Medicina Nautica: An Essay on the Diseases of Seamen* (London, 1803).

—, *A View of the Nervous Temperament* (London, 1807).

—, *An Essay Medical, Philosophical, and Chemical on Drunkenness and its Effects on the Human Body* (1804), ed. R. Porter (London: Routledge, 1988).

Trusler, J., *The London Adviser and Guide* (London, 1786).

Turgenev, I., *Fathers and Sons*, trans. R. Matlaw (New York: Norton, 1966).

Walker, S., *A Treatise on Nervous Diseases* (London, 1796).

—, *Observations on the Constitution of Women and on some of the Diseases to which they are more Especially Liable* (London, 1803).

Warner, R. (ed.), *Original Letters from Richard Baxter, Matthew Prior, etc.* (Bath, 1817).

Webster, J., *A True and Brief Account (With Directions for the Use) of the* CEREVISIA ANGLICANA (London, n.d.).

Wesley, J., *The Desideratum: or, Electricity Made Plain and Useful* (London, 1760).

—, *Primitive Physic*, 20th edn (London, 1781).

Whytt, R., *Observations on the Nature, Causes, and Cure of those Disorders which have been Commonly Called Nervous, Hypochondriac, or Hysteric*, 2nd edn (Edinburgh, 1765).

Willan, R., *Reports on the Diseases in London, particularly During the Years 1796, 97, 98, 99, and 1800* (London, 1801).

Willis, T., *London Practice of Physick* (London, 1685).

Wilson, A., *Rational Advice to the Military, When Exposed to the Inclemency of Hot Climates and Seasons* (London, 1780).

Winslow, F., *Physic and Physicians: A Medical Sketch Book, Exhibiting the Public and Private Life of the Most Celebrated Medical Men of Former Days*, 2 vols (London, 1839).

Wollstonecraft, M., *A Vindication of the Rights of Woman* (London, 1792).

Secondary Works

Alberiti, F. B. (ed.), *Medicine, Emotion and Disease, 1700–1950* (London: Palgrave Macmillan, 2006).

Armstrong, D., *Herbs that Work: The Scientific Evidence of their Healing Powers* (Berkeley, CA: Ulysses Press, 2001).

Barfoot, M., 'On William Cullen and Mr. Adam Smith: A Case of Hypochondriasis?', *Proceedings of the Royal College of Physicians Edinburgh*, 21 (1991), 204–14.

Barker-Benfield, B., 'The Spermatic Economy: A Nineteenth Century View of Sexuality', *Feminist Studies*, 1:1 (1972), pp. 45–74.

Barker-Benfield, G. J., *The Culture of Sensibility: Sex and Society in Eighteenth-Century Britain* (Chicago, IL: Chicago University Press, 1992).

Barnes, B. and S. Shapin, *Natural Order: Historical Studies of Scientific Culture* (Beverley Hills, CA: Sage Publications, 1979).

Baur, S., *Hypochondria: Woeful Imaginings* (Berkeley, CA: University of California Press, 1988).

Berrios, G., 'Hypochondriasis: History of the Concept', in V. Starcevic and D. Lipsitt (eds), *Hypochondriasis: Modern Perspectives on an Ancient Malady* (Oxford: Oxford University Press, 2001), pp. 3–10.

Berry, C., *The Idea of Luxury: A Conceptual and Historical Investigation* (Cambridge: Cambridge University Press, 1994).

Bertucci, P., 'Revealing Sparks: John Wesley and the Religious Utility of Electrical Healing', *British Journal of the History of Science*, 39:3 (2006), pp. 341–62.

Bertucci, P., and Pancaldi, G. (eds), *Electric Bodies: Episodes in the History of Medical Electricity* (Bologna: Università di Bologna, 2001).

Bettany, G. T., *Eminent Doctors: Their Lives and Their Work*, 2 vols (London, 1885).

Borsay, A., *Medicine and Charity in Georgian Bath: A Social History of the General Infirmary, c. 1739–1830* (Aldershot: Ashgate, 1999).

Borsay, P., The *Image of Georgian Bath, 1700–2000* (Oxford: Oxford University Press, 2000).

Boss, J., 'The Seventeenth-century Transformation of the Hysteric Affection, and Sydenham's Baconian Medicine', *Psychological Medicine*, 9 (1979), pp. 221–34.

Bresadola, M., 'Early Galvanism as Technique and Medical Practice', in P. Bertucci and G. Pancaldi (eds), *Electric Bodies: Episodes in the History of Medical Electricity* (Bologna: Universita di Bologna, 2001)

Brown, P. S., 'Medicines Advertised in Eighteenth-Century Bath Newspapers', *Medical History*, 20:2 (1976), pp. 152–68.

Bynum, W. F., *Science and the Practice of Medicine in the Nineteenth Century* (Cambridge: Cambridge University Press, 1994).

Bynum, W. F., and R. Porter (eds), *William Hunter and the Eighteenth-Century Medical World* (Cambridge: Cambridge University Press, 1985)

—, *Medical Fringe and Medical Orthodoxy, 1750–1850* (London: Croom Helm, 1987).

—, *Brunonianism in Britain and Europe* (London: Wellcome Institute for the History of Medicine, 1988).

—, *Medicine and the Five Senses* (Cambridge: Cambridge University Press, 1993).

Bynum, W. F., R. Porter, and M. Shepherd (eds), *The Anatomy of Madness: Essays in the History of Psychiatry*, 2 vols (London: Tavistock Publications, 1985).

Cantor, G. N. and Hodge, M. J. S. (eds), *Conceptions of Ether: Studies in the History of Ether Theories, 1740–1900* (Cambridge: Cambridge University Press, 1981).

Chandler, J. (ed.), *The Cambridge History of English Romantic Literature* (Cambridge: Cambridge University Press, 2009).

Clarke, E. and C. D. O'Malley, *The Human Brain and Spinal Cord: A Historical Study Illustrated by Writings from Antiquity,* 2nd edn (San Francisco, CA: Norman Publishing, 1996).

Cohen, M., *Fashioning Masculinity: National Identity and Language in the Eighteenth Century* (London: Routledge, 1996).

Colburn, G. (ed.), *The English Malady: Enabling and Disabling Fictions* (Cambridge: Cambridge Scholars Press, 2008).

Colley, L., *Britons: Forging the Nation, 1707–1837* (London: Vintage, 1992).

Conway, S., *War and National Identity in the Mid-Eighteenth-Century British Isles* (Oxford: Oxford University Press, 2001).

Corfield, P., *Power and the Professions* (London: Routledge, 1995).

Cunningham, A. and R. French, *The Medical Enlightenment of the Eighteenth Century* (Cambridge: Cambridge University Press, 1990).

De Belecourt, W. and Usborne, C. (eds), *Cultural Approaches to the History of Medicine* (London: Palgrave Macmillan, 2004).

Deutsch, H., 'Symptomatic Correspondences: The Author's Case in Eighteenth-Century Britain', *Cultural Critique,* 42 (1999), pp. 35–80.

Di Trocchio, F., 'The Vital Principle in Therapy: Barthez and the Theory of Fluxions', in G. Cimino and F. Duchesneau (eds), *Vitalisms from Haller to the Cell Theory* (Firenze: Leo S. Olshki Editore, 1997), pp. 83–110.

Dickinson, H. T. (ed.), *A Companion to Eighteenth-Century Britain* (Oxford: Basil Blackwell Publishers, 2002).

Dingwall, H., '"To Be Insert in the Mercury": Medical Practice and the Press in Eighteenth-Century Edinburgh', *Social History of Medicine*, 13:1 (2000), pp. 23–44.

Doig, A., J. P. S. Ferguson, I. A. Milne and R. Passmore (eds), *William Cullen and the Eighteenth-Century Medical World* (Edinburgh: Edinburgh University Press, 1993), pp. 133–51.

Donovan, A. L., *Philosophical Chemistry in the Scottish Enlightenment* (Edinburgh: Edinburgh University Press, 1975).

Dwyer, J., *Virtuous Discourse: Sensibility and Community in Late Eighteenth-Century Scotland* (Edinburgh: John Donald Publishers, 1985).

Earle, P., *The Making of the English Middle Class: Business, Society and Family Life in London 1660*–1730 (Berkeley, CA: University of California Press, 1989).

Ellis, M., *The Politics of Sensibility: Race, Gender, and Commerce in the Sentimental Novel* (Cambridge: Cambridge University Press, 1996).

Emerson, R., *Professors, Patronage and Politics: The Aberdeen Universities in the Eighteenth Century* (Aberdeen: Aberdeen University Press, 1992).

Estes, J. W., *Dictionary of Protopharmacology: Therapeutic Practices, 1700–1850* (Canton: Science History Publications, 1990).

Fara, P., *Sympathetic Attractions: Magnetic Practices, Beliefs, and Symbolism in Eighteenth-Century England* (Princeton, NJ: Princeton University Press, 1996).

Fawcett, T., 'Selling the Bath Waters: Medical Propaganda at an Eighteenth-Century Spa', *Somerset Archaeology and Natural History*, 134 (1990), pp. 193–206.

Fissell, M., *Patients, Power and the Poor in Eighteenth-Century Bristol* (Cambridge: Cambridge University Press, 1991).

Forth, C. and Carden-Coyne, A. (eds), *Cultures of the Abdomen: Diet, Digestion and Fat in the Modern World* (New York: Palgrave Macmillan, 2005).

Foust, C., *Rhubarb: The Wondrous Drug* (Princeton, NJ: Princeton University Press, 1992).

French, R. and Wear, A., *British Medicine in an Age of Reform* (London: Routledge, 1991).

Gaul, M., *English Romanticism: The Human Context* (London: W. W. Norton, 1988).

Gijswijt-Hofstra, M. and Porter, R. (eds), *Cultures of Neurasthenia from Beard to the First World War* (Amsterdam: Rodopi, 2001).

Gilman, S., *Hysteria Beyond Freud* (Berkeley, CA: University of California Press, 1993).

Gouk, P. and Hills, H., *Representing Emotions: New Connections in the Histories of Art, Music and Medicine* (Aldershot: Ashgate, 2005).

Grinnell, G., *The Age of Hypochondria: Interpreting Romantic Health and Illness* (New York: Palgrave Macmillan, 2010).

Guerrini, A., 'Case History as Spiritual Autobiography: George Cheyne's "Case of the Author"', *Eighteenth-Century Life*, 19 (1995), pp. 17–27.

—, 'A Diet for a Sensitive Soul: Vegetarianism in Eighteenth-Century Britain', *Eighteenth Century Life*, 23:2 (1999), pp. 34–42.

—, *Obesity and Depression in the Enlightenment: The Life and Times of George Cheyne* (Oklahoma City: University of Oklahoma Press, 1999).

Habermas, J., *The Structural Transformation of the Public Sphere: An Inquiry into a Category of Bourgeois Society*, trans. T. Burger (Cambridge: MIT Press, 1989).

Hamlin, C., 'Predisposing Causes and Public Health in Early-Nineteenth-Century Medical Thought', *Social History of Medicine*, 5 (1992), pp. 43–70.

Haycock, D. B. and P. Wallis (eds), *Quackery and Commerce in Seventeenth-Century London: The Proprietary Medicine Business of Anthony Daffy* (London: Tavistock, 2005).

Heberden, E., *William Heberden: Physician in the Age of Reason* (London: Royal Society of Medicine Services, 1989).

Hitchcock, T., and M. Cohen (eds), *English Masculinities, 1660–1800* (London: Longman Ltd., 1999).

Howes, A. (ed.), *Sterne: The Critical Heritage* (London: Routledge, 1974).

Hutt, M., 'Medical Biography and Autobiography in Britain, 1780–1920' (D.Phil Dissertation, University of Oxford, 1995).

Ingram, A., *Boswell's Creative Gloom: A Study of Imagery and Melancholy in the Writings of James Boswell* (New Jersey: Barnes and Noble Books, 1982).

Jackson, S., 'Melancholia and Mechanical Explanation', *Journal of the History of Medicine and Allied Sciences* 38 (1983), pp. 298–319.

Jacyna, L. S., *Philosophic Whigs: Medicine, Science and Citizenship in Edinburgh, 1789–1848* (London: Routledge, 1994).

Jenner, M., 'The Politics of London Air: John Evelyn's FUMIFUGIUM and the Restoration', *Historical Journal*, 38:3 (1995), pp. 535–551.

Jewson, N., 'Medical Knowledge and the Patronage System in 18th Century England', *Sociology*, 8:3 (1974), pp. 369–85.

Jordanova, L., 'The Social Construction of Medical Knowledge', *Social History of Medicine*, 8:3 (1995), pp. 361–81.

Knott, S., *Sensibility and the American Revolution* (Chapel Hill, NC: University of North Carolina Press, 2009).

Lane, J., *A Social History of Medicine: Health, Healing and Disease in England, 1750–1950* (London: Routledge, 2001).

Lawlor, C., *Consumption and Literature: the Making of a Romantic Disease* (New York: Palgrave Macmillan, 2006).

Lawlor, C. and A. Suzuki (eds), *Science of Body and Mind: Literature and Science, 1660–1843*, vol. 2: *Sciences of Body and Mind* (London: Pickering and Chatto, 2003).

Lawrence, C., 'Medicine as Culture: Edinburgh and the Scottish Enlightenment' (Phd Dissertation, UCL, 1984).

—, 'The Nervous System and Society in the Scottish Enlightenment', in B. Barnes and S. Shapin (eds), *Natural Order: Historical Studies of Scientific Culture* (Beverley Hills, CA and London: Sage, 1979), pp. 19–40.

—, *Medicine in the Making of Modern Britain, 1700–1920* (London: Routledge, 1994).

Lawrence, S., *Charitable Knowledge: Hospital Pupils and Practitioners in Eighteenth-Century London* (Cambridge: Cambridge University Press, 1996).

Logan, P., *Nerves and Narratives: A Cultural History of Hysteria in Nineteenth-Century British Prose* (Berkeley, CA: University of California Press, 1997).

Loudon, I., *Medical Care and the General Practitioner, 1750–1850* (Oxford: Clarendon Press, 1986).

Lutz, T., *American Nervousness: An Anecdotal History* (Ithaca, NY: Cornell University Press, 1991).

Mangan, J. A. and Walvin, J., *Manliness and Morality: Middle-Class Masculinity in Britain and America, 1800–1940* (Manchester: Manchester University Press, 1987).

McCalman, I. (ed.), *An Oxford Companion to the Romantic Age: British Culture 1776–1832* (Oxford: Oxford University Press, 1999), pp. 170–8.

McIntyre, S., 'The Mineral Water Trade in the Eighteenth Century', *Journal of Transport History*, 2:1 (1973), pp. 1–19.

McKendrick, N., J. Brewer, and J. H. Plumb (eds), *The Birth of a Consumer Society: The Commercialization of Eighteenth-Century England* (London: Europa Publications, 1982).

Micale, M., *Hysterical Men: The Hidden History of Male Nervous Illness* (Boston, MA: Harvard University Press, 2008).

Mullan, J., *Sentiment and Sociability: The Language of Feeling in the Eighteenth Century* (Oxford: Oxford University Press, 1988).

Murch, J., *Biographical Sketches of Bath Celebrities* (London 1893).

Nutton, V. and Porter, R. (eds), *The History of Medical Education in Britain* (Amsterdam: Rodopi, 1995).

Oppenheim, J., *'Shattered Nerves': Doctors, Patients, and Depression in Victorian England* (Oxford: Oxford University Press, 1991).

Pickstone, J., 'Establishment and Dissent in Nineteenth-Century Medicine: An Exploration of Some Correspondence and Connections Between Religious and Medical Belief Systems in Early Industrial England' in W. J. Shiels (ed.), *The Church and Healing* (Oxford: Basil Blackwell, 1982), pp. 165–89.

Plasha, W., 'The Social Construction of Melancholia in the Eighteenth Century: Medical and Religions Approaches to the Life and Work of Samuel Johnson and John Wesley' (D.Phil Dissertation, University of Oxford, 1993).

Porter, D., and Porter, R., *Patient's Progress: Doctors and Doctoring in Eighteenth-Century England* (Oxford: Clarendon Press, 1989).

Porter, I. A., 'Thomas Trotter, M.D., Naval Physician', *Medical History*, 7:2 (1963), pp. 154–64.

Porter, R., 'The Sexual politics of James Graham', *British Journal of Eighteenth-Century Studies*, 5 (1982), pp. 199–206.

—, 'Lay Medical Knowledge in the Eighteenth Century: The Evidence of the Gentleman's Magazine', *Medical History*, 29 (1985), pp. 138–68.

—, *George Cheyne: The English Malady (1733)* (London: Routledge 1991).

—, 'Addicted to Modernity: Nervousness in the Early Consumer Society', in J. Melling and J. Barr (eds), *Culture in History: Production, Consumption and Values in Historical Perspective* (Exeter: University of Exeter Press, 1992), pp. 180–94.

—, *Doctor of Society: Thomas Beddoes and the Sick Trade in Late-Enlightenment England* (London: Routledge, 1992).

—, *Quacks: Fakers and Charlatans in English Medicine* (Stroud: Tempus Publishing, 2000).

—, *Flesh in the Age of Reason* (London: Allen Lane, 2003).

Porter, R. (ed.), *Patients and Practitioners: Lay Perceptions of Medicine in Pre-Industrial Society* (Cambridge: Cambridge University Press, 1985).

—, *The Popularization of Medicine* (London: Routledge, 1992).

—, *Medicine in the Enlightenment* (Amsterdam: Rodopi, 1995).

—, *Drugs and Narcotics in History* (Cambridge: Cambridge University Press, 1995).

Porter, R., and Porter, D. (eds), *In Sickness and in Health: The British Experience, 1650–1850* (London: Fourth Estate, 1988).

Porter, R., and Shepherd, M. (eds), *The Anatomy of Madness: Essays in the History of Psychiatry*, vol. 1 (London: Tavistock Publications, 1985).

Quinlan, S., 'Sensibility and Human Science in the Enlightenment', *Eighteenth Century Studies*, 37:2 (2004), pp. 296–301.

—, 'Inheriting Vice, Acquiring Virtue: Hereditary Disease and Moral Hygiene in Eighteenth-Century France', *Bulletin of the History of Medicine*, 80:4 (2006), pp. 649–76.

Raven, J., *Judging New Wealth: Popular Publishing and Responses to Commerce in England, 1750–1800* (Oxford: Clarendon Press, 1992).

Rey, R., 'Vitalism, Disease and Society' in R. Porter (ed.), *Medicine in the Enlightenment* (Amsterdam: Rodopi, 1995), pp. 274–88.

Richetti, J. (ed.), *The Cambridge Companion to the Eighteenth-Century Novel* (Cambridge: Cambridge University Press, 1996).

Risse, G., 'The Brunonian System of Medicine: Its Theoretical and Practical Implications', *Clio Medica*, 5 (1970), pp. 45–51.

—, 'Brunonian Therapeutics: New Wine in Old Bottles?', in W. Bynum and R. Porter, *Brunonianism, Brunonianism in Britain and Europe* (London: Wellcome Institute for the History of Medicine, 1988), pp. 46–62.

—, *Hospital Life in Enlightenment Scotland: Care and Teaching at the Royal Infirmary of Edinburgh* (Cambridge: Cambridge University Press, 1986).

—, 'The History of Therapeutics', in W. Bynum and V. Nutton (eds), *Essays in the History of Therapeutics* (Amsterdam: Rodopi, 1991), pp. 3–12.

—, 'Cullen as Clinician: Organisation and Strategies of an Eighteenth-Century Medical Practice', in A. Doig, J. P. S. Ferguson, I. A. Milne and R. Passmore (eds), *William Cullen and the Eighteenth Century Medical World* (Edinburgh: Edinburgh University Press, 1993), pp. 133–51.

—, *Mending Bodies, Saving Souls: A History of Hospitals* (Oxford: Oxford University Press, 1999).

—, *New Medical Challenges during the Scottish Enlightenment* (Amsterdam: Rodopi, 2005).

Risse, G., and J. H. Warner, 'Reconstructing Clinical Activities: Patient Records in Medical History', *Social History of Medicine*, 5 (1992), pp. 183–205.

Robertson, J., *The Scottish Enlightenment and the Militia Issue* (Edinburgh: John Donald Publishers, 1985).

Rocca, J., 'William Cullen (1710–90) and Robert Whytt (1714–66) on the Nervous System', in H. Whitaker, C. U. M. Smith and S. Finger (eds), *Brain, Mind and Medicine: Essays in Eighteenth-Century Neuroscience* (New York: Springer, 2007), pp. 85–98.

Rosner, L., *Medical Education in the Age of Improvement* (Edinburgh: Edinburgh University Press, 1991).

Rousseau, G. S., 'Science Books and Their Readers in the Eighteenth Century' in I. Rivers (ed.), *Books and Their Readers in Eighteenth-Century England* (Leicester: Leicester University Press, 1982), pp. 197–255.

—, *Nervous Acts: Essays on Literature, Culture and Sensibility* (New York: Palgrave Macmillan, 2004).

—, 'John Hill, Universal Genius Manqué: remarks on his life and times, with a checklist of his works', in J. A. Leo and G. S. Rousseau, *The Renaissance Man in the Eighteenth Century* (Los Angeles, CA: Clark Memorial Library, 1978), pp. 45–129.

Rousseau, G. S. (ed.), *The Letters and Papers of Sir John Hill, 1714–1775* (New York: American Medical Society, 1982).

—, *Nervous Acts: Essays on Literature, Culture and Sensibility* (New York: Palgrave Macmillan, 2004).

Rousseau, G. S., and Haycock, D. B., 'Framing Samuel Taylor Coleridge's Gut: Genius, Digestion, Hypochondria' in Rousseau, G.S., Gill, Miranda, Haycock, David, and Herwig, Malte (eds), *Framing and Imagining Disease in Cultural History* (New York: Palgrave Macmillan, 2003), pp. 231–65.

Rowbottom, M. and C. Susskind, *Electricity and Medicine: History of Their Interaction* (San Francisco, CA: San Francisco Press, Inc., 1984).

Ruberg, W., 'The Letter as Medicine: Studying Health and Illness in Dutch Daily Correspondence, 1770–1850', *Social History of Medicine*, 23:3 (2010), pp. 492–508.

Schiller, R., 'Yawning?' *Journal of the History of Neurosciences*, 11:4 (2002), pp. 392–401.

Schmidt, J., *Melancholy and the Care of the Soul: Religion, Moral Philosophy and Madness in Early Modern England* (Aldershot: Ashgate, 2007).

Schofield, R., *Mechanism and Materialism: British Natural Philosophy in an Age of Reason* (Princeton, NJ: Princeton University Press, 1970).

Shoemaker, R., *Gender in English Society, 1650–1850: The Emergence of Separate Spheres?* (London: Longman, 1998).

Shorter, E., *From Paralysis to Fatigue: A History of Psychosomatic Illness in the Modern Era* (New York: The Free Press, 1992).

Shuttleton, D., '"Pamela's Library": Samuel Richardson and Dr. Cheyne's "Universal Cure"', *Eighteenth Century Life*, 23 (1999), pp. 59–79.

Smith, L. W., '"An Account of an Unaccountable Distemper": The Experience of Pain in Early Eighteenth-Century England and France', *Eighteenth-Century Studies*, 41 (2008), pp. 459–80.

Steinke, H., *Irritating Experiments: Haller's Concept and the European Controversy on Irritability and Sensibility, 1750–90* (Amsterdam: Rodopi, 2005).

Stephanson, R., 'Richardson's "Nerves": The Physiology of Sensibility in Clarissa', *Journal of the History of Ideas*, 49:2 (1998), pp. 267–85.

Taylor, B. and S. Knott (eds), *Women, Gender and Enlightenment* (New York: Palgrave Macmillan, 2005).

Thackray, A., *Atoms and Powers* (Cambridge, MA: Harvard University Press, 1970).

Todd, J., *Sensibility: An Introduction* (London: Methuen, 1986).

Turner, E. S., *Taking the Cure* (London: Michael Joseph, 1967).

Van Sant, A. J., *Eighteenth-Century Sensibility and the Novel: The Senses in Social Context* (Cambridge: Cambridge University Press, 1993).

Vaughan, L., '"Improvements in the Art of Healing": William Heberden (1710–1801) and the Emergence of Modern Medicine in Eighteenth-Century England' (D.Phil Dissertation, University of Oxford, 2005).

Veith, I., *Hysteria: The History of a Disease* (Chicago, IL: Chicago University Press, 1965).

Vila, A., *Enlightenment and Pathology: Sensibility in the Literature and Medicine of Eighteenth-Century France* (Baltimore, MD: Johns Hopkins University Press, 1998).

Vrettos, A., *Somatic Fictions: Imagining Illness in Victorian Culture* (Stanford, CA: Stanford University Press, 1995).

Walton, J., *The English Seaside Resort: A Social History 1750–1914* (Leicester: Leicester University Press, 1983).

Wallis, P., 'Medicines for London: The Trade, Regulation and Lifecycle of London Apothecaries, *c.* 1610–*c.*1670' (D.Phil Dissertation, University of Oxford, 2002).

Wand-Tetley, J. I., 'Historical Methods of Counter-Irritation', *Rheumatology*, 3 (1956), pp. 90–8.

Webster, C. (ed.), *Health, Medicine and Mortality in the Sixteenth Century* (Cambridge: Cambridge University Press, 1979).

Whitaker, H., C. U. M. Smith and S. Finger (eds), *Brain, Mind and Medicine: Essays in Eighteenth Century Neuroscience* (New York: Springer, 2007).

Whyman, S., 'Letter Writing and the Rise of the Novel: The Epistolary Literacy of Jane Johnson and Samuel Richardson', *Huntington Library Quarterly*, 70:4 (2007), pp. 577–606.

Wild, W., *Medicine-by-Post: The Changing Voice of Illness in Eighteenth-Century British Consultation Letters and Literature* (Amsterdam: Rodopi, 2006).

Williams, E., *A Cultural History of Medical Vitalism in Enlightenment Montpellier* (Aldershot: Ashgate Publishing, 2003).

—, 'Stomach and Psyche: Eating, Digestion, and Mental Illness in the Medicine of Philippe Pinel', *Bulletin of the History of Medicine*, 84:3 (2010), pp. 358–86.

Williams, K., 'Hysteria in Seventeenth-Century Case Records and Unpublished Manuscripts', *History of Psychiatry,* 1 (1990), pp. 383–401.

Wilson, K., *The Sense of the People: Politics, Culture and Imperialism in England, 1715–1785* (Cambridge: Cambridge University Press, 1998).

Wiltshire, J., *Samuel Johnson in the Medical World: The Doctor and the Patient* (Cambridge: Cambridge University Press, 1991).

—, *Jane Austen and the Body: 'The Picture of Health'* (Cambridge: Cambridge University Press, 1992).

Withers, C., and P. Wood (eds), *Science and Medicine in the Scottish Enlightenment* (East Linton: Tuckwell Press, 2002).

Wolfson, S. (ed.), *The Cambridge Companion to Keats* (Cambridge: Cambridge University Press, 2001).

Wrigley, R., and G. Revill (eds), *Pathologies of Travel* (Amsterdam: Rodopi, 2000).

INDEX

For Product Safety Concerns and Information please contact our EU
representative GPSR@taylorandfrancis.com
Taylor & Francis Verlag GmbH, Kaufingerstraße 24, 80331 München, Germany

www.ingramcontent.com/pod-product-compliance
Ingram Content Group UK Ltd.
Pitfield, Milton Keynes, MK11 3LW, UK
UKHW021004180425
457613UK00019B/803

9 781138 664609